TEAS V PREP
STRATEGIES, PRACTICE & REVIEW

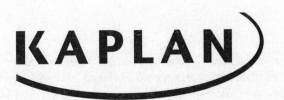

Published by Kaplan Publishing, a division of Kaplan, Inc.
750 Third Avenue
New York, NY 10017

Printed in the United States of America

10 9 8 7 6 5 4 3 2 1

ISBN-13: 978-1-62523-714-9

Kaplan Publishing books are available at special quantity discounts to use for sales promotions, employee premiums, or educational purposes. For more information or to order books, please call the Simon & Schuster special sales department at 866-506-1949.

CONTENTS

Unit 4: Science

Unit 6: Plan for Success

KapSnap

Reading

Math

Science

Grammar

Introduction

Congratulations! Preparation is the key to success, and you've taken the first step in preparing yourself for a rewarding and challenging health care career. This workbook contains the information you'll need to achieve success on school entrance exams such as the Test of Essential Academic Skills, version 5 (TEAS V).

When weighing the qualifications of applicants, school admissions offices use student performance on exams such as the TEAS as a standardized indicator of ability. It is important to become comfortable with both the content and the structure of the exam to ensure that you have your choice of school.

Structure of This Book

To get you off to the right start, the Introduction section of this book outlines the structure of the TEAS V, including item counts per section and the format of each item type, and identifies additional resources that will be of help to you as you complete the lessons in the rest of the book.

The first section is an abbreviated Diagnostic Test. This practice test will give you insights into your strengths and weaknesses so that you can focus on your weaker areas and use your study time most efficiently. It will also give you a sense of the exam as a whole, which is important in establishing a level of comfort with the material and format of the TEAS.

Unit 1 covers the critical skills you'll need not only to adequately prepare for the entrance exams, but also to achieve success while in school. Kaplan's classroom-tested study strategies and test-taking hints are outlined here.

Units 2, 3, 4, and 5 offer targeted lessons on the individual sections of the exam: Reading, Math, Science, and Grammar (known as English Language Arts, or ELA, on the TEAS). Each lesson has six subsections: Learn, Strategize, Apply, Guided Practice, Independent Practice, and ReKap.

Each Guided Practice section gives you an inside peek into the thought process involved in applying the concepts and strategies. The Independent Practice sections then allow you to gauge your understanding of the material and the process. By combining teaching and practice, the lessons in these units will prepare you for success. Plus, the ReKap feature at the end of each lesson encapsulates the key learning points you've just studied to enhance your recall.

Finally, our exclusive KapSnap section summarizes all the skills, terms/formulas, strategies, and quick steps you learned in the lessons, and reminds you the common errors to avoid. When you think you know the material in each lesson, review that KapSnap to test yourself.

By using Kaplan's *TEAS V Prep: Strategies, Practice & Review,* you're embarking on the comprehensive preparation necessary to achieve the best score possible and start a successful career in health care. Good luck!

Introduction to the TEAS

Commonly referred to as the TEAS, the Test of Essential Academic Skills is administered by the Assessment Technologies Institute (ATI) of Stilwell, Kansas. There have been several iterations of this exam, the current one being the TEAS V. This book will focus on getting you familiar with that exam's format, as it is most likely what you'll experience on exam day. Designed by a panel of health care experts, the TEAS is widely accepted by programs across the country. However, you should inquire as to which entrance exam the school of your choice requires before you begin your study regimen.

The TEAS exam is administered at a number of testing locations for a fee. The exam dates are set based on application deadlines for local nursing schools. The TEAS exam is offered in both paper-and-pencil and computerized formats. The format of the exam is chosen by the site where the exam is administered. Some sites offer only one format, while others offer both. Should you have more than one TEAS administration site in your location, consider which exam format you are most comfortable with when registering.

The TEAS must be registered for in advance of the test date.

Structure of the TEAS

The TEAS is divided into four areas: Reading, English Language Arts (ELA), Science, and Math. The following chart details the number of items in each section and the time allotted for each.

Content	Item Count	Allotted Time (minutes)
Reading	48	58
English Language Arts	34	34
Science	54	66
Math	34	51
Total	**170**	**209**

After taking the exam, you receive an individual score for each of the four test areas. Additionally, you receive scores on 16 content categories.

About the TEAS Reading Section

The reading section of the TEAS measures student comprehension of paragraphs, passages, and informational sources. These sources may be graphic, such as charts, maps, graphs, scientific instruments, or diagrams. After reading or interpreting the given information, you will answer two or three questions that assess targeted skills.

Skills that are commonly tested in the reading section of the TEAS exam are:

- Identifying the author's purpose or intent
- Distinguishing among topic, main idea, theme, and supporting details
- Distinguishing fact from opinion
- Identifying genre
- Identifying text features/structure
- Drawing conclusions, making inferences and predictions
- Identifying the author's tone
- Identifying the meaning of a word based on context
- Reading scientific instruments accurately

About the TEAS English Language Arts (ELA) Section

The ELA section of the TEAS measures student knowledge of definitions, grammar, spelling, punctuation, and sentence structure.

The skills that are commonly tested in the ELA section of the TEAS are:

- Parts of speech
- Rules of capitalization
- Plural form
- Simple, compound, and complex sentences
- Commonly misspelled and/or misused words
- First and third-person point of view
- Subject-verb agreement
- Multiple-meaning words
- Capitalization
- Passive and active voice

About the TEAS Science Section

The science section of the TEAS assesses student knowledge of scientific areas including taxonomy, ecology, chemical reactions, states of matter, energy, human body systems, genetics, and heredity.

The skills that are commonly tested in the science section of the TEAS are:

- Identifying steps of the scientific method
- Identifying functions of cell organelles
- DNA/RNA functions
- Human demographics
- Reading the periodic table
- Phase changes and identifying a state based on properties

About the TEAS Math Section

The math section of the TEAS helps schools evaluate a prospective student's understanding of numbers, equations, operations, algebra, as well as data interpretation.

The skills that are commonly tested in the math section of the TEAS are:

- Ordering and comparing numbers
- Square roots
- Absolute value
- Converting between fractions and decimals
- Long division
- Ratio
- Metric prefixes
- Units
- Circles, squares, composite figures, volume
- Data displays
- Roman numerals

The Next Steps

Now that you've familiarized yourself with the TEAS, you're ready to move on to critical skills that you'll be able to apply to these exams and throughout your career in health care. Familiarity with the format of every item on both of these exams coupled with useful strategies will ensure a calm and successful test day!

Diagnostic Test

Use the text in the graphic below to answer questions 1 and 2.

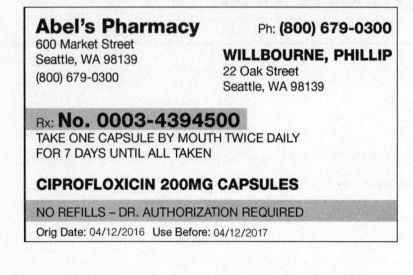

Abel's Pharmacy
600 Market Street
Seattle, WA 98139
(800) 679-0300

Ph: **(800) 679-0300**

WILLBOURNE, PHILLIP
22 Oak Street
Seattle, WA 98139

Rx: **No. 0003-4394500**
TAKE ONE CAPSULE BY MOUTH TWICE DAILY
FOR 7 DAYS UNTIL ALL TAKEN

CIPROFLOXICIN 200MG CAPSULES

NO REFILLS – DR. AUTHORIZATION REQUIRED

Orig Date: 04/12/2016   Use Before: 04/12/2017

1. **This passage is an example of which type of writing?**

   A) Technical
   B) Narrative
   C) Expository
   D) Persuasive

2. **Certain information is highlighted and in bold. What is the purpose of utilizing these text features?**

   A) The bold text tells the patient when the medication will expire.
   B) The bold text tells the pharmacist who the prescribing doctor is.
   C) The bold text makes it easy for the patient or pharmacist to identify the prescription.
   D) The bold text separates the important information from the unimportant information.

3. Read the following index excerpt. Then answer the question.

Senegalese customs, 27–29
Senghor, Leopold Sedar, 113, 122
Slave trade
    American slave traders, 27–30
    Gorèe Island in slave trade, 21, 23–24, 35
    Middle Passage, 30
    Portuguese slave traders, 21–24
    role of signares, 25–26, 31

According to the index excerpt above, on which pages of this book can one find the best information about the kind of food the Senegalese ate?

A) Pages 21–24

B) Pages 23–24

C) Pages 25–26

D) Pages 27–29

4. Cesar Chavez became a national hero for his leadership in organizing migrant farm workers to fight for higher wages and better living conditions. Within his own organization, the National Farm Workers, he had to prove that his nonviolent methods would be as effective as the violence that some people advocated.

Chavez's testing ground was the 1968 struggle to gain union representation and fair pay for workers in the California vineyards. He supported the striking grape workers by organizing a nationwide boycott of grapes and by leading a protest march through 350 miles of California farmland to the state capitol at Sacramento. When workers at some vineyards used physical force, Chavez began to fast as a protest. His action caused the violence to end.

Which of the following is a logical conclusion based on the text?

A) Cesar Chavez was a man of conviction.

B) Cesar Chavez was a laborer in the grape industry.

C) Cesar Chavez was worried about grape production.

D) Cesar Chavez was someone who wanted to gain fame.

5. Memo
To: Students in Chemistry 302
Re: Exam

The final exam will be given on Tuesday, May 27, at 9 a.m. Please bring only yourself. You will be asked to check your personal belongings prior to entering the exam room. All questions will be multiple choice. Be sure to highlight the correct answer and then click on it. Good luck!

Based on the text, what prediction can be made?

A) The exam will be three hours long.

B) The exam will consist of experiments.

C) The exam will be taken on a computer.

D) The exam will have two-part questions.

Use the text in the graphic at right to answer questions 6 and 7.

6. Which of the following is the topic of the passage?

A) A job opening

B) Nursing tasks

C) Hospice care compensation

D) Job requirements for nursing

7. Which sentence is the main idea of the paragraph labeled "Job Description"?

A) Our RNs are shining examples of skill, training, leadership, and compassion.

B) RN will perform physical assessment on patients in hospice care.

C) RN will develop a plan for the care of patients based on their specific needs.

D) RN will work closely with physicians to determine best type of care for patients nearing the end of their lives.

Richard White Memorial Hospital System

RWMHS   *Always Caring*

TITLE: RN Case Manager
PROGRAM: RWMHS Hospice Care
LOCATION: Manhattan Campus

Job Description

RN Case Manager

Our RNs are shining examples of skill, training, leadership, and compassion. RN will perform physical assessment on patients in hospice care. RN will develop a plan for the care of patients based on their specific needs. RN will work closely with physicians to determine best type of care for patients nearing the end of their lives. RN will be responsible for the training and supervision of aides and physical therapists.

Job Requirements

Associate's Degree/Diploma from an accredited school of Nursing; BSN preferred. Three years experience in Medical, Surgical, or Community Health preferred. New York State RN license and a valid New York State driver's license are both required for this position. Teaching or training experience much appreciated!

Compensation

- Employee health coverage
- Family health coverage options
- Pension plan
- 3 weeks paid vacation
- Employee tuition reimbursement

We are an equal opportunity employer.

APPLY TODAY!

8. Which sentence expresses an opinion?

A) Patients feel that Cincinnati City Hospital is in need of more nurses.

B) Cincinnati City Hospital has reduced their nursing staff by 12 percent since 2009.

C) Eighty-four percent of doctors polled reported that Cincinnati City Hospital is in need of more nurses.

D) Studies show that Cincinnati City Hospital received better ratings prior to their nursing staff reduction.

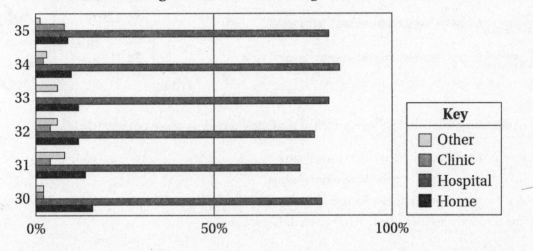

Arizona Birthing Locations: Women Ages 30-35

9. According to the graph above, what is the most popular birthing location for women in Arizona between ages 30 and 35?

A) Other

B) Clinic

C) Hospital

D) Home

DIAGNOSTIC TEST — READING

Use the text in the graphic below to answer questions 10 and 11.

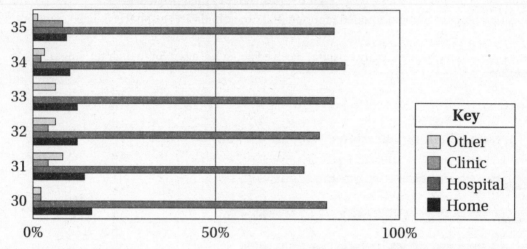

Arizona Birthing Locations: Women Ages 30-35

Key
- Other
- Clinic
- Hospital
- Home

10. Based on the information in the graph, which of the following is true about home births?

A) Home births are less popular than clinic births.

B) Home births are more popular with older women.

C) Home births are more popular with younger women.

D) Home births are less popular than other birthing locations.

11. According to the graph above, approximately what percentage of women age 30 chose to have home births?

A) 10%

B) 20%

C) 50%

D) 75%

Use the text in the graphic below to answer question 12.

Drug Facts

Active Ingredient (in each tablet) — Purpose

Active Ingredient (in each tablet)	Purpose
Diphenhydramine HCL 10 mg	Antihistamine
Acetaminophen 400mg	Pain Reliever

Uses

- Temporarily relieves symptoms of common allergies, including:
- Runny nose • Headache • Itchy, watery eyes
- Itchy Throat • Fever

Warnings

Do not use this medication if you have had previous allergic reactions to its ingredients.

When using this product, follow the recommended dosage exactly. Do not take more than directed for your age.

If rash occurs, **stop use of product and contact your doctor immediately**.

If you are pregnant or **breast-feeding**, ask your doctor before taking this medication.

This medication not intended for children. In case of overdose, contact a Poison Control Center right away. ▶

Directions

AGE	TABLETS
Adults and children 12 years of age and older	1 tablet every 24 hours
Children under 12 years of age	Do not use
Adults over 65 years of age	Consult your doctor

12. When using this product, follow the <u>recommended</u> dosage exactly. Do not take more than directed for your age.

   Based on context, which of the following is the definition of the underlined word in the sentence above?

   A) applied

   B) cautioned

   C) instructed

   D) encouraged

13. Writers tend to fall into two camps: those who outline their work and those who do not. The benefits of outlining are numerous and well documented, but there is certainly something to be said for writing directly from passion, burning through ideas so quickly that the story seems to explode onto the pages, regardless of what any preconceived outline may have looked like.

    Which inference can logically be made based on the paragraph?

    A) The author of the paragraph is a writer who chooses to outline.

    B) Writers will not feel passionate about work that they have outlined in advance.

    C) The author of the paragraph writes from passion and does not believe in the benefits of outlining.

    D) Writers who have outlined their work might disregard their outline and write from passion in the moment.

14. A poet has written a poem in AABB form. In the last verse, he finds that he cannot think of the final rhyme he needs to complete the poem. Which source of information would be most appropriate for him to use in this situation?

    A) a thesaurus

    B) a dictionary

    C) an online atlas

    D) an online newspaper

DIAGNOSTIC TEST — MATH

1. Which shows the following set of numbers arranged in descending order?

   $8, -4, |-7|, \sqrt{9}$

   A) $\sqrt{9}, 8, -4, |-7|$
   B) $\sqrt{9}, 8, |-7|, -4$
   C) $8, |-7|, \sqrt{9}, -4$
   D) $-4, |-7|, \sqrt{9}, 8$

2. $8 - 4 \div 4 + 6$

   Simplify the expression above. Which of the following is correct?

   A) 1
   B) 7
   C) 13
   D) 14

3. What is the sum of $6\frac{2}{3}$ and $9\frac{5}{6}$?

   A) $15\frac{7}{9}$
   B) $16\frac{1}{2}$
   C) $15\frac{3}{4}$
   D) $16\frac{1}{6}$

4. The 750 window decals Patrick ordered for his company last month were shipped in 25 boxes. This month Patrick ordered 450 window decals. If the same number of decals is always shipped in each box, how many boxes will be needed to ship this month's order of decals?

    A) 12

    B) 15

    C) 17

    D) 18

5. A painting has a value of $206. After one year, the value of the painting increases by 15%. What is the new value of the painting?

    A) $30.90

    B) $209.09

    C) $236.90

    D) $309.00

6. Which of the following is the number of feet in 12 yards?

    A) 1

    B) 4

    C) 36

    D) 144

7. Find the sum of the expressions $8x - 1$ and $2x + 5$.

A) $6x + 4$

B) $6x - 6$

C) $10x + 4$

D) $10x + 6$

8. $2x - 15 = 19$

Solve the equation above. Which of the following is correct?

A) 2

B) 8

C) 17

D) 23

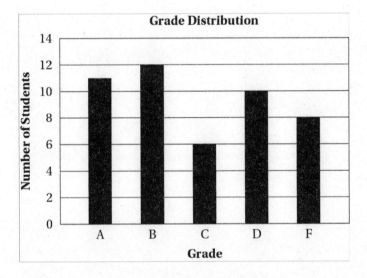

9. The chart above shows the grade distribution for a class of college students. Which grade did the largest number of students receive?

A) A

B) B

C) C

D) F

10. Taxes of $152.50, insurance premiums of $98, and a retirement contribution of $75 are deducted from a nutritionist's pay each month. If the nutritionist earns $1842.50 each month, what is his monthly take-home pay after deductions?

A) $1442.00

B) $1517.00

C) $1690.00

D) $2168.00

DIAGNOSTIC TEST — SCIENCE

1. A scientist is studying the effect of a new medicine on appetite control. The scientist has a group of 500 participants. Half receive the new medicine; half receive a placebo.

   What is the control in this experiment?

   A) 500 people

   B) appetite control

   C) the new medicine

   D) the placebo

2. A scientist is studying the effect of using 50 grams of fertilizer X every week on the growth of corn plants.

   What data should the scientist record every day?

   A) the type of fertilizer used weekly

   B) the number of corn plants grown

   C) the growth of the corn plants

   D) the species of corn plants

3. Where is genetic material stored in cells?

   A) in the nucleus

   B) in the ribosomes

   C) in the mitochondria

   D) in the cell membrane

4. Which of the following make up proteins?

   A) DNA

   B) RNA

   C) amino acids

   D) nucleotides

5. Anemia is a condition that arises when the body cells do not get enough oxygen. Which system is affected by anemia?

   A) circulatory

   B) digestive

   C) excretory

   D) lymphatic

6. Symptoms of pancreatitis include weight loss and nausea. Which system is most affected by pancreatitis?

   A) circulatory

   B) digestive

   C) excretory

   D) reproductive

7. Which system is most affected in a patient with cancer in the trachea?

   A) circulatory

   B) digestive

   C) lymphatic

   D) respiratory

8. Which systems help maintain balance in body systems through communication?

   A) nervous and digestive

   B) nervous and endocrine

   C) digestive and excretory

   D) endocrine and excretory

9. The scientific name for the pathogen that causes malaria is *Plasmodium falciparus.* Which two categories of classification are present in the scientific name?

A) genus and species

B) genus and phylum

C) kingdom and species

D) kingdom and phylum

10. Which of the following statements about elements is accurate?

A) All atoms of a given element have the same atomic mass.

B) All atoms of a given element have the same atomic charge.

C) All atoms of a given element have the same number of protons.

D) All atoms of a given element have the same number of electrons.

11. How many atoms of oxygen are present in tricalcium phosphate $Ca_3(PO_4)_2$?

A) 1

B) 2

C) 4

D) 8

12. Which of the following is an acid-base reaction?

A) $Zn + 2\,HCl \rightarrow ZnCl_2 + H_2$

B) $2\,S_2O_3^{-2} + I_2 \rightarrow S_4O_6^{-2} + 2I^-$

C) $HBr + NaOH \rightarrow NaBr + H_2O$

D) $C_{10}H_8 + 12\,O_2 \rightarrow 10\,CO_2 + 4\,H_2O$

13. Which phase transition will occur if heat energy is added to a solid?

A) condensing

B) evaporating

C) freezing

D) melting

14. Which energy conversion occurs when a toaster oven is used to make toast?

A) electrical to heat

B) electrical to chemical

C) mechanical to electrical

D) mechanical to light

15. Which of the following describes a country with a high emigration rate?

A) More people are being born than dying.

B) More people are dying than being born.

C) More people are leaving than entering the country.

D) More people are entering than leaving the country.

16. Which of the following is an example of conduction?

A) A person burns his hand when he touches a hot toaster.

B) A person gets warmed standing in front of a heating vent.

C) A person gets warmed after turning on the heat in his car.

D) A person burns her scalp when using a hot setting on a hair dryer.

DIAGNOSTIC TEST — GRAMMAR

1. My <u>favorite</u> stuffed animal was <u>completely</u> destroyed after the dog absconded with it.

   Which of the following correctly identifies the parts of speech in the underlined portions of the sentence above?

   A) adverb; verb
   B) adverb; adverb
   C) adjective; adverb
   D) adjective; adjective

2. While we ate _____ we discussed our upcoming trip to the beach.

   Which of the following correctly punctuates the sentence above?

   A) colon
   B) semicolon
   C) hyphen
   D) comma

3. Which sentence is correctly punctuated?

   A) "When I told him about the news," Wanda said, "he said "Wow!""
   B) 'When I told him about the news,' Wanda said, 'he said 'Wow!"
   C) 'When I told him about the news,' Wanda said, 'he said '"Wow!"'
   D) "When I told him about the news," Wanda said, "he said 'Wow!'"

4. Which of the following sentences provides an example of correct subject-verb agreement?

   A) The group, after meeting for three weeks, have decided to move forward on the proposal.
   B) Neither Sarah nor Mical, despite having tried it several times, enjoy fishing.
   C) The twins or their brother are generally home by three o'clock.
   D) Both Nancy and Patrice were first year students.

5. Jerry and Mike held _____ annual chili cook-off once again this week

Which of the following correctly completes the sentence above?

A) their

B) his

C) its

D) there

6. Whether I attend the party tonight _____ .

Which of the following completions for the above sentence results in a compound sentence structure?

A) depends on my work schedule this evening.

B) is still undecided for now.

C) depends on you, and you haven't said whether you are coming.

D) or I stay home with a movie will determine my level of energy tomorrow.

7. Which of the following sentences is an example of a complex sentence?

A) I waited in line, but the tickets had already sold out.

B) Tonight, I am trying to choose between two of my favorite meals.

C) Neither of the boys managed to hear the doorbell this morning.

D) Although I did not see the lunar eclipse, Mary said it was fantastic.

8. Which of the following words is spelled correctly?

A) permissable

B) conceivible

C) convertable

D) credible

9. Tim had left his colleagues in a <u>precarious</u> situation, with nobody knowing quite what to say to management or whom they would upset with the news.

Based on the sentence above, what does <u>precarious</u> most likely mean?

A) irresponsible

B) offensive

C) uncertain

D) unforeseen

10. Everyone came to the barbecue. The barbecue was a great success. The food was delicious. The games were entertaining.

To improve sentence fluency, which of the following best states the information above in a single sentence?

A) The barbecue had delicious food and entertaining games and was a great success, so everyone came.

B) Everyone came to the barbecue, which was a great success with delicious food and entertaining games.

C) Everyone came to the successful barbecue, where there was delicious food and entertaining games and it was a great success.

D) At the barbecue, which was a great success, the delicious food was eaten and people were entertained by the games, and everyone came.

DIAGNOSTIC TEST — ANSWERS

Answer Key

Reading

1. A
2. C
3. D
4. A
5. C
6. A
7. A
8. A
9. C
10. C
11. B
12. C
13. D
14. A

Math

1. C
2. C
3. B
4. B
5. C
6. C
7. C
8. C
9. B
10. B

Science

1. D
2. C
3. A
4. C
5. A
6. B
7. D
8. B
9. A
10. C
11. D
12. C
13. D
14. A
15. C
16. A

Grammar

1. C
2. D
3. D
4. D
5. A
6. C
7. D
8. D
9. C
10. B

Answers — Reading

1. **A**
   A. KEY. The passage is a sample prescription label, which offers specific information on the patient, prescription, dosage, and doctor. This is an example of technical writing.
   B. The passage is a sample prescription label. It is not an example of narrative writing, which relates a story.
   C. The passage is a sample prescription label and is not an example of expository writing. Expository writing explains a topic.
   D. The passage is a sample prescription label. It is not an example of persuasive writing, which attempts to convince the reader of something.

2. **C**
   A. The highlighted, bold text does not tell the patient when the medication will expire. That information is not in bold.
   B. The highlighted, bold text does not tell the pharmacist who the prescribing doctor is. That information is not in bold.
   C. KEY. The highlighted, bold text indicates the prescription number, which makes it easy for both the patient and pharmacist to track it.
   D. The highlighted, bold text does not separate the important information from the unimportant information, as its importance is relative to the role of the person reading the label.

3. **D**
   A. These pages would not give information about the kind of food the Senegalese ate, but about Portuguese slave traders.
   B. These pages would not give information about the kind of food the Senegalese ate, but about Gorée Island and the slave trade.
   C. These pages would not give information about the kind of food the Senegalese ate, but about the role of signares.
   D. KEY. These pages would give information about the kind of food the Senegalese ate; the food people eat is part of their customs

4. **A**
   A. KEY. This conclusion is supported by the evidence in the text; Cesar Chavez believed in changing conditions through peaceful means, not violent means.
   B. This conclusion is not supported by the text; there is nothing to suggest that Cesar Chavez was a laborer in the grape industry.
   C. This conclusion is not supported by the evidence in the text; there is no mention of his being concerned about grape production.
   D. While Cesar Chavez did become nationally known, this is not what his goal was; this conclusion is not supported by the text.

5. **C**

   A. This prediction is not supported by the evidence in the text; there is no reason to believe that the test will be three hours long.

   B. This prediction is not supported by the evidence in the text; there is no reason to think that the exam will consist of experiments.

   C. KEY. This prediction is correct; there is evidence that the exam will be taken on a computer.

   D. This prediction is not supported by the evidence; there is no reason to think the exam will have two-part questions.

6. **A**

   A. KEY. This passage is a job posting for a nursing position at a hospice care facility. The topic, which is the most general information included in the passage, is a job opening.

   B. This passage is a job posting for a nursing position at a hospice care facility. The topic, which is the most general information included in the passage, is not nursing tasks. The tasks described are supporting details.

   C. This passage is a job posting for a nursing position at a hospice care facility. The topic, which is the most general information included in the passage, is not hospice care compensation. This is a supporting detail.

   D. This passage is a job posting for a nursing position at a hospice care facility. The topic, which is the most general information included in the passage, is not job requirements for nursing. These requirements are included as supporting details.

7. **A**

   A. KEY. The main idea of the paragraph specifically reflects and summarizes the information contained in that paragraph.

   B. This sentence is a supporting detail, included in the paragraph to expand on the main idea.

   C. This sentence is a supporting detail, included in the paragraph to expand on the main idea.

   D. This sentence is a supporting detail, included in the paragraph to expand on the main idea.

8. **A**

   A. KEY. This statement reflects a feeling shared by patients of the hospital. Opinions are judgments that are not based in fact. The other choices reflect information that is proven.

   B. This statement is a fact that can be verified with data.

   C. This statement is a fact that can be verified by the results of the poll.

   D. This statement is a fact that can be verified by the ratings that were included in the studies.

9. **C**

   A. Some people prefer to give birth in other locations, but this is not the most popular choice for these women.

   B. While some women do prefer to give birth in a clinic, the data does not indicate that this is the most popular option.

   C. KEY. The hospital is the most popular birthing location across all ages represented in the graph.

   D. More women choose to give birth at home than in clinics; however, it is not the most popular birthing location.

10. **C**
    A.   The graph indicates that home births are more popular, not less popular, than clinic births.
    B.   According to the graph, home births are more popular with younger women than with older women.
    C   KEY. Home births are more popular with the youngest women represented on the graph. The popularity of this choice decreases with age
    D.   Home births are less popular than hospital births; however, they are more popular than clinics and other locations.

11. **B**
    A.   The bar showing the percentage of home births would be shorter if 10% of women chose this option.
    B.   KEY. Home births are more popular with the youngest women represented on the graph. The popularity of this choice decreases with age.
    C.   If 50% of women had chosen home births, the bar for this option would reach the 50% line in the center of the graph.
    D.   If 75% of women had chosen home births, the bar for this option would reach halfway between 50% and 100% on the graph.

12. **C**
    A.   This medication is taken in tablet form, so the dosage would not be applied. This word does not make sense in the context of the sentence.
    B.   This word does not makes sense in the context of the sentence.
    C.   KEY. The passage is a sample prescription label. The excerpt warns the reader to follow directions. To safely use the medication, patients must follow the instructions.
    D.   The proper dosage must be followed exactly, so the manufacturer would not simply encourage patients to take it correctly. This word would not make sense in the context of the text.

13. **D**
    A.   The author includes several reasons for not using an outline, so this answer is not supported by the text.
    B.   While writers who do feel passionate may not use an outline, the passage does not suggest that using an outline will prevent writers from feeling passionate.
    C.   The writer states that there are numerous benefits of outlining, so this answer is not supported by the text.
    D.   KEY. The final sentence of the paragraph implies that outlines are sometimes disregarded when a writer is working on a story.

14. **A**
    A.   KEY. The most appropriate source for the poet to turn to for a rhyme that fits his form is a thesaurus.
    B.   A dictionary might offer a few synonyms but would not be the most appropriate source to use.
    C.   An atlas is a book of maps and would not be helpful in this situation.
    D.   A newspaper would not include a list of words that have the same meaning that might rhyme with the word in the poem.

Answers — Math

1. C

   A. These numbers are arranged in descending order if the square root and absolute value signs are ignored.

   B. These numbers are arranged in descending order if the square root, absolute value, and negative sign are ignored.

   C. KEY. Numbers arranged in descending order are arranged from greatest to least. $|-7|$ is the distance between -7 and 0 on the number line, so $|-7| = 7$. $\sqrt{9}$ represents the number, that when multiplied by itself, equals 9, so $\sqrt{9} = 3$. Since negative numbers are always less than positive numbers, -4 must be the least number. Therefore, 8 has the greatest value, followed by $|-7|$, followed by $\sqrt{9}$, and finally, -4.

   D. These answers are arranged in ascending order, from least to greatest.

2. C

   A. This is the result of first dividing correctly, but then performing addition before subtraction instead of recognizing that they should be performed from left to right.

   B. This is the result of performing the operations in order from left to right instead of using the proper order of operations.

   C. KEY. The operations must be done using the proper order of operations. Use the acronym PEMDAS to remember the order of the steps Parentheses, Exponents, Multiplication and Division (from left to right), Addition and Subtraction (from left to right). Since there are no parentheses or exponents, the first step would be to do the division. Dividing 4 by 4 gives a result of 1 and the expression is now $8 - 1 + 6$. Addition and subtraction are grouped together and performed from left to right, so the next step is to subtract 8 minus 1, which is 7. Lastly, add the 7 to the 6 to get a final result of 13.

   D. This is the result of incorrectly calculating $4 \div 4$ as 0 instead of 1, and then performing the other steps in the correct order.

3. B

   A. When adding two fractions, you must find equivalent fractions with a common denominator before combining the numerators. Further, the two denominators are never added together.

   B. KEY. Adding the whole number parts of the mixed numbers yields 15. Adding the fractional parts yields $\frac{2}{3} + \frac{5}{6} = \frac{4}{6} + \frac{5}{6} = \frac{9}{6}$, or $1\frac{1}{2}$. Combining this with 15 results in the final answer of $16\frac{1}{2}$.

       Another method would involve writing both mixed numbers as improper fractions. $6\frac{2}{3} = \frac{20}{3}$ and $9\frac{5}{6} = \frac{59}{6}$. Adding these two improper fractions yields $\frac{99}{6}$, which can be written as the mixed number $16\frac{1}{2}$.

   C. After getting common denominators, the two denominators should be added together.

   D. The whole numbers were added to yield 15, and then the numerators in the fractions were added to yield 7 and were then incorrectly used over the denominator of 6 instead of finding a common denominator before adding the fractions.

4. B

A. This is the result of subtracting 750 – 450 and dividing the difference by 25.

B. KEY. The proportion $\frac{750 \text{ decals}}{25 \text{ boxes}} = \frac{450 \text{ decals}}{x \text{ boxes}}$ can be used to solve this problem. Cross-multiplying to solve the proportion gives that $450(25) = 750x$ or $11250 = 750x$. Then dividing by 750 gives that $x = 15$. Another way to solve would be to determine how many decals are in each box. Divide the 750 decals by the 25 boxes: $\frac{750}{25} = 30$, so there are 30 decals in each box. Now divide 450 by 30 to determine how many boxes are need for this month's shipment: $\frac{450}{30} = 15$.

C. This is the result of dividing 750 by 450, making an error while placing the decimal point, and then rounding the quotient up to the nearest whole number.

D. This is the result of dividing 450 by 25.

5. C

A. $30.90 represents 15% of the painting's initial value, but the question asks for the value of the painting after a 15% increase. $30.90 only represents the first step in solving the problem.

B. When converting 15% into a decimal, we must calculate $15 \div 100 = 0.15$. It is easy to miscalculate this decimal as 0.015. This leads to an increase of 1.5%:
$206 \times (1.015) = \$209.09$

C. KEY. Converting 15% into a decimal yields the number 0.15. By multiplying $206 by 0.15, we see that a 15% change in price is a difference of $30.90. Since the value of the painting increases, $30.90 should be added to the original price: $206 + \$30.90 = \$236.90$.

D. 15%, as a decimal, is 0.15. Since this problem asks for an increase in the painting's value, it is easy to miscalculate 15% as 1.5. Multiplying $206 by 1.5 yields the incorrect answer $309.00.

6. C

A. This is the result of dividing the number of yards by 12. This would be the method for converting inches to feet. A yard is 3 feet, not 12 feet.

B. This is the result of dividing by 3 or incorrectly setting up the conversion factor as $12 \text{ yards} \times \frac{1 \text{ yard}}{3 \text{ feet}}$. If the conversion factor is set up in this way, the yards units will not cancel out. The unit in the denominator of the conversion factor should match the original unit in order for the units to cancel out.

C. KEY. 1 yard = 3 feet so the conversion factor $\frac{3 \text{ feet}}{1 \text{ yard}}$ can be used. By multiplying $12 \text{ yards} \times \frac{3 \text{ feet}}{1 \text{ yard}}$ the units, yards, cancel out. This leaves the unit feet.

D. This is the result of multiplying the number of yards by 12. This would be the method for converting feet to inches.

7. C

A. The difference in the x-terms' coefficients was found, rather than the sum.

B. The difference in the two expressions was found.

C. KEY. Add to find a sum. When adding two algebraic expressions, the coefficients of the like terms must be added. Therefore, $8x$ added to $2x$ must be $10x$. The two constant terms are also like terms. The sum of -1 and 5 is 4. Therefore, the expression representing the sum of $8x - 1$ and $2x + 5$ is $10x + 4$.

D. The constant terms were added incorrectly. The constant term in $8x - 1$ is -1, not positive 1.

8.   C

   A.   This is the result of subtracting 15 from each side, rather than adding, and then dividing by 2. To solve an equation, you must use the inverses of the operations in the given equation in order to isolate the variable. So, the first step is to add 15 to each side of the equation.

   B.   This is the result of subtracting 15 from each side and then multiplying by 2. Again, to solve an equation, you must use the inverses of the operations in the given equation in order to isolate the variable. So, the first step is to add 15 to each side of the equation and the second step is to divide by 2 on each side.

   C.   KEY. To solve the equation, isolate the variable by using the reverse order of operations (SADMEP). First, perform the inverse of –15 by adding 15 to each side to get the new equation $2x = 34$. To cancel out the multiplying by 2, divide both sides of the equation by 2 to get $x = 17$.

   D.   This is the result of substituting 19 into the expression $2x - 15$. To solve for x, you must perform the inverse operations in order to get the variable alone on one side of the equation.

9.   B

   A.   While A represents the highest grade, this question focuses on how many people received each of these grades. Since the bar for A is shorter than the bar for B, that means that fewer people received As than people who received Bs.

   B.   KEY. This question asks which group has the largest number of students. "Number of Students" is represented on the vertical axis, so we must identify which grade has the tallest bar. The grade with the largest group must be B, as its bar, which represents the number of students receiving that grade, is the tallest.

   C.   The group of people who received Cs is the smallest among the four grades, but this question asks for the largest group.

   D.   This may be an appealing answer since the bar for F is farthest to the right on the horizontal axis. If numbers are shown along the horizontal axis in a graph, then the largest value would be shown on the right. However, the horizontal axis here shows categories, people receiving each grade, rather than numbers. This question asks for the largest-sized group, which is strictly measured by the height of the bars. Since the height of the bar representing the Fs group is shorter than that of the Bs group, the number of students receiving Bs is greater.

10.   B

   A.   This is the result of subtracting the retirement contribution twice. To determine the take-home pay, each deduction should be subtracted once from the pay.

   B.   KEY. To determine the take-home pay, all the deductions should be subtracted from the pay. Another way to solve this is to add up all the deductions first, and then subtract that total from the pay to determine take-home pay.

   C.   This is the result of only subtracting the taxes. All the deductions must be subtracted to determine the take-home pay.

   D.   This is the result of adding all the numbers in the problem. To determine take-home pay, all the deductions should be subtracted from the pay.

Answers — Science

1. **D**
   A. The 500 people are the participants in this experiment.
   B. Appetite control is what the scientist is studying; it is not the control.
   C. The new medicine is the variable or the thing that changes in this experiment.
   D. KEY. The placebo is the control because it should not have an effect on appetite control and will therefore serve as something to compare the results to.

2. **C**
   A. The type of fertilizer is important, but does not need to be recorded at regular intervals since it does not change in the experiment.
   B. The number of corn plants should not change during the experiment and therefore does not need to be recorded daily.
   C. KEY. The growth of the corn plants is what the scientist is studying, and it will change during the course of the experiment; therefore, this should be recorded every day.
   D. The species of corn plant is not something that will change during the course of the experiment.

3. **A**
   A. KEY. The nucleus is where genetic material is stored.
   B. The ribosomes are the site of protein synthesis.
   C. The mitochondria are where cellular respiration occurs; genetic material is not stored here.
   D. The cell membrane regulates what passes into and out of the cell.

4. **C**
   A. DNA carries the codes for proteins, but does not make up proteins.
   B. RNA carries the DNA code and is involved with protein synthesis, but does not make up proteins.
   C. KEY. Amino acids combine to form proteins.
   D. Nucleotides form the codes for amino acids, but do not make up proteins.

5. **A**
   A. KEY. The circulatory system includes the red blood cells which are responsible for transporting oxygen to the body cells.
   B. The digestive system is involved with digesting or breaking down food, not the transport of oxygen in the body.
   C. The excretory system is responsible for the removal of wastes, not the transport of oxygen in the body.
   D. The lymphatic system is responsible for removing excess fluids in the body, not transporting oxygen to the body cells.

6. **B**

 A. The circulatory system includes the blood vessels, heart, and blood. Symptoms of a disorder in this system would not necessarily include weight loss. Additionally, the pancreas is not part of this system.

 B. KEY. The pancreas is part of the digestive system, so this system would be affected in a person with pancreatitis. Additionally, symptoms of a disorder in this system may include weight loss and nausea as the role of the digestive system is to break down food.

 C. The excretory system includes the bladder, kidneys, ureters, and urethra; the pancreas is not part of this system. Additionally, symptoms of a disorder in this system would not necessarily include weight loss and nausea.

 D. The pancreas is not part of the reproductive system. Additionally, symptoms of a disorder in this system would not necessarily include weight loss or nausea.

7. **D**

 A. The trachea is part of the respiratory system, not the circulatory system.

 B. The trachea is part of the respiratory system, not the digestive system.

 C. The trachea is part of the respiratory system, not the lymphatic system.

 D. KEY. The trachea is part of the respiratory system; it is also called the windpipe because it is the vessel through which air moves from the mouth or nasal passages to the bronchi, which lead to the lungs.

8. **B**

 A. The digestive system is involved with breaking down food, not maintaining balance in the body.

 B. KEY. The nervous and endocrine systems are involved in communicating with the body through electric and chemical signals that help to maintain the best working conditions in the body.

 C. The digestive system is involved with breaking down food, not maintaining balance in the body. The excretory system, while important in keeping the proper balance of materials in the blood, does not do so through communications with the body.

 D. The excretory system, while important in keeping the proper balance of materials in the blood, does not do so through communications with the body.

9. **A**

 A. KEY. The scientific name is comprised of an organism's genus and species.

 B. The phylum is not part of the scientific name of an organism.

 C. The kingdom is not part of an organism's scientific name.

 D. The kingdom and phylum are not part of an organism's scientific name as these two categories are very broad.

10. **C**

    A.   Atoms of a given element can have different atomic mass as mass is determined by the number of protons and neutrons, and the number of neutrons in an atom can change.

    B.   Atoms of a given element can have a different charge because the charge is determined in part by the number of electrons in an atom and this number can change.

    C.   KEY. All atoms of a given element will have the same atomic number, which is determined by the number of protons in a given element. If the number of protons in an atom changes, it becomes a different element.

    D.   Atoms of a given element can have a different number of electrons.

11. **D**

    A.   There is one molecule of tricalcium phosphate, but there is more than one atom of oxygen in this molecule.

    B.   There are two molecules of phosphate in one molecule of tricalcium phosphate, but there is more than one atom of oxygen per molecule of phosphate.

    C.   There are four atoms of oxygen in a molecule of phosphate, but there are two molecules of phosphate in tricalcium phosphate.

    D.   KEY. There are eight atoms of oxygen in tricalcium phosphate; there are four atoms in each molecule of phosphate, and two molecules of phosphate. Two times four equals eight atoms altogether in tricalcium phosphate.

12. **C**

    A.   While an acid is part of the reactants, there is no base in the reactants, so this is not an acid-base reaction.

    B.   There are no acids or bases in the reactants of this reaction, so it is not an acid-base reaction.

    C.   KEY. HBr is an acid, and NaOH is a base; additionally, the products of this reaction are a salt and water, indicating that this is an acid-base reaction.

    D.   This is a combustion reaction, not an acid-base reaction. There are no acids or bases present in the reactants of this equation.

13. **D**

    A.   Condensing involves the removal of heat. Gas → liquid.

    B.   Evaporating involves the addition of heat energy. Liquid → Gas

    C.   Freezing involves the removal of heat. Liquid → solid

    D.   KEY. Melting involves the addition of heat energy. Solid → liquid.

14. **A**

    A.   KEY. Electrical energy moves through the electrical cord and is converted to heat energy to warm items in a toaster oven.

    B.   In a toaster, the energy that cooks the bread is not chemical energy.

    C.   Mechanical energy is the energy of movement, and the energy that cooks bread is not electrical energy.

    D.   Light energy is not the type of energy that cooks bread to make toast.

15. C

    A.   If more people are being born than dying, then the population rate would be increasing, but this does not affect the emigration rate.

    B.   If more people are dying than being born, the population rate would be decreasing, but this does not affect the emigration rate.

    C.   KEY. Emigration is the movement of people out of a country, so if more people are leaving rather than entering a country, the emigration rate would be high.

    D.   Immigration is the movement of people into a country, so if more people were entering rather than leaving a country, the immigration, not emigration, rate would be high.

16. A

    A.   KEY. This is an example of conduction because the transfer of heat is directly from the matter—the toaster—to the person's hand.

    B.   This is radiation because the person feels the heat energy as it moves through space.

    C.   This is radiation because the person feels the heat energy as it moves through the space of the car.

    D.   This is convection because the person feels the heat as it moves through the air flowing from the hair dryer.

Answers — Grammar

1. **C**
   A. Favorite precedes an adjective, *stuffed*, but it is modifying the noun *animal*. Only adjectives can modify nouns. The verb in the sentence is *destroyed*.
   B. This answer does correctly identify completely as an adverb, but it cannot be correct due to incorrectly identifying *favorite* as an adverb.
   C. KEY. *Favorite* is modifying the noun *animal*, therefore it is an adjective. *Completely* is a classic *–ly* adverb modifying the verb *destroyed*.
   D. This answer correctly identifies *favorite* as an adjective, but it incorrectly identifies the adverb *completely* as an adjective.

2. **D**
   A. "While we ate" is introductory information, but is not an independent clause. After information like this, a sentence requires a comma.
   B. A semicolon separates two independent clauses (clauses that could exist as separate sentences). Since "while we ate" cannot exist independently, it needs a comma to connect it to the rest of the sentence.
   C. A hyphen connects the parts of compound words and numbers. "While we ate" is introductory information, so it should be connected to the main part of the sentence with a comma, not a hyphen.
   D. KEY. As introductory information, "while we ate" should have a comma placed between it and the main part of the sentence.

3. **D**
   A. Because the sentence is a direct quotation, it needs double quotation marks. However, within the sentence, the speaker quotes someone else's dialogue. Therefore, this dialogue requires single quotation marks.
   B. Within this sentence, the speaker quotes someone else's dialogue, which correctly uses single quotation marks. However, because the sentence itself is a direct quotation, it needs double quotation marks.
   C. Because the sentence is a direct quotation, it needs double quotation marks, not single ones. In addition, within the sentence, the speaker quotes someone else's dialogue. Therefore, this dialogue requires single quotation marks, not double ones.
   D. KEY. Because the sentence is a direct quotation, it correctly uses double quotation marks. However, within the sentence, the speaker quotes someone else's dialogue. Therefore, this dialogue correctly uses single quotation marks.

4. **D**
   A. The subject of the sentence is *the group*. Therefore, the verb should be singular: has, not *have*.
   B. The subject of the sentence is *neither*, an indefinite pronoun. Therefore, it should take a singular verb: *enjoys*, not *enjoy*.
   C. When the subject of a sentence includes *or*, the verb should correspond to the noun nearest the verb: in this case, *is*, not *are*, to match *brother*.
   D. KEY. The compound subject *both Nancy and Patrice* is plural, so the verb is also plural.

5. **A**

A. KEY. The subject of the sentence is *Jerry and Mike*. Because the subject is plural, the proper possessive pronoun is *their*.

B. *Jerry and Mike* is a plural noun, so the correct possessive pronoun is *their*, not *his*.

C. Because *Jerry and Mike*, the subject of the sentence, is plural, the possessive pronoun describing *annual chili cook-off* should be *their*, not *its*.

D. *Jerry and Mike* the plural pronoun their, not the commonly confused word *there*.

6. **C**

A. This is a simple sentence structure, with a subject phrase (*whether I attend*) and a verb (*depends*).

B. This is a simple sentence structure, with a subject phrase (*whether I attend*) and a verb (*is*).

C. KEY. This sentence contains two independent clauses joined by the coordinating conjunction *and*.

D. This is a simple sentence structure, with a compound subject and a single verb.

7. **D**

A. This is a compound sentence, because it contains two independent clauses joined with a coordinating conjunction.

B. This is a simple, although long, sentence, containing one subject and one verb.

C. This is a simple sentence containing a compound subject.

D. KEY. This is a complex sentence. It contains one dependent clause joined to an independent clause with the subordinating conjunction although.

8. **D**

A. This is incorrect, because *permissible* ends with *–ible*, not *–able*.

B. This is incorrect, because *conceivable* ends with *–able*, not *–ible*.

C. This is incorrect, because *convertible* ends with *–ible*, not *–able*.

D. KEY. When changing *credit* to *credible*, the suffix used is *–ible*.

9. **C**

A. Although *irresponsible* may describe Tim's behavior, the context clues suggest that the *precarious* situation is one in which it is difficult to know how to act diplomatically. *Uncertain* offers the best synonym for this.

B. Although *offensive* may describe the results of saying the wrong thing in this situation, the context clues suggest that the *precarious* situation is one in which it is difficult to know how to act diplomatically. *Uncertain* offers the best synonym for this.

C. KEY. The context clues suggest that the *precarious* situation is one in which it is difficult to know how to act diplomatically. Uncertain offers the best synonym for this.

D. Although *unforeseen* may be a quality of this situation, the context clues suggest that the *precarious* situation is one in which it is difficult to know how to act diplomatically. *Uncertain* offers the best synonym for this.

10. B

    A.   This sentence adds the sense that the barbecue's success causes people to come to it, which is not suggested by the original information.

    B.   KEY. This sentence combines the information concisely without adding wordiness or awkwardness.

    C.   This sentence is awkwardly worded and repetitive, and could be made more concise by combining information more efficiently.

    D   This sentence uses passive voice unnecessarily.

DIAGNOSTIC TEST — SCORES

Now that you have completed the Diagnostic Test, let's see how well you did. Analyzing your scores can help you to identify your areas of strength and determine the subjects on which you should focus your study time. After checking your responses against the answer key, record the number of questions you answered correctly below. Then, use the fraction to determine the percentage of the items you answered correctly in each subject.

Reading	**Math**
$\dfrac{\text{Number correct}}{\text{Number of items} \quad 14} = \rule{2cm}{0.4pt}$	$\dfrac{\text{Number correct}}{\text{Number of items} \quad 10} = \rule{2cm}{0.4pt}$
_____% correct	_____% correct
Science	**Grammar**
$\dfrac{\text{Number correct}}{\text{Number of items} \quad 16} = \rule{2cm}{0.4pt}$	$\dfrac{\text{Number correct}}{\text{Number of items} \quad 10} = \rule{2cm}{0.4pt}$
_____% correct	_____% correct

What percentage of items did you answer correctly? Rank your scores from lowest to highest by subject below.

1. _____

2. _____

3. _____

4. _____

UNIT

Critical Skills

1 CRITICAL SKILLS · LESSON 1
Preparation

Events are almost always less stressful when we know what to expect. This is especially true for exams. Being prepared will reduce your stress level and allow you to feel that you are in control of the outcome of the test. In order to enter an exam situation with a clear and focused mind, it is essential to be able to anticipate what will be asked of you.

In this lesson, you will familiarize yourself with the critical skills needed to create and execute a study plan, allowing you to master not only the content of TEAS, but the structure and timeframe of the test as well.

Know What to Expect

In the previous pages of this book, we looked at the structure of the TEAS. To perform your absolute best, you will need to become comfortable with each type of item you will encounter on the test that you will take.

Knowing in advance the various types of items you can expect on the test you are preparing for is a great advantage. When you know in advance what to expect, you can strategize and use the most efficient approach for finding the correct answer.

Applying a predetermined strategy to each item type will also help you save time. This will help to ensure that you won't be racing the clock on exam day.

Analyze Your Strengths and Weaknesses

The TEAS requires students to recall and apply an extensive amount of information in a short period of time. To study efficiently, it is important to identify the areas where you excel, and the areas that need your attention prior to test day. Once you determine the topics on which to focus your attention, you can set up a study plan and a study timeline to help you strengthen your skills.

You have already taken the provided Diagnostic Test. Recreating test conditions as closely as possible not only allowed you to experience your emotions on test day but also to gain a realistic idea of your strengths and weaknesses.

Now that you have scored your Diagnostic Test, take some time to reflect on your performance and how it relates to your feelings about each section. Did you score very highly on a particular section? Did you notice that it took you less time than allotted to finish those items? If so, you can identify this subject area as a strength.

Using the results of your own Diagnostic Test, list the four test sections, reading, grammar, science, and math, in order of your personal performance from weakest to strongest. This will help to form your study schedule.

_____

_____

_____

_____

Your least successful section should now become the main focus of your preparation. Save your strongest section for the time closest to test day and you will end your studying on a high note!

Establish a Timeline for Extra Practice

The way in which you prepare for an admissions test will depend heavily on the amount of time you have to review. This book has been designed to give you enough time to review the most important content featured in each section of the TEAS. When you reach the end of unit, you will have gained knowledge, confidence, and speed; however, it is important to set aside time to practice the strategies you have learned.

Make an assessment of the amount of time you have before the exam to devote to extra studying. Keeping in mind that you will work through this entire book; decide how much time you can allocate to reviewing each section of the test. Use the list we just completed, and start with the section you struggled with the most on the Diagnostic Test. Remember, you will learn both content and strategies to apply to the various item formats you'll be presented with. This time will be used to review content and practice the strategies you are learning.

If you have one month or less before the exam, read the lessons associated with all of the items you answered incorrectly, focusing on the types of items you struggled with. This book will help you apply strategies that will increase your speed and accuracy.

What is your test date?

_____

How many hours per week can you study outside of classes?

_____

Set Up a Practice Plan

Now that you know what you need to work on and how long you have to work on it, you can make a schedule that will ensure well-paced, targeted practice.

If you have more than one month before the exam, begin with the section of the diagnostic test that you struggled the most with and work your way through that section of this book and the remaining lessons in the Critical Skills unit. Once you have done so, repeat that section of the diagnostic test. Is there a difference in your score? Be sure to study the answer explanations. Revisit the lessons that correlate to the items you answered incorrectly. Repeat both the guided and independent practice sections of those lessons. The more you apply the approaches set forth in the lessons to practice items, the more confident you'll become.

After you feel you're comfortable with your results on that section, move on to the next section that you found to be difficult. Approach that section the same way – thoroughly and patiently. Time is on your side. Relax and focus on the lessons.

The remaining two sections should cover the content you feel the most confident with. It will be beneficial for you to review these sections. Even if you have a firm grasp on the content, you can always improve your speed and accuracy.

When you have completed all of the units in the book, go back to the initial diagnostic test. Hopefully, some time has passed and you can look at the questions with fresh, practiced eyes! Re-do the exam under proctored and timed conditions just like you did when starting your review journey.

Congratulate yourself for having improved your score and revisit any lessons you feel you need more work on.

If you have less than one month to the exam, your practice plan will be similar, but condensed.

Starting with the section you struggled with the most on the diagnostic test, you'll complete all of the lessons in the unit pertaining to that subject as well as the guided and independent practice items. Reassess your knowledge by completing this section of the diagnostic test again. Pay close attention to which items you answer incorrectly the second time you take the test.

Compare the items you answered incorrectly to the guided practice section and study the answer explanations and the strategy applied to answering the item correctly. Challenge yourself to apply the strategies to correct your diagnostic test.

As your results improve, move on to the next subject area that you feel needs your attention. Review the lessons and guided and independent practice items. Spend the remainder of your practice time steadily working through the sample items you have at your disposal, including items that you feel confident answering. The extra practice will improve your speed and accuracy.

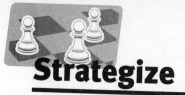

Strategize

If test day is just days away, you will approach your practice differently. Instead of focusing on one area that you struggled with on the Diagnostic Test, you will complete the test and then take a step back. Take some time to observe patterns – is there one type of item that gives you trouble?

Work through the guided practice items in the corresponding lesson and then try the independent practice. If you find that you haven't scored well, review the lessons and then redo that portion of the diagnostic test.

Because you don't have an extended time to practice, you should focus on getting comfortable with the items and the exam structure. While there is still time to learn content, you may benefit most by practicing based on item type instead of content section.

Pay close attention to the test-taking strategies put forth in this unit. For example: On the TEAS, there is no penalty for guessing and getting an answer wrong. The strategies you'll find in this book will help you use this to your advantage. If you pair the strategies with the online item bank, you'll find that if you re-take the diagnostic test, your score will be improved.

Practice

Now that you've identified the areas where you need extra practice and have a plan in motion, you need to know how to practice effectively! There are many ways to practice something. In basketball, players repeat the same shots hundreds of times until their muscles can successfully score the points without much forethought.

Repetition is one form of practicing. People learning new languages often sit with native speakers and have full conversations. Of course, they can't understand every word, but they learn to pick out the words they do understand and string together their knowledge until the sentence makes sense. Isolating the important information is another technique you'll use.

Strategies are plentiful, but how do you know which will work best for you? How do you know if that method will work for the exam you've scheduled? Answering these questions is what will differentiate practicing from practicing *effectively*.

Break Down the Material

The variety of material covered on any exam can seem overwhelming. This book breaks down all of the material you'll need to review in easy-to-manage sections. With content sorted into lessons, you can easily review the topics covered in class when you're on your own. You'll find that the lessons are easily digestible—if you narrow down the areas in which you need extra practice, you'll find that you won't feel overwhelmed.

Analyze the Item Types

Each test section of TEAS has a limited number of ways to test your knowledge of specific information. The format of all items on this exam is multiple choice, meaning that the answer to every question is on the page in front of you. If you are intimidated by the content, remember that part of these exams involves learning to pick out the right answer.

Each section of the exam will use the multiple-choice format to present information to you in various ways. The easiest way to get to know the item types you can expect is to practice. Look for patterns within each subject area. Is there a particular way the items addressing vocabulary are presented? If so, those items can be approached the same way each time. Opportunities to practice strategies will be given in each lesson, first within in the lesson with detailed explanation and examples, then on your own in a guided review and independent practice.

Focus on the Stem

Multiple-choice items will present you with a direct question. Sometimes there is additional information for you to absorb. This is called a stimulus. A stimulus can be presented in the form of a graph, a reading passage, or another piece of information. While it may be tempting to absorb the information presented in the stimulus first, it will be most beneficial to read the stem first. The stem is the actual question the item requires you to answer. By reading the stem first, you're giving yourself context with which to look at the stimulus.

For example, if you see a graph with axes labeled "Rainfall" and "Year," you do not yet know what you should be concluding from the graph. If you read the stem first, though, it will tell you exactly what you should be focusing on. The stem might say something like *How does the amount of rainfall in 2001 compare to the amount of rainfall in 2012?* By reading the stem first, you can automatically focus your attention on just two years on the graph. This method will save you time and help you eliminate incorrect answer choices.

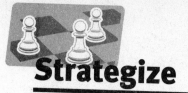

Strategize

Choose a Memorization Method

To be successful on an exam, you need to use both forms of memory—short- and long-term. You'll use your long-term memory to recall content that you've learned across years of schooling; for example, basic grammar and math that you have used repeatedly across multiple grades exists in your long-term memory. Your short-term memory holds information that you've learned recently. During your test, you will likely pull strategies and content covered in your review sessions from your short-term memory.

There are several different ways to commit information to your short-term memory when you don't have a lot of time before an exam. Think about how you have studied for tests in the past. Most likely, you already know what method works best for you.

The most common memorization technique is repetition. You can utilize repetition to commit a large amount of material to your short-term memory in a condensed period of time. If you've ever used flash cards, you are already aware of how helpful they can be, but it is important that you choose carefully which types of content are best suited to this type of memorization. Grammar, vocabulary, mathematical equations, and scientific terms are best suited to flash cards because this type of information is brief and can be cycled through quickly. Shuffle your cards regularly so that you can be sure that you're memorizing the content and not the order.

Longer math strategies and science concepts are better suited to memorization through a study guide, like this book. The more items you work through—especially items that come along with an explanation—the more you can train your mind to approach similar items in the same way.

Some students are auditory learners, meaning that they learn best when hearing information and speaking it out loud. Can you recall your teachers' voices speaking certain pieces of information in class? If so, you may benefit from this type of memorization. Try reading both your notes and the lessons in this book out loud several times. Putting the words into your own voice may make them easier for you to understand and recall under test circumstances. If you decide to use flash cards, make sure to read them aloud.

Another excellent way to memorize information is to summarize it as you learn or review. Some students find it challenging to stay engaged when learning certain subjects. Building a summarization step into your review will keep your mind focused. In your own words, repeat what you just learned. If you can't explain what the lesson has taught you, go back and start again. Putting a concept in your own words will allow it to feel natural and familiar. Talking an item through will allow you to teach yourself, which will build your confidence and help you memorize at the same time.

Isolate Important Information

Most items you will encounter on the TEAS contain more information than is necessary to answer the question. As a nurse, you'll need to be able to identify pieces of information that are more important than others. For example, if a patient lists his or her symptoms, your training will allow you to absorb the entire list while zeroing in on anything that may be particularly alarming. Test questions function in much the same way.

As mentioned earlier, you should always read the stem of an item first. This will help you to identify the task that the item is asking you to complete, and the information you're expected to use in solving the problem. The stem is also where you'll find important key words. Ask yourself what the stem is really asking you. Try rephrasing it to eliminate any unnecessary words.

If the item is accompanied by a stimulus, you'll want to look for the same key words in that information, or look for synonyms. It may be helpful to you to underline or highlight the key words. This will keep you focused when absorbing other information that may be interesting but not critical to answering the item correctly. On an exam, time is of the essence. Skimming a stimulus to look for the key words or phrases from the stem will help you move forward quickly but accurately.

Read Inquisitively

As tempting as it may be to race through a test, it is important to ask yourself several questions when working on each item. First and most important is, *What is this question asking me to do?* It seems simple but requires you to trim the item down to its most basic information. Asking yourself this question will help you eliminate answer choices that are not applicable to the core of the item. Because the TEAS is multiple choice, any question you can ask yourself that will help you eliminate an answer choice increases your probability of answering the question correctly by 25% purely based on the process of elimination.

Another question you should ask yourself is, What information do I need to answer this? Knowing what to look for will help you navigate stimuli that purposefully include unnecessary information. By mindfully answering this question, you can be very specific in your hunt for the correct answer. After reading a stem associated with a passage, if you can say to yourself, *Okay, I'm looking for the percentage of patients who experience a relapse of symptoms*, you can automatically skip information pertaining to the primary onset of symptoms and focus on numbers located later in the passage.

For items that require you to solve a problem rather than recall or interpret information, ask yourself, *Is there a formula or rule that can help me solve this problem?* This question requires you to think about ways you may have solved this type of item in the past. If there is a formula or strategy that you recall from your review sessions, write it down on scrap paper. Refer to it as you work through the problem.

Pace Yourself

Knowing how much time you'll have to answer every item at a comfortable pace is a crucial aspect of knowing what to expect from a test. Because there is no penalty on the TEAS for answering items incorrectly, being able to finish every item will work to your advantage.

Manage Stress

Although stress management isn't directly related to the content you can expect to see on an exam, it is almost equally important. Being able to strategically work through your exam with a clear mind will improve your speed and accuracy exponentially. A low stress level will keep you from making easy-to-avoid mistakes like choosing an answer that looks very similar to the correct answer but is slightly different, or misgridding your answer.

Preparation is key to stress management, but studying frantically isn't beneficial. Consider your mood when you're reviewing. Are you feeling calm and positive, or are you rushing through the lessons and practice tests? Are you feeling nervous? No need! If you're taking the time to prepare, you deserve to feel calm and confident. Take deep breaths and feel positive about the work you're putting into your preparation—good things come to those who work hard, and that's you!

Before your exam, pay attention to your diet and exercise. Both of these factors play a big role in stress management and brain function. Hunger is a huge distraction, so make sure to eat regularly, not only the day of your exam, but also when you're studying. It's hard to retain information when your stomach is growling! Proteins, complex carbohydrates, veggies, and plenty of water are key. Exercise is a great stress reliever and also helps to increase your attention span and ability to focus. Although you may be tempted to study at your desk for days on end, getting the recommended amount of exercise per week will boost the faculties you need to do well on your test.

A good diet and plenty of exercise may be important, but perhaps more important than both of those habits is getting a good night's sleep. Simple but effective, sleep has a hand in keeping you refreshed and alert, and also plays a big role in memory retention. You've been absorbing a lot of information while getting ready for your test, and sleeping will help you keep that information in your mind on test day.

The day before your test, relax. Have a good meal. Exercise. Go to bed early. You're ready!

CRITICAL SKILLS · LESSON 2
Test-Taking Strategies

Taking an exam is sometimes about more than demonstrating a strong grasp of the content. Your performance can be affected by how well you respond to the format of the exam, the amount of time you're given for each section, and the strategies you can apply to help you move through the items quickly and accurately.

The TEAS is multiple choice in format and is available in either computer-based or paper-based formats, depending entirely on the policy of the school(s) to which you apply. Regardless of the format of your test, there are numerous strategies that you can apply to help you solve each item correctly. If you consider the general strategies detailed in this lesson to be the primary tools in your toolbox, you'll be ready to work through every problem, whether it appear on paper or on a computer screen.

Process of Elimination

Process of elimination allows you to use the format of a test to your advantage. There is only one correct answer, meaning that the other three choices have been added because they look like they could be correct. If you can eliminate choices that you know are incorrect, you will have statistically improved your chances of answering the item correctly, even if you're unsure of the correct response.

There is no penalty for incorrect answers on the TEAS. What does this mean, exactly? When you answer a question correctly, you receive points toward your overall score. When you answer a question incorrectly, you don't receive points, but you do not lose points, either. This makes it worthwhile to answer every question on the exam, regardless of your confidence as to the right answer. If you can eliminate one answer choice as incorrect, you have a 1 in 3 chance of answering correctly. If you can eliminate two answer choices, you have a 1 in 2 chance. Those are good odds—do not be distracted by the answer choices. Use the information you do know on the topic to make your most educated guesses.

When using the process of elimination, always predict the answer before you read the answer choices. By generating your own response, you avoid the confusion that comes along with answers that all seem similar. When you have an answer in your mind, you can read the answer choices to find one that best matches your organic response. This should, at the very least, help you eliminate incorrect answer choices and take a confident guess.

Predict Before You Peek

Predict Before You Peek is a strategy you'll see reiterated throughout this book. Often times, multiple choice tests feature choices for each item that look very similar to the right answer. When you look at the distractors before you read the question or before you decide for yourself what you think the right answer is, your judgment can be influenced by the incorrect choices.

Predicting the answer before you peek at the answer choices will ensure that you remain in control of your own thoughts. Work through the problem from start to finish before looking at the answer choices.

Is the answer you found one of your options? If so, choose it and move on to the next question confidently.

If you don't see the answer that you found as an option, the next strategy may come in handy!

Working Backwards

Working backwards from the answer choices can help you if you're feeling stuck. Let's assume that you worked through the problem using the Predict Before You Peek strategy above. If none of the answer choices look like what you had in mind, try choosing an answer choice and plugging it into the thought process you used to determine your first answer.

This strategy is especially helpful with math problems. If you know what the question is asking and you know the formula needed to solve the problem, working backwards can be very efficient.

Because numerical answer choices are often ordered by size, A being the lowest value and D being the highest, it is beneficial to work backwards starting from answer choice C. If the result you get when working through the problem backwards is too large, you can eliminate answer choice D and instead move on to focus on answer choices A and B. This will help you save time.

Plugging the answer choices into grammar and vocabulary items can also help you find the correct answer. Try plugging in each answer choice and reading the sentence silently to yourself. Go with your gut as to what sounds correct.

Making an Educated Guess

If you were not able to eliminate the incorrect answer choices or work backwards to the correct answer, it is time to make an *educated* guess. This does not mean that you should choose at random—an educated guess involves processing the information that you understand and using it to rule out the choices that you can.

To make sure that your guess really is an educated one, think back to questions that you saw earlier in the exam or during your review process at home. Can you remember how you solved that question? Using that experience may help you predict the correct answer in your current situation.

At this point, you may be over-analyzing. Reread the question. Have you followed all of the clues? Look at the wording of the item to make sure you're not missing a simple solution.

Of the answer choices you were unable to rule out, choose the answer that looks most like the answer you found when you applied the Predict Before You Peek strategy.

During the Exam

First Things First

Before you leave your house on test day, ask yourself, *Do I have everything I need to take this exam?* If you don't have the tools you're used to using, such as sharpened pencils and erasers, now is the time to get them! You don't need the stress of broken pencils when you're sitting in the exam room. Simply forgetting something at home can set you up to feel like you're behind, and that can adversely affect your performance.

Note that you will need a government-issued form of identification, such as a driver's license or passport, in order to take the exam. A student ID card or credit card will not be accepted. If you do not have a government-issued form of identification, you should look into this right away. Occasionally, it can take time to receive these types of documentation. You want to make sure there is ample time before your exam to receive your ID.

If you are taking the test at an unfamiliar location on campus or at a testing center in a neighboring town, drive to the location at least once before the real test day—and at approximately the same time. Time yourself and make notes on traffic conditions or parking issues that you may encounter. If taking the test at your prospective school, ask the test administrator before the start of the test about any parking requirements such as a fee or visitor's tag. You must plan ahead to avoid using test time to remedy parking issues.

Keep a Positive Attitude

Keeping a positive attitude is sometimes easier said than done. People usually don't respond favorably to tasks they're being graded on, and even less favorably when a clock is ticking. These factors make it that much more important to keep a firm grip on your outlook.

To keep a positive outlook during an exam, remind yourself: *I am prepared*. When you work through a problem and feel confident in your answer, smile. Smiling is a natural mood booster, and it will help you feel like you're in an enjoyable situation, which you are. After all, you're about to do very well on the TEAS!

UNIT 2 Reading

Reading Fundamentals

When you pick up something to read, do you ask yourself what kind of text it is? As you read, you can use strategies that will help you determine the type of text you are reading. Let's begin by reviewing some of these concepts and strategies.

Common Uses in Health Care

- instructions for medications
- patients' charts
- doctors' orders

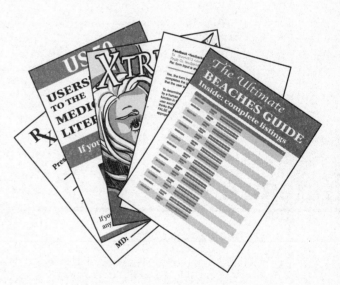

Key Terms/Formulas

- **cause-effect** – text structure that discusses an event and its results

- **compare-and-contrast** – text structure that compares two or more things, people, events, or ideas

- **expository text** – text that explains a topic

- **fiction** – made-up text

- **informational text** – factual text

- **narrative** – text that tells a story

- **persuasive text** – text that tries to convince

- **problem-solution** – text structure that presents a problem and then resolves it

- **sequence** – text structure that organize text in chronological order

- **technical text** – text that contains precise and technical information

- **text features** – headings, subheadings, italicized or boldfaced words

- **text structure** – way in which text is organized

Recall that all writing is divided into two types: fiction and informational. **Informational text** is factual, like a newspaper, a speech, or a textbook. **Fiction** is made up, although parts of it may have happened.

Different Kinds of Passages

The TEAS requires comprehension and analysis of passages, paragraphs, and informational sources. There are various kinds of passages. The chart lists the main types. Passages and paragraphs can be categorized by their purposes, content, and format.

What type of passage?	Why write this passage?	What are some examples?
Narrative	To tell a story by relating a series of events	• Short story • Personal letter • Autobiography
Persuasive	To convince the reader of something	• Letters to the editor • Speeches • Advertisements
Expository	To explain a topic	• Academic papers • History books • Art books
Technical	To give specific technical information	• Computer manuals • Scientific papers • Medical literature

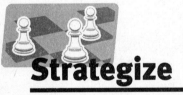

Strategize

Analyze and Decide

As you read a passage, look for clues that will tell you what type of text it is. Seek out characteristics of each type of text as you read that will help you decide. For example, you may ask yourself:

- *What is the author trying to do?*

- *Is the author trying to convince me of something?*

- *Is the author trying to explain a subject?*

- *Is the author trying to give me instructions on how to operate something?*

Predict Before You Peek

Any time you answer a Reading question on the admissions test, take a few moments to predict before you peek. If you encounter a question asking you to identify a passage's type or purpose, first skim through the passage. Use the content to decide the passage's type before you read through the answer choices. Then, test each answer choice against your own determination to find which one best matches your prediction.

Why do this? Making your own decision without considering the answer choices means that those tempting wrong answer choices will seem less tempting.

Apply

How might these strategies help you on the admissions test? Let's look at a passage and try to determine its type.

The following letter appeared in a local newspaper's editorial page.

Dear Editor,

The city is now facing one of the most critical decisions it will have to make in this decade: whether to build a new performance arena. A new performance arena would go far in putting this city on the map. It would bring touring companies to town, which would create many side benefits.

People who go to plays or musicals tend to go out to eat before the performance, for example. Therefore the restaurant industry in town would thrive. The theater would also draw people from surrounding communities, bringing new money into town.

I implore everyone to attend Wednesday evening's council meeting to support the new performance center. I will see you there.

Sincerely,

Andrew Lang

STEP 1: Scan.

Look for clues and key words that show characteristics of each type of writing.

STEP 2: Analyze.

Think about words and phrases such as *Dear Editor* and *implore*. What do these suggest about the passage's type?

STEP 3: Decide.

The author wants to convince the reader to think and act a certain way. This must be a persuasive text.

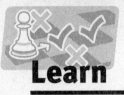

Text Features

Informational text often makes use of text features. These include boldface or italic type, headings, subheadings, and bulleted lists. Often, these features are helpful to your understanding of the text. They can also help you find information quickly by indicating the main content of a particular section of the text.

What are some common text structures?

There are several different ways that text can be structured, or organized.

What kind of text structure?	What is its purpose?	What are some examples?	Key Words
Sequence	To relate events or steps of instructions in the order that they happen or should be done	• Instructions • Autobiography • Short stories or novels	• First • Next • Then • Last • Later
Problem-solution	To present a problem and then give a solution	• Medical or scientific papers • Computer manuals • Technical papers	• Problem • Solution • Resolve • Since • In order to
Cause-effect	To present a problem and the effects that it will have	• Medical information • Letters to the editor • Environmental literature	• Because • Therefore • Thus • Since • Due to
Compare-and-contrast	To compare and/or contrast one thing or person to another thing or person	• Reviews • Academic papers • Scientific papers	• But • Similarly • However • As opposed to • On the other hand

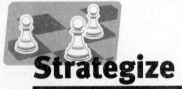
Strategize

Scanning or skimming your text

Before you start to read, quickly scan or skim through the text. You can get a good idea about what is in the text from doing this.

- Identify any text features. Pay close attention to titles, headings, subheadings, and emphasized words. These features usually highlight the main points of a text.

- Look for key words that show text structure, such as *first*, *next*, *problem*, or *as a result*.

- Read sections with key words more closely. Remember, some key words may apply to more than one type of text structure.

Apply

Let's practice using text features and key words to identify the structure of a text.

First, open the bottle of glue by squeezing down on the top and turning.

Then apply the glue thoroughly to the two pieces of wood that you need to glue together.

Next, carefully place one piece of wood on top of the other with the glued areas facing each other.

Finally, clamp the two pieces of wood together.

After 24 hours, the glue has set and the wood can be used.

STEP 1: Scan

Scan the text, looking for any text features that may help you identify text structure. Look closely at headings, titles, boldface or italicized words, and/or key words that give hints about the text's structure.

STEP 2: Analyze

Analyze any important words or phrases that you have identified. What do these words or phrases suggest about the text?

In this case, you might notice that all of the time-ordered words such as *First, Then, Next, Finally,* and *After* are boldfaced. This is a clue to the text's structure. The directions are in sequential order, listed in the order that they need to be done.

 WATCH OUT!

Some key words may trick you. For instance, the word ***then*** could indicate sequential order, but it could also be a sign of cause-effect structure. You will need to read the passage carefully to ensure you have made the correct choice.

Guided Practice

Let's work through a few examples together. Review the lesson content to help you apply the concepts and strategies you learned.

1. The annual "Race for Food" fundraiser will take place next Saturday at 8 a.m. at Greenfield Park. This four-mile race raises money for the Samara Food Pantry, where demand has risen significantly in the past few months. Those interested in participating are asked to call 555-9097 before Wednesday to reserve a spot. Runners must be sponsored by individuals or businesses. Organizers are suggesting that sponsors pledge $10 per mile, but any donation is welcomed.

   The passage is reflective of which of the following types of writing?

   A) narrative

   B) persuasive

   C) expository

   D) technical

   STEP 1: Scan

   What is the question asking?

   _____

   _____

   STEP 2: Analyze

   What is the general idea of the passage?

   _____

   _____

   STEP 3: Decide

   What type of text is this?

   _____

   _____

2. Dear Mrs. Cantarella:

Thank you for contacting me about your software problems. I know they must be extremely annoying to you. My staff and I can help you find what needs to be done to resolve the situation. A technician will call you later today and walk you through the steps you need to improve the software's performance. If this does not work we will send another copy of the software. We certainly want to do everything we can to support you. Thank you for your business.

Most sincerely,

Robert Ruiz

General Manager

COMEX

This letter is reflective of which of the following types of text structure?

A) sequence

B) compare-and-contrast

C) cause-effect

D) problem-solution

STEP 1: Read

Read the question. What does it ask you to determine?

_____

_____

STEP 2: Analyze

Scan through the text. What key words can you find?

_____

_____

STEP 3: Predict

Based on the key words you found, what is the text structure of this letter?

_____

_____

Guided Practice

3. Federal Youth Work Regulations

Youths Under 16

Federal regulations dictate that 14- or 15-year-olds may work as long as the job does not interfere with school. They are also not allowed to operate heavy or dangerous machinery or work after 10:00 p.m.

Youths 16 to 17

Federal regulations dictate that 16- or 17-year-olds may work until midnight with parental consent.

Youths 18 and Over

No parental consent form needed for those aged 18 or over.

Consent Forms

Consent forms may be obtained from the federal government website or from the unemployment office in your area.

A 14-year-old boy wants to get a job. Which section of the article would be mostly likely to provide him with information on relevant regulations?

A) Youths Under 16

B) Youths 16 to 17

C) Youths 18 and Over

D) Consent Forms

STEP 1: Read

Read the question. What skill does it ask you to apply?

_____

_____

STEP 2: Scan

Scan through the text. What text features do you see?

_____

_____

STEP 3: Analyze

Which text feature most likely provides the information requested in the item?

_____

_____

Independent Practice

1. Clean the lint filter before each load.
Put only one washer load into the dryer at a time.
Use the regular cycle to dry towels, bed linens, jeans, and other regular fabrics.
Use the permanent press cycle to dry nylons, acrylics, polyesters, and blends.
Remove permanent press items as soon as the dryer stops to prevent wrinkling.
Use the air-fluff cycle to freshen pillows, throw rugs, etc. (items that have not been washed).
When drying small loads, set the timer to the number of minutes desired.

The passage is most reflective of which type of writing?

A) descriptive

B) narrative

C) persuasive

D) technical

HINT   *What kind of process does this passage tell about?*

2. Reggie Jackson has always been a natural athlete. As a kid, he was a star in track and football as well as in baseball. He spent long hours practicing hitting after school.

Professional Player
After two years in college at Arizona State, Reggie accepted an offer to play professional baseball with the Kansas City Athletics organization. He did so well in the minor league that the Athletics, or A's, let him play in the majors at the end of the season.

Before the '68 season began, the A's moved to Oakland, California. Charlie Finley, their owner, kept the team's promise, and Reggie became a regular team member. The year was full of ups and downs.

Success
Reggie spent the winter of '71 playing baseball in Puerto Rico and learning to be patient. It paid off. All next season he played good baseball. The A's had become the best team in the country. Three years in succession, they won the World Series. In 1973, Reggie was named Most Valuable Player in the American League. Twenty years later, he was inducted into the Baseball Hall of Fame.

This passage is reflective of which type of text structure?

A) compare-contrast

B) problem-solution

C) sequence

D) narrative

HINT   *What do key words such as* before, later, *and in succession* *suggest about the passage's text structure?*

Independent Practice

3. One hundred and fifty million years ago, dinosaurs roamed the western United States. They could be found in Colorado, Montana, Utah, and Wyoming. The west was very different then. It was hot and moist, dotted with many lakes and swamps, and the dinosaur inhabitants were many and variegated. Prominent among them was the large brontosaurus, a plant eater that had a long neck enabling it to reach the top of vegetation, and the allosaurus, a fierce carnivore with sharp teeth and a large head. The allosaurus was a successful predator with short front limbs probably used to grasp prey and strong back legs for speed.

Which characteristic helps you to know this is an informational text?

A) It explains a topic.

B) It tries to persuade readers.

C) It is in a sequential order.

D) It has advanced vocabulary.

HINT ⟩ *Ask yourself what the passage is doing.*

ReKap

In this lesson, you learned about different types of writing and their characteristics. You learned the difference between fiction and informational text. You also learned about the various types of writing that are used to achieve different purposes.

Types of everyday texts encountered by nurses:
Doctor's orders; prescription literature; patients' charts. These may be instructional or informational texts.

You learned that there are many ways a text can be structured, such as sequentially, problem-solution, cause-effect, and compare-contrast.

You learned about text features, including boldfaced and italicized words, headings, and subheadings. You learned about looking for key words to help you determine the type of writing or text structure.

You learned strategies to help you answer test items. These strategies are:

- Scan and Skim

- Predict Before You Peek

- Analyze and Decide

> **?** **What are three examples of texts that are you likely to encounter in your day-to-day work as a health care professional? What types of texts are these?**
>
> _____
>
> _____
>
> _____
>
> _____

Answers

Guided Practice

1. Step 1: The question asks one to identify the type of writing in the paragraph.

   Step 2: In general, the paragraph includes facts about the fundraiser.

   Step 3: The text is expository.

   Answer: (C) expository

2. Step 1: The question asks about the text structure.

   Step 2: Key words include *problem* and *resolve*.

   Step 3: The text structure is problem-solving.

   Answer: (D) problem solving

3. Step 1: One needs to use text features to answer the question.

   Step 2: Text features include a title, headings, and boldfaced words.

   Step 3: The heading *Youths Under 16* is the section that provides the needed information.

   Answer: (A) Youths Under 16

Independent Practice

1. **Answer: (A) descriptive**

   This passage gives a set of directions to operate a machine, so it is a technical text. The text lacks the main characteristics of any of the other types listed.

   TIP: It may help to predict the type before reading answer choices.

2. **Answer: (C) sequence**

   This biography provides a series of important events in an athlete's career in order. Therefore, it uses the sequence text structure.

3. **Answer: (A) It explains a topic.**

   Informational text provides facts and details about a particular topic, as this text provides facts and details about dinosaurs. This text is not persuasive, nor is it organized using a sequence text structure.

ReKap

Three common examples of text are narrative (telling a series of events), expository (explaining a topic), and technical (giving specific technical information).

2

Paragraph and Passage Fundamentals

Do you enjoy reading different kinds of passages? What are your favorites? You will find a wide variety of passage types on the TEAS exam, everything from texts about historical events to stories about strange things that have happened to medical texts that explain the use of various medicines. When you read, it is important to think about the kind of text you are reading and its purpose, or why the text was written.

Common Uses in Health Care

- case studies
- clinical trials
- medical histories

	Author's intent
✓	Author's purpose
	Main idea
✓	Supporting detail
	Theme
✓	Topic

Key Terms/Formulas

- **author's intent** – what the author hopes to accomplish with the text

- **author's purpose** – why the author writes a text

- **main idea** – what a text is specifically about

- **supporting details** – information that tells more about the main idea

- **theme** – a subject that the text touches upon more than once

- **topic** – what a text is generally about

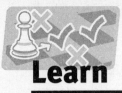

Learn

The **author's purpose** and the **author's intent** are what the author hopes to accomplish by writing a text. A writer may want to

- entertain

- express feelings

- inform

- persuade

Author's Purpose for Writing	Type and Examples of Texts	What the Author Wants the Reader to Take Away from the Passage
to entertain	• Fiction (poetry, stories, folktales, mysteries)	• a lesson, an experience, entertainment
to express feelings	• Fiction or nonfiction (stories, poems, letters, articles)	• a feeling or thought
to inform	• Nonfiction (how-to articles, brochures, recipes, lab reports, technical writing)	• information, instructions
to persuade	• Nonfiction (advertisements, editorials, essays)	• a thought, belief, or action; agreement with the writer's ideas or perspective

While many authors clearly show readers the text's purpose or intent, others write in a way that makes this information more difficult to discern. For example, someone who wants to persuade may hide the real purpose of what is being said. That is why it is important to ask yourself, *Why did the author write this text? What is the author's purpose for sharing his or her ideas?* Once you understand a text's purpose, you will more easily understand its meaning.

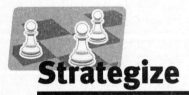

Strategize

Scan and Skim

Skim through a text and look for key words or expressions that express an opinion, or for facts that are unique. These could help you determine the author's purpose for writing the text.

Read and Decide

Read through the text and decide whether there is an obvious purpose. Ask yourself why the author wrote the text.

Check Your Response

As you read a text, check to see what your personal response to it is. Does it make you laugh? Does it teach you something? Does it persuade you to believe something? These are clues to the author's purpose.

Sample Passages

To Persuade

The idea of school uniforms is not new. Faculty, administrators, and students all have concerned themselves with this issue at one time or another. Yet, few conclusions have been adopted on whether such a requirement is beneficial to the education process. The pros and cons have been bandied about, but there is no clear-cut answer. The truth is, in today's world the idea of school uniforms is an anachronism that has outgrown its usefulness. That is why we are coming together as a group to oppose the latest attempt to regulate the clothes that students wear to school. To be sure, we are in favor of dress that is within the guidelines of good taste, but we refuse to approve the notion that all students should look alike. We should not be required to be carbon copies of one another. We deserve to be able to express ourselves as individuals. Join us in our pledge to put an end to this initiative.

To Inform

Many experts say that bananas were the first fruit cultivated by humans. Unfortunately some people fear that bananas may completely disappear in the near future. This is because they are prone to disease. Fungus organisms can infect the banana plant fairly easily. Since all bananas are grown from plants, the disease would likely be transmitted from one to the other very quickly. Scientists are trying to engineer banana plants that are more resistant to disease.

To Entertain

An Ant went to the bank of a river to quench its thirst, and being carried away by the rush of the stream, was on the point of drowning. A Dove sitting on a tree branch overhanging the water plucked a leaf and let it fall into the stream close to her. The Ant climbed onto it and floated in safety to the bank. Shortly afterward, a bird catcher came and stood under the tree and laid his lime-twigs for the Dove, which sat in the branches. The Ant, perceiving his design, stung him in the foot. In pain, the bird catcher threw down the twigs, and the noise made the Dove take wing.

To Express Feelings

At times I
Wonder at my
Path through
Life.
Not bold as I
Desired as a
Child.
More like a wave
That comes and goes
Seeking to fill in
The empty spots
Seeking to find
A home,
But endless.

Sample Passages

Recipe

Banana Milkshake
First pour twelve ounces of milk into a blender.
Peel a banana and cut it into pieces.
Put banana into blender.
Add ½ teaspoon of vanilla.
Blend the mixture on slow and then on frappe.

Letter to the Editor

To the Editor:

Even though the Great United Supermarket employs over 200 people, there is no reason that it should remain open. Some people may argue that it offers a wide selection of food at low prices. But Great United sells spoiled food that makes people ill. Health inspectors have issued complaints about it, and our local hospital is concerned. More than a dozen patients have been admitted for care after eating food purchased there. This supermarket must be closed. Until then, no one should buy anything at Great United.

Janet Rojo

Speech

Ladies and Gentlemen:

I have come here today to let you know what my administration will be focusing on in the next two years. We are intent upon solving some problems that have been with us for a long time, but which we have somehow ignored. Let me say, this is not what will be happening in the future.

Informational Text

The armadillo is like a little tank because it is covered with plates. Its name in Spanish means the "little one all covered in armor." When necessary, it can curl into a tight ball, completely covered by its shell, safe from most predators who cannot get at its soft belly. However, it's not likely that you'll ever see a curled up armadillo, because it's a fast runner, too swift for most of its enemies. It's also a strong digger that will usually dig to safety.

The gray whale is one of nature's most majestic creatures. The migration habits of these creatures are unique as well. From April to November, the gray whale lives in the Arctic waters of the Bering and Beaufort Seas. The whale then travels to the warm waters off the coast of Baja California, Mexico, where they mate. The females birth and nurse their young in Baja. The baby whales, which are called calves, grow very quickly. The whales return north, after the young have become strong, in late winter. They are so wonderful to see.

Apply

Let's practice using these strategies to determine the author's purpose for writing a few passages similar to those you would see on the admissions test.

A giant bridge was built connecting the tip of the San Francisco peninsula to the adjoining land. Named the Golden Gate Bridge, its construction was started in 1933 and finished in 1937.

Everyone was very excited on the first day after the bridge was completed, but no celebration was planned for that day. Only one person was allowed on the bridge on that whole day. A blind woman and her dog were the first pedestrians.

The next day 200,000 people crossed the bridge. It was a colorful event and some people did strange things. One guy walked the whole way on stilts. One woman crossed with her tongue sticking out while another woman crossed wearing a big wooden hat. Of course, most of those who crossed did nothing unusual. The day after the bridge was completed was one of the most exciting days in San Francisco history.

In deciding what the author's purpose is, it is helpful to use the strategies that we reviewed.

STEP 1: Scan and Skim

We can quickly tell the text is about the building of the Golden Gate Bridge. But this does not tell us its purpose. Looking further, you can see a lot of information about the opening of the bridge. This is one clue to the purpose.

STEP 2: Read and Decide

Read the text in full. Why did the author write this text? Is it entertaining, informative, expressing feelings, or trying to persuade you of something?

STEP 3: Check Your Response

Review the kind of details that are in the text. Did they make you laugh? Did they persuade you to feel or believe something? Your reaction is key to figuring out what the author's purpose is.

While you might think the purpose of the passage is to inform, it is more likely that the author's purpose is to entertain, since he tells funny stories about what people did to celebrate the opening of the bridge. Did you think the stories were funny?

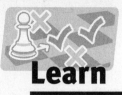
Every text has various elements. These elements help the reader to better understand what the text is about. This chart lists the main elements of paragraphs.

What is the element?	What is its definition?	What is an example?
Topic	What the text is generally about	*Medicine*
Main Idea	What the text is specifically about	*There are a number of medicines available for the treatment of diabetes.*
Supporting Details	Information that tells more about the main idea	*The effectiveness and side effects of each medicine*
Theme	Subjects frequently touched upon	*Medical improvements*

When you read a text, think about each of the different elements that make up a passage. Ask yourself what the text is about in general. That will give you the text's **topic**. Ask yourself what the text is about specifically. That will give you the **main idea**. Then look to see what information there is in the text that talks about, or helps to explain, the main idea. These are the **supporting details**. Finally, decide if there is a subject that is touched on over and over. That would bring you the **theme** of the text.

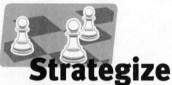

Strategize

Scan and Skim

Quickly read over the passage to find the topic. Notice what the passage is mainly about.

Read and Decide

Next, read the passage carefully. As you read, look for what specific information is given about the topic.

Make a Chart

When you read a text, it can be helpful to make a chart similar to the one above. In the first column, fill in the names of the text elements. In the middle column, write the following questions: What is the text generally about? What is the text specifically about? What information supports the main idea? Is there a subject that the text touches on repeatedly? In the last column, write your answers. You won't have much time to do this on the nursing admissions test, so just make a rough chart.

Apply

Now, let's practice identifying the topic, main idea, supporting details, and theme of a text.

Modern art has puzzled many people. One reason is that often modern art does not present a realistic picture. Instead the painting may just consist of patterns of color and shapes. Some of the greatest works of modern art were ridiculed when they were first shown to the public. Even now that modern art is widely accepted, there have been problems.

Once, a painting by Matisse, a great modern artist, was hung upside down in a museum. Over 116,000 people saw the painting, many of them experts in art, before someone noticed that the painting was hung the wrong way. At another exhibit for an unknown artist, the paintings were highly praised by experts. Imagine their embarrassment when the experts found out that the show was a trick. The paintings had been done by a chimpanzee playing around with brushes and paint.

What is the element?	What is the question?	What is the answer?
Topic	What the text is generally about	
Main Idea	What the text is specifically about	
Supporting Details	What information tells more about the main idea?	
Theme	What subject is frequently touched upon?	

Now we can answer the questions. The topic seems clear enough. By quickly scanning and skimming the text, we can tell that the topic is art. By reading the whole passage, we can decide that the specific subject is the fact that modern art is puzzling. This is the main idea. There are a number of supporting details: Matisse's painting was hung upside down; paintings praised by experts were a trick. The theme is more difficult to pin down. But the subject of art being difficult to assess could be the theme.

Guided Practice

Now, let's practice using what you have learned by working through a few examples together.

1. It was July 4, 1989, at about 8 P.M. The fireworks were ready, but no one wanted to go out on the beach and begin the celebration. Everyone was waiting for a turtle to finish laying her eggs on the beach. The turtle mother was quite slow in digging a hole for the eggs to hatch in because her back flippers were badly injured. Perhaps a shark had bitten them off. Still, she struggled to dig the hole, although she made little progress.

    Our local naturalist, Mr. Harvey, decided to come to her aid. He crawled over to the turtle carefully so as not to alarm her. Every time she pushed her flippers in the sand, he helped her out by scooping some sand from the hole. Within a few minutes, the job was completed. As soon as the turtle was satisfied that the hole was deep enough, she laid her eggs, covered them, and headed back into the ocean. All the spectators applauded. Then they came pouring out onto the beach, and the fireworks began. Everyone agreed that it was the best Fourth of July celebration the town ever had.

    What is the main idea of the passage?

    A) The fireworks on July fourth were great.

    B) People were worried about a turtle laying eggs.

    C) A naturalist helped a turtle lay her eggs in the sand.

    D) A wounded turtle was having trouble laying her eggs in the sand.

    STEP 1: Scan and Skim

    What is the text generally about?

    _____

    _____

    STEP 2: Read and Decide

    What is the text specifically about?

    _____

    _____

    STEP 3: Make a Chart

    Make an elements chart and see how you answer each question.

    What belongs under the main idea in the chart?

    _____

    _____

2. At the beginning of the 20th century, few scientists suspected that there was a world of living plants and animals on the bottom of the ocean. All life that we knew of then was dependent on the energy of the sun. Essentially, plants made food from sunlight and water and animals ate plants. The sun was the ultimate power source.

But beginning in 1977, scientists began to discover that volcanic springs on the bottom of the seas were the source of energy for totally different forms of life. These volcanic sources produced a chemical like hydrogen sulfide, a substance which stinks like rotten eggs and is poisonous to most life we know. But down on the ocean bottom, new forms of life have evolved which can live and grow with energy provided by hydrogen sulfide. One of these unexpected life forms is the tube worm, a long, white, worm-like creature which stands upright and has a red top that looks like the top of a lipstick tube.

These strange creatures have no eyes, no mouths, and no way to travel. They seem to just stand there on the bottom of the ocean.

Is the following sentence a topic, main idea, supporting detail, or theme?

These strange creatures have no eyes, no mouths, and no way to travel.

A) Topic

B) Main idea

C) Supporting detail

D) Theme

STEP 1: Scan and Skim

Look through the passage quickly to find out what it is about and to look for key words.

What is the passage about?

_____

_____

STEP 2:

What strategy goes here and what will it help you do?

_____

_____

STEP 3: Read and Decide

Based on your analysis, how would you classify this sentence?

_____

_____

Guided Practice

3. To the Editor:

I was dismayed to read of the disgraceful behavior of a few members of one high school team at the All-Star Playoffs. They were anything but representative of the spirit of good sportsmanship. Defacing property and displaying temper is too childish for representatives at an All-Star meet. I hope that their coach will punish the offenders and force them to make restitution for what they have done. The amount of damage is not the issue. What I see as important is the need to make it clear to these young people, and all young people, that such actions will not and should not be tolerated. We must make a stand for good sportsmanship now or it will slowly be eroded in years to come.

Sincerely,

Mickey Schwitz

What is the author's main purpose in writing the letter?

A) To inform

B) To entertain

C) To persuade

D) To express feelings

STEP 1: Scan and Skim

Skim through the text. What kind of text is this?

_____

_____

STEP 2: Read and Decide

Read through the text and decide whether there is an obvious purpose. Why did the author write the text?

_____

_____

STEP 3:

What strategy would you use here to determine the author's purpose, and how would this strategy help you?

_____

_____

Independent Practice

1. The train was pulling in. This would be hard for Eric. It had been five years since he had seen his father. And even now, he wasn't sure he was doing the right thing by coming home. There had been so many things that had happened between them--things that were said that shouldn't have been. He wanted to forget. He put his head in his hands. It was aching and he was breathing heavily. He couldn't apologize. It hadn't been his fault. He was just following his instinct for survival, which had told him to get away.

   Is the following a topic, main idea, supporting detail, or theme of the paragraph?

   Life is not always easy.

   A) Topic

   B) Main idea

   C) Supporting detail

   D) Theme

   HINT Ask yourself the four questions about paragraph elements to help find the answer.

2. Eggplant parmigiana isn't that hard to make. Simply heat your oven to 375 degrees. Fry the eggplant in hot oil after slicing and peeling it. Then layer the slices in a small casserole. Prepare the cheese sauce according to the directions. Pour over the eggplant, dot with butter, and bake 45 minutes until golden brown on top. Cool before serving and you have a delicious dish.

   What is the author's intention in the passage?

   A) To inform

   B) To entertain

   C) To persuade

   D) To express feelings

   HINT *Why would you read this paragraph? What does it do?*

3. Most sugar comes from two plants, sugar cane and sugar beets. Sugar cane is like a tall grass. It needs hot sun and rain in order to grow. As sugar cane grows, it fills with a dark green juice, which is squeezed out when the cane is ripe. Sugar is made from the juice. Sugar beets do not need heat and rain to grow. Sugar is made from juice squeezed from the beets.

   Which sentence is a supporting detail for the paragraph?

   A) Sugar is sweet.

   B) Sugar comes from two sources.

   C) Sugar is made from vegetation.

   D) Sugar beets do not need heat to grow.

   HINT *Which choice supports the main idea?*

ReKap

In this lesson, you learned about the author's purpose and intent as well as the different elements of a text. You learned the difference between topic and main idea and how to tell them apart.

You also learned about supporting details and themes.

You learned that while there are always a topic, main idea, and supporting details, not all texts have a theme.

You learned strategies to help you answer test items. These strategies are:

- Scan and Skim

- Check Your Response

- Read and Decide

- Make a Chart

> **?** **What are four purposes that an author may have for writing a text? Why are most texts written?**
>
> _____
>
> _____
>
> _____
>
> _____

Answers

Guided Practice

1. Step 1: In general, the text is about a turtle.

   TIP: Remember, the main idea is a broad statement.

   Step 2: Specifically, the text notes a turtle has injured flippers. She (the turtle) needs to lay her eggs. Someone helps her dig a hole.

   TIP: Supporting details provide facts and add interest.

   Step 3: The main idea is that a wounded turtle struggles to dig a hole in which to lay her eggs.

   Answer: (C) A naturalist helped a turtle lay her eggs in the sand.

2. Step 1: The passage is about tube worms.

   Step 2: Making a chart can help you find the topic, theme, main idea, and supporting details in the text.

   Step 3: The identified sentence is a supporting detail.

   Answer: (C) Supporting detail.

3. Step 1: The text is a letter to the editor.

   Step 2: The author wrote the text to convince others to share his opinion.

   Step 3: Using the strategy *Check Your Response* would help to determine how the text makes you feel.

   Answer: (C) To persuade

Independent Practice

1. **Answer: (D) Theme**

   This sentence is the theme of the passage. Although it is not stated in the text, it is hinted at by the problems that the narrator has had in the past and is expecting in the future. It is not the topic of the passage; the topic is seeing a relative. The main idea is that a person is seeing his father after a falling out.

2. **Answer: (A) To inform**

   This passage is clearly meant to inform the reader. It is a recipe and teaches the reader how to make the dish. It is not entertaining, and no feelings are expressed. It is obviously not trying to persuade the reader about anything either.

3. **Answer: (D) Sugar beets do not need heat to grow.**

   Choice A and C are both broad statements and are similar to main ideas, but they are not in the text itself, so they can be eliminated. Choice D is the only one that tells more about sugar. Choice B is the main idea that Choice D supports.

ReKap

An author may have four purposes for writing a text: to entertain, to express feelings, to inform, and to persuade. Most textbooks are written to inform.

2 READING • LESSON 3
Informational Fundamentals

If you want to know the time a movie will start, you read a movie schedule. If you want to find out when the train leaves to go to your work site, you read a train schedule. Many things that we read are functional texts. They provide information. There is a wide variety of functional, or everyday, texts. When you read functional texts, you probably have a good reason. Nurses especially need to be skilled at reading functional texts to ensure patients receive the treatment they need.

Common Uses in Health Care

- nutritional labels
- prescription labels
- instructions

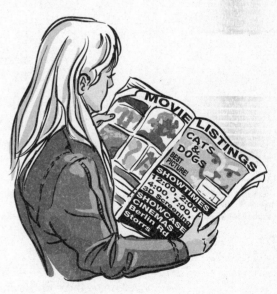

Key Terms/Formulas

- **fact** – information that can be proven

- **functional text** – text that contains everyday information

- **index** – text in the back of a book that lists topics in a book alphabetically

- **instructions** – step-by-step directions on how to do something

- **label** – text that tells you what is in food or medication, or tells you how to use a product

- **opinion** – a personal statement or feeling that cannot be proven

- **primary source** – text that is original

- **reliability** – extent to which content is from a credible source

- **table of contents** – text in the front of a book that outlines what is in the book

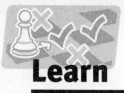

Labels and instructions are types of functional text. Functional texts' main purpose is to inform the reader. They do not entertain, persuade, or express feelings. Their intention is always to inform. But they have individual purposes as well. Labels are often put on medication bottles to remind those administering the medication of the dosage and frequency. Labels can also list what is in a particular food. Even clothing has labels that tell how to care for the items. Labels are important to read. Their purpose is to provide pertinent and vital information.

Instructions are important as well. There are many different kinds of instructions. Some can indicate how to use a particular medicine; others may tell how to do something. On the admissions test, you may be asked questions that are not related to health care in any way. You might be asked to follow instructions and see what new word you make. You might be asked to put different shapes together in a particular order and see what results.

This chart can help you remember what these functional texts do and why they were written.

Type of Functional Text	Information That May Be Contained
Labels	• The composition of medications • The nutritional value of a food • How to care for clothes
Instructions	• How to use medications • How to assemble or fix something • How to solve a puzzle
Schedules	• When movies start • When trains or buses run • When services are available • Days and times an employee is expected to work • Days and times patients are expected for their appointments
Advertisements	• Why a product should be bought • Why a person should go to an event

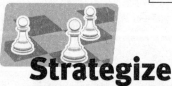

Strategize

Scan and Skim

Look for key words that tell you what the text is mostly about. Knowing this will help you determine the purpose of the text. It will also help you figure out the answer to a question that is asked about a functional text on the nursing admissions test.

The Learning Curve

When you read through the functional text, ask yourself the following questions:

• How will the information help you?

• What is the text mostly about?

• Will this main idea help you make a judgment about a product?

• Will the text help you learn how to do something?

Read and Decide

Read through the text and decide whether there is an obvious purpose. Ask yourself what purpose the text serves.

Organize

Keep track of the details in a set of instructions or directions; take some notes to remind yourself what to do.

Sample Passages:

Guacamole recipe	Clothes label	**SISTER CITY FUNDRAISER** volunteer schedule
Cut an avocado in half. *Pull out the stone from the center.* *Peel the avocado pieces.* *Mash in a small bowl.* *Add lemon juice and chopped cilantro.* *Mix well.* *For spicier guacamole, add flaked red peppers.*	*Wash in cold water.* *Use gentle cycle.* *Use lowest dryer setting.* *Iron if needed.*	**8:30 am to 10:30 am:** *Robert Winchell* *Adrianna Hovel* **10:30-12:30** *Philip Dugan* *Anna Guida* ***Please arrive five minutes before your shift.***

 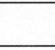

Start with the shapes pictured above. Follow the directions to arrange the shapes.

1. Put the square on top of the rectangle.

2. Put the circle on top of the square.

3. Put the triangle below the rectangle.

4. Turn the final shape upside down.

What does the assembled shape look like?

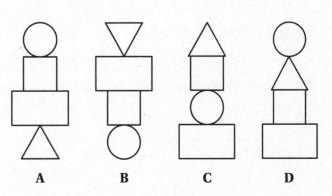

Choice B is correct.

Apply

Let's practice using these strategies to determine what this nutritional label tells the reader. It is similar to the nutritional labels you would see on the admissions test.

A1. Suppose a person needs to eat a low-salt diet. She can have no more than 1500mg of salt each day. What does the nutrition label tell you?

Nutrition Facts

Serving Size 1 cup (228g)
Servings per Container 2

Amount Per Serving	
Calories 280	**Calories from Fat** 120

	% Daily Value*
Total Fat 13g	20%
Saturated Fat 5g	25%
Trans Fat 2g	
Cholesterol 2mg	10%
Sodium 990mg	28%
Total Carbohydrate 31g	10%
Dietary Fiber 3g	0%
Sugars 5g	
Protein 5g	

Vitamin A 4%	•	Vitamin C 2%
Calcium 15%	•	Iron 4%

*Percentage Daily Values are based on a 2,000-calorie diet. Your daily values may be higher or lower depending on your calorie needs.

Let's use the strategies to figure this out.

STEP 1: Scan and Skim

You can look through the nutritional label to find key words. On the label, you see the word *sodium*, which means the same thing as salt. That is an important key word.

STEP 2: The Learning Curve

Look through the label and see what you can learn. You can learn how much sodium or salt there is in one serving of the product.

STEP 3: Read and Decide

Now you are ready to make a decision about the issue of salt. Knowing that the person can only have 1500mg of salt a day, you make the decision that this product contains too much salt for her. She would be allowed very little salt in the other foods she ate in a day if she consumes just one serving of this food.

Take a look at the label below. What can you determine about this item by reading the label?

Nutrition Facts	
Serving Size 1 cup (240mL)	
Servings per Container About 16	
Amount Per Serving	
Calories 90	**Calories from Fat** 0
	% Daily Value*
Total Fat 0g	0%
Saturated Fat 0g	0%
Trans Fat 0g	
Cholesterol Less than 5mg	1%
Sodium 130mg	5%
Potassium 420mg	12%
Total Carbohydrate 13g	4%
Dietary Fiber 0g	0%
Sugars 12g	
Protein 9g	
Vitamin A 10% •	Vitamin C 4%
Calcium 30% •	Iron 0%
Vitamin D 25% •	Phosphorus 25%
*Percentage Daily Values are based on a 2,000-calorie diet. Your daily values may be higher or lower depending on your calorie needs.	

All nutritional labels list the amount of sodium that a product contains along with the amount of fat, fiber, carbohydrates, cholesterol, and protein. Nutrition labels also show the kind of fat in the product, whether it is trans or saturated fat. Vitamins are also listed.

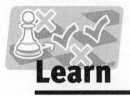

Learn

The **table of contents** and **index** (or **indices** if more than one is included) are both valuable tools for helping you quickly find the information you are looking for in a text. When you open a book, you can look at the table of contents to find out what information the book contains, such as chapter or section titles. It also tells you the page on which you will find the information.

Indices are helpful when you want to know about a certain topic that may not be listed in the table of contents. The index will alphabetically list all topics covered in the book and the pages on which that the topic is found.

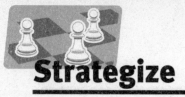

Strategize

Look for Key Words

Looking for key words will help you find the information you need quickly. Just skim through the table of contents to find your key words. You can also find key words in the index, which is in alphabetical order, making the key words easy to locate.

Apply

Let's practice using these strategies to locate information in a table of contents.

A2. Suppose you wanted to find information on career counseling as a profession. How would you go about finding out what pages you should read?

STEP 1: The Learning Curve

Look through the table of contents. Figure out what kind of book this must be.

STEP 2: Look for Key Words

Ask yourself what the key words might be. *Career* is one. Another key word is *counseling*. A third is *profession*. Do you find these key words in the table of contents?

STEP 3: Read and Decide

Now you are ready to make a decision about where you should look. There is a reference to the word *career* in the chapter called "Choosing the Right Career in Psychology," so that is a possibility. However, the other two key words are found in chapter 6, "Counseling: A Growing Profession." You need to decide which chapter is most likely to have information about career counseling as a profession. If you chose page 103 to start reading, you were correct.

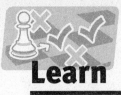

Learn

Suppose you are reading medical instructions on how to deal with a certain disease. While you are reading, you should ask yourself if the instructions are a **primary source**. This means that they are the direct source of information or a report, not someone else's interpretation of a text or report. You need to do this in order to check the **reliability** of what you read. Something that is a primary source will usually be reliable, or credible. While you read, you should also check for statements that are based on a **fact** and statements that are based on an **opinion**.

For instance, if you are reading about a medical procedure, does the text provide documentation for the statistics it cites? Is the documentation reliable?

When looking for statements that are based on opinion rather than fact, you should scan the text to find words that suggest a statement of opinion. These include such words as *should*, *best*, *worst*, and *probably*.

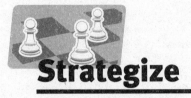

Strategize

Facts Can Be Checked

Whenever you are in doubt about whether a statement is based on fact or opinion, ask yourself if the statement can be checked to see if it is true or not. Facts can be proven or verified. If the statement cannot be proven, it is most likely based on an opinion.

Apply

Now let's use the strategies on the following passage to answer the next question.

FORMABEX is indicated for the relief of the signs and symptoms of rheumatoid arthritis and for the management of acute pain in adults.

Important Safety Information

*All prescription NSAIDs, like FORMABEX, have the same warning for cardiovascular patients. They may all increase the chance of heart attack or stroke. This chance increases if you have heart disease or high blood pressure.

Serious skin reactions, or stomach and intestine problems, such as bleeding and ulcers, can occur without warning.

Tell your doctor if you have:

- **a history of ulcers or bleeding in the stomach or intestines**
- **high blood pressure**
- **kidney or liver problems**

**All information is based on controlled studies done by FICCE Laboratories and endorsed by MDC, a federal government agency.

A3. **Suppose you read this text on the admissions exam and were asked whether the claims are based on fact or not. Here is one way you could figure out the answer.**

STEP 1: The Learning Curve

Look through the text. Figure out what it is telling you. What is the main idea?

STEP 2: Facts Can Be Checked

Look through the claims that the text makes. Are they based on fact or opinion? Look at the citation for the claims. Is it a reliable source?

STEP 3: Read and Decide

Now you are ready to make a decision about whether the statements or claims are based on fact. You must decide whether the source for these claims is a reliable one. The fact that these were findings from a laboratory and have been endorsed by a federal agency suggests that the claims are based on fact. Do you agree?

Guided Practice

Now, let's practice using what you have learned about reading information texts by working through a few examples together.

1. **Read the following set of directions. Then answer the question.**

   1. Start with the word "FUN."

   2. Add the letter "D" to the end of the word.

   3. Add the letter "S" to the end of the word.

   4. Add the letter "E" to the beginning of the word.

   5. Add the letter "R" to the beginning of the word.

   A) FUND

   B) FUNDS

   C) REFUND

   D) REFUNDS

   STEP 1: Skim and Scan

   What are the instructions for?

   _____

   _____

   STEP 2: Organize

   What notes will you write down to help you remember the order of instructions?

   _____

   _____

   STEP 3: Read and Decide

   What decision do you make?

   _____

   _____

Guided Practice

2. There has been a traffic accident on the Sands River Bridge. Traffic is worse than I can ever remember. It is backed up for miles on Third Street. It is best to take alternative routes if at all possible. The Sturgeon Bridge is open and there are no traffic delays there. Also, you can bypass the Sands River Bridge by taking Route 16 to Route 25. We expect that traffic will be backed up for at least an hour. After that the Sands River Bridge should be clear.

Which sentence from the text is an opinion?

A) Traffic is worse than I can ever remember.

B) It is backed up for miles on Third Street.

C) The Sturgeon Bridge is open and there are no traffic delays there.

D) Also, you can bypass the Sands River Bridge by taking Route 16 to Route 25.

STEP 1: Skim and Scan

What do you think the passage is about?

_____

_____

STEP 2:

What strategy should be used next, and what will it help you do?

_____

_____

STEP 3: Read and Decide

Can you figure out which statement is based on opinion?

_____

_____

3. Read the passage below.

```
┌─────────────────────────────────────────────────────────┐
│ Canter's Pharmacy      Ph: (800) 343-7000               │
│ 600 Dawson Street                                        │
│ Wilmington, NC 28403   HOUSTON, CHARLES                 │
│ (800) 343-7000         310 Anne Street                  │
│                        Wilmington, NC 28401             │
│                                                          │
│ Rx: No. 1151-018175                                     │
│ TAKE ONE TABLET BY MOUTH THREE TIMES                    │
│ A DAY FOR 10 DAYS                                       │
│                                                          │
│ ACYCLOVIR 400MG TABLET                                  │
│                                                          │
│ NO REFILLS – DR. AUTHORIZATION REQUIRED                 │
│ Orig Date: 10/15/2016    Use Before: 08/12/2017         │
└─────────────────────────────────────────────────────────┘
```

What is the intent of the passage?

A) to inform

B) to entertain

C) to persuade

D) to express feelings

STEP 1: Skim and Scan

What do you think the passage is about?

_____

_____

STEP 2: Look for Key Words

What words help you figure out the intent of the passage?

_____

_____

STEP 3:

What strategy would you use here to determine the author's intent?

_____

_____

Independent Practice

1. A person has been told by his doctor to increase the amount of fiber in his diet. Which of the following is true?

Nutrition Facts

Serving Size 2 crackers (14g)
Servings per Container About 21

Amount Per Serving	
Calories 60	**Calories from Fat** 15
	% Daily Value*
Total Fat 1.5g	2%
Saturated Fat 0g	0%
Trans Fat 0g	
Cholesterol 0mg	0%
Sodium 70mg	3%
Total Carbohydrate 10g	3%
Dietary Fiber Less than 1g	3%
Sugars 0g	

A) This food should not be eaten at all.

B) This is not a good food option for the person.

C) This food should be eaten three times a day.

D) This is an excellent food for the person to consume.

HINT *Which part of the label do you need to look at?*

2. Three eyewitnesses are cited in the article below: John Freeman, Freeman's son Christian, and Fire Chief William Blair.

Yesterday evening John Freeman reported a fire at an abandoned building, a former factory, down the street from where he lived. "I was taking my dog for a walk when I first saw the flames," Freeman told this reporter. "It looked terrible. I dialed 911 and told them and they said they would alert the fire department. I stayed here until they arrived."

Emergency fire vehicles reached the scene at 8:05 P.M. and started to spray the building to attempt to get the fire under control, but were unable to contain it. After ten hours, the fire was finally out, but the building was basically destroyed.

"It was a terrible fire," said Fire Chief William Blair. "We just could not get it under control. My men worked very hard, but by the end they were totally exhausted. They are hard workers. I am just glad there was no loss of life."

Freeman's son, Christian Freeman, said that he could smell smoke before his father saw the flames. "It was very noticeable," he said. "I knew something was wrong. When I saw my father and he told me, I went to check out the fire itself. It was terrible. I stayed for about an hour and then came home."

This reporter contacted the person listed as the owner of the building, but he had no comment.

Which statement best describes the eyewitness accounts in the article?

A) None of them are primary sources.

B) All of them are primary sources.

C) Fire Chief William Blair and John Freeman are primary sources; Christian Freeman is not.

D) Christian Freeman is a primary source; Fire Chief William Blair and John Freeman are not.

HINT *What is the definition of a primary source?*

3. Where in the index would you find information about an allergy to metals?

Allergy...pp.105–140

   definition ....pp. 106–107

   types ....pp. 107–126

      to food types ....pp. 108–110

      to animals...pp. 111–120

      other...pp. 121–130

   treatments..pp. 130–140

A) pages 106–107

B) pages 108–110

C) pages 121–130

D) pages 130–140

HINT *What listing is most important to answering the question?*

4. Which of the following would most likely be a reliable source for learning more about metal allergies?

A) the results of an allergy study published by an accredited medical school

B) an editorial in a newspaper about the problems associated with metal allergies

C) a brochure by a pharmaceutical company to advertise a new allergy medication

D) a review of an article discussing innovative new treatment options for those with allergies

HINT *Which choice is most reliable?*

ReKap

In this lesson, you learned about functional text and its various purposes. You learned about labels and instructions and other kinds of text.

You learned to determine the reliability of a text as well as how to tell the difference between statements based on fact and those based on opinion.

You also learned to recognize primary sources.

You learned strategies to help you answer test items. These strategies are:

- Scan and Skim
- The Learning Curve
- Read and Decide
- Organize
- Look for Key Words
- Facts Can Be Checked

What are four different functional texts?
What are their purposes?

_____

_____

_____

_____

Answers

Guided Practice

1. Step 1: The instructions are for you to make a new word.

    Step 2: Notes may include: add D to end of FUN; add S to end of word; add E to beginning of word; add R to the beginning of word.

    Step 3: The end result is that the word is REFUNDS.

    Answer: (D) REFUNDS

2. Step 1: The passage is about a traffic tie-up.

    Step 2: *Facts Can Be Checked* can help you determine which statements are based on facts, not opinions.

    Step 3: The statement – the traffic is worse that I can ever remember – is based on opinion.

    Answer: (A) Traffic is worse than I can ever remember.

3. Step 1: The passage is a prescription label.

    Step 2: Words such as *take tablet* and *no refills* help to figure out the intent of the passage.

    Step 3: *Read and Decide* can help you determine the author's intent.

    Answer: (A) to inform

Independent Practice

1. **Answer: (B) This is not a good food option for the person.**

    The food does not have very much fiber in it; it would not be the best nutritional option for a person who needs a large amount of fiber.

2. **Answer: (B) All of them are primary sources.**

    The passage gives three eyewitness accounts. A primary source is something or someone who has first-hand knowledge of an event. These three people were all at the fire, so they are primary sources.

3. **Answer: (C) pages 121–130**

    It is easy to eliminate some of the answer choices since Choice A is about definitions and Choice B is about food allergies. Choice D is about treatments, but that is not what the question asks. The information you would need is under *Other*.

4. **Answer: (A) the results of an allergy study published by an accredited medical school**

    This is the primary source and the most reliable source of the ones that are given. Choice B is a text that is based on opinion; Choice C cannot be trusted because the pharmaceutical company is attempting to sell its product. Choice D is not a primary source. The information in the article may not be verified.

ReKap

Functional texts include labels (nutrition label, clothing wash label), instructions (steps of assembly), schedules (start and end times), and advertisements (why a product should be bought).

2 READING · LESSON 4
Reading Technical Documents and Tools

There are a number of different kinds of passages on the admissions test. Some of these passages may be mostly visuals, rather than just being text. Diagrams, drawings of medical instruments, maps, graphs, scales, and pie charts are all tools that provide information. It is important to know how to interpret this information.

Common Uses in Health Care

- reading temperatures
- weighing medication
- understanding medical graphs

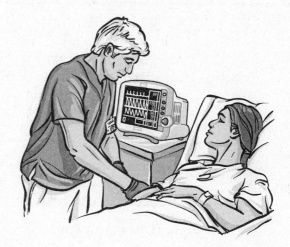

Key Terms/Formulas

- **bar graph** – graph that presents numerical information by the length of lines or rectangles

- **compass rose** – graphic that shows directions on a map

- **distance scale** – a means to measure distance on a map

- **legend** – explanation of the symbols on a map

- **line graph** – graph that presents numerical information by using a line

- **map** – diagrammatic representation of an area showing cities, roads, and other sites

- **pie chart** – circle divided into sectors that each represent a portion of the whole

- **scale** – instrument that weighs items or people

- **scientific instruments** – tools used in science and medicine

- **table** – graphic that organizes and displays information

- **visual information** – image such as a chart, graphic, or map used to present information

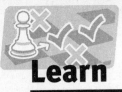

Learn

Scientific tools and medical instruments display important information. Being able to interpret this information is vital. The kinds of instruments and tools that you will find on the admissions test are varied. This chart lists some instruments that you may be asked questions about and what they are used for.

Instrument	Purpose
Scales	• To measure weight • To measure medication
Blood pressure monitor	• To measure the diastolic and systolic levels of the blood pressure • To measure pulse rate
Thermometers	• To measure the temperature of the body • To measure temperature of the air

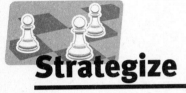

Strategize

Study the Visual

What does it look like? When you see a visual representation of a scientific or medical instrument, you will need to be able to figure out what it is quickly. You will need to look at the visuals for clues to what it is. If there are numbers, look to see if they are labeled. The labels will be a clue to what the instrument is used for.

Find the Purpose

Ask yourself what the instrument is used for. Ask yourself if you have ever seen this instrument and what it was used for. Think about the type of information that the instrument provides, and why this information is important.

Figure Out How It Works

Ask yourself what kind of information the instrument displays and whether you know how it works. If you are not sure what kind of instrument it is, just look at the readings and labels on the visual. That should help you figure out what it is and how it works.

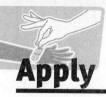

Apply

Let's practice using these strategies to determine the answer to the following question, which is similar to questions you would see on the admissions test.

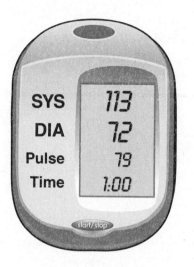

A1. Based on the blood pressure monitor, what is the patient's systolic pressure?

A) 72

B) 79

C) 113

D) 1229

STEP 1: Study the Visual

What is this a picture of? According to the question, it is a blood pressure monitor. Think about what you know about blood pressure monitors. What information is visible on the machine?

STEP 2: Find the Purpose

What does a blood pressure monitor do? What do the numbers on the monitor mean?

STEP 3: Figure Out How It Works

Why are there three numbers? Notice the labels indicating what information is given by each number. Think about how the machine works and what it is measuring. Look for the number next to the SYS label. That will give you the answer.

▶Based on this information you can figure out that the number of the systolic pressure is Choice C, 113.

Scales are another instrument that the admissions test will have questions about. There are many different kinds of scales. Some are used to measure the weight of a person; others measure amounts of medication or other substances. Some are used to weigh produce. You have probably seen this kind of scale in the supermarket.

Apply

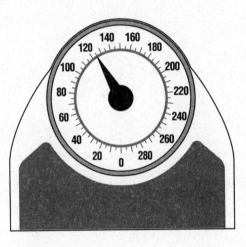

A2. A measurement of approximately how many pounds is represented on the above scale face?

A) 119

B) 124

C) 129

D) 131

STEP 1: Study the Visual

Look at the visual. The question tells you it is a scale. You will need to look at all its parts. What do the numbers mean? What does the arrow mean?

STEP 2: Find the Purpose

The question tells you that the scale is weighing something, but what is it weighing? Is it a person who is being weighed?

STEP 3: Figuring Out How It Works

Look at the numbers. They go up, but they do not go up in increments of 5 or 10. You need to figure out that the scale goes up in increments of 20. To read the scale correctly, you must understand how it works. Based on this information, you can figure out that the scale face indicates 124 pounds, Choice B.

 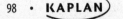

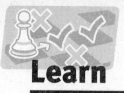

When you take the admissions test, do not be surprised to see maps of places with questions. The questions that you may be asked about a map are based more on logic than anything else. They also assess how well you pay attention to details. You could be asked what you will pass if you go down Street A and turn onto Street B. Or you could be asked how many times you will run into road work if you drive from your starting point to another destination.

Maps are made up of many components. This table explains the different components.

Map Component	Purpose
Legend	• A legend tells what the symbols on a map mean. Symbols could stand for things such as buildings, campsites, road work, or anything else that is important on the map.
Compass rose	• A compass rose helps to orient you as to the direction of everything on a map. It shows where north, south, east, and west are. It may be found in the legend.
Distance scale	• A distance scale gives you a means to measure the distance on a map. For example, it could show an inch-long line and indicate that each inch on the map equals five miles. This may be found in the legend.

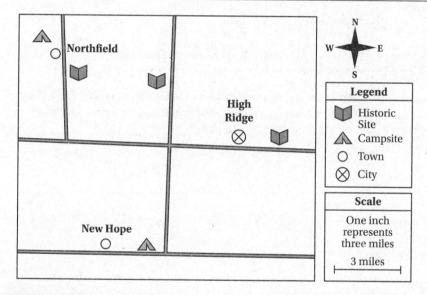

Strategize

Pay Attention to Details

When you look at a map, make sure to use all of the components of a map. They can help you interpret the information that the map presents. Be sure to study all the symbols, any legend or compass rose, and the distance scale if present. Try to orientate yourself to the map. Ask yourself what the map shows.

Map of Greenkill Park

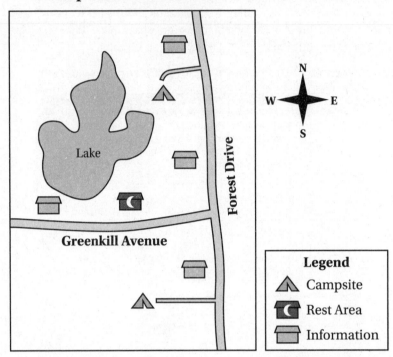

A3. A family is planning to camp at the camp site closest to the lake in Greenkill Park. They enter the park on Greenkill Avenue and proceed to the campsite. How many information booths will they pass on the way to their campsite?

A) 1

B) 2

C) 3

D) 4

STEP 1: Study the Visual

Take a good look at the visual. You can identify it quickly as a map. Look at the different symbols in the legend on the map. Find the locations mentioned in the question.

STEP 2: Find the Purpose

Ask yourself what the purpose of the map is. What does it show? It has a title. It is a map of a park. It shows the locations of the campsites.

STEP 3: Pay Attention to Details

Make sure to study the legend to figure out what the symbols mean. They will be important to answer the question, which asks how many information booths the family will pass on the way to the campsite nearest the lake. You need to locate that campsite and trace their route to it. Count the number of information booths. If you come up with Choice B, 2, you are correct.

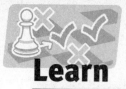
There will be other kinds of visual passages on the admissions test as well. This chart introduces these passage types and identifies the purpose of each.

The chart below is an example of one kind of visual passage on the test. This chart organizes information about visual passages for easy access to information.

Visual Passages	What They Do
Bar graphs or charts	• Diagrams in which the numerical values of variables are represented by the height or length of lines or rectangles of equal width
Line graphs	• Diagrams in which the numerical values of variables are represented by a line that tracks the changes
Pie charts	• Circles divided into sectors that each represent a portion of the whole
Tables	• Charts that organize information for making comparisons

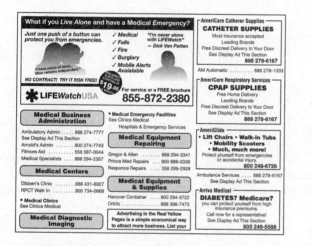

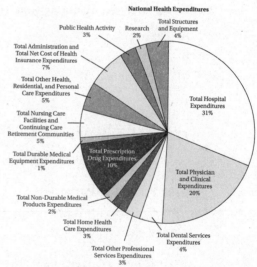

Above you find text from the yellow pages and an example of a pie chart.

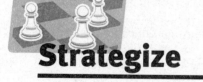

Strategize

Read the Question Carefully

The question will help you understand what the visual is and what it is showing. Be sure to read the question before making any assumptions about the visual. The question will tell you which information you should focus on.

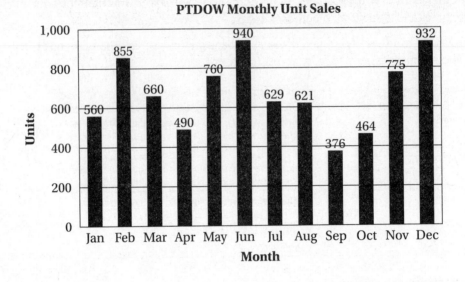

PTDOW Monthly Unit Sales

A4. Based on the chart, during which month did PTDow make the least amount of money?

A) January

B) April

C) September

D) October

STEP 1: Study the Visual

Look closely at the visual. Ask yourself what it looks like. Does it look like a bar chart?

STEP 2: Find the Purpose

Look at the other information in the chart. What is the title? Is this a clue about what the chart represents?

STEP 3: Figure Out How It Works

By looking at the labels below each bar on the chart, you can figure out that the bars represent monthly unit sales. The bars go up and down each month, so you know that this is a visual representation of how well the company has done financially during the months of the year. Look for the shortest bar. That will give you the answer to the question. Which month has the shortest bar? September, Choice C.

Guided Practice

	Plan 1	Plan 2	Plan 3	Plan 4
Disk Space	Unlimited	Unlimited	Unlimited	Unlimited
Bandwidth	Unlimited	Unlimited	Unlimited	Unlimited
Domains Allowed	1	10	20	Unlimited
Free Dedicated IP	✗	✓	✓	✓
Free Private SSL	✗	✓	✓	✓
Site Builder	✗	✓	✓	✓
24x7 Support	✓	✓	✓	✓
99.9% Uptime Guarantee	✓	✓	✓	✓
Price	$5.95/ month	$10.95/ month	$20.95/ month	$30.95/ month

1. The owner of a start-up company wants to improve the company's presence online and must decide which kind of service would be best. The company does not have a need for many domains, but does need more than one. Which plan would be best?

A) Plan 1

B) Plan 2

C) Plan 3

D) Plan 4

STEP 1: Study the Visual

What does the visual look like?

_____

_____

STEP 2: Find the Purpose

What purpose does the visual serve?

_____

_____

STEP 3: Answer

What do the checks mean?

_____

_____

Guided Practice

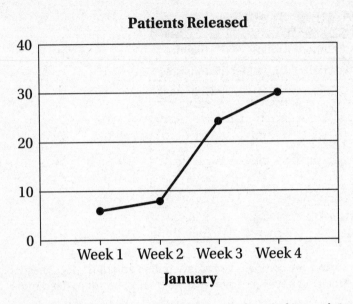

Patients Released

January

2. How many patients were released from the hospital in week 3 of January?

A) about 16

B) about 19

C) about 24

D) about 31

STEP 1: Find the Purpose

What does the visual look like?

_____

_____

STEP 2:

What strategy goes here and what will it help you do?

_____

_____

STEP 3: Make Sure to Read the Question

What do the dots or bullet points mean?

_____

_____

Body Mass Index

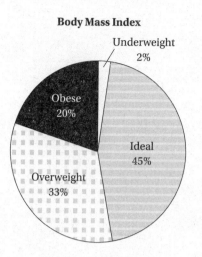

3. This pie chart shows the body index of the group of patients. Which type of body mass has the fewest number of patients?

   A) Ideal

   B) Obese

   C) Overweight

   D) Underweight

STEP 1: Find the Purpose

What is the purpose of the pie chart?

_____

_____

STEP 2: Pay Attention to the Details

What are the details telling you?

_____

_____

STEP 3:

Which strategy should be used next, and how will it help you?

_____

_____

Independent Practice

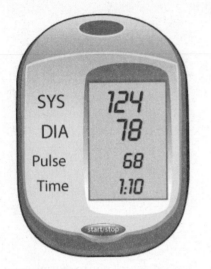

1. Based on the blood pressure monitor, which is the patient's pulse rate?

   A) 68

   B) 78

   C) 110

   D) 124

   HINT *Which number represents the pulse rate?*

Store	Price	Shipping and Handling
Furniture Forever	$210	$35
Hardwoods Only	$190	$20
S & B Furniture	$200	$50
The Final Touch	$225	Shipping included

2. A consumer wants to buy a chair. The table above shows price quotes from four online retailers. Which retailer offers the best buy?

   A) Furniture Forever

   B) Hardwoods Only

   C) S & B Furniture

   D) The Final Touch

   HINT *What would be the total cost of the chair if it was bought from each company listed?*

Map of Downtown Oak Ridge

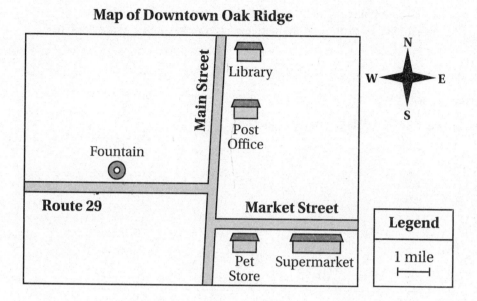

3. A woman is driving east on Route 29 into Oak Ridge to do some errands. She drives to the library first to return some books. She drops off some letters at the post office. Then she goes to the supermarket, then to the pet store, and then home. How many times would she see the fountain on her trip?

A) 1

B) 2

C) 3

D) 4

HINT ▸ *Pay attention to the details of her trip.*

ReKap

In this lesson, you learned about the many different kinds of visual passages that will be on the nursing school admissions test. You learned their purposes and how to interpret them, as well as how to use the information to respond to specific questions.

You learned to read maps, charts, and tables.

You learned what a yellow page consists of.

You learned strategies to help you answer test items. These strategies are:

- Study the Visual
- Find a Purpose
- Figure Out How It Works
- Pay Attention to Details
- Read the Question Carefully

? What are four ways information can be compared?

_____

_____

_____

_____

Answers

Guided Practice

1. Step 1: The visual looks like a table or chart.

    Step 2: The table compares services.

    Step 3: The checks show what each plan offers. Plan 2 has more than one domain, but is the least expensive of the three that offer this plan.

    Answer: (B) Plan 2

2. Step 1: The visual is a line graph that shows how many patients were released from a hospital during the weeks of January.

    Step 2: *Pay Attention to Details* will help you figure out how many patients were released each week.

    Step 3: The dots or bullets are located at the number of patients discharged for each week. The question asks about week 3, so you need to look at the dot for week 3.

    Answer: (C) About 24

3. Step 1: The pie chart shows the percentage of patients with each body mass type.

    Step 2: The details tell that most students have an ideal body mass.

    Step 3: *Make Sure to Read the Question.* This will tell you what part of the chart on which to focus.

    Answer: (D) Underweight

Independent Practice

1. **Answer: (A) 68**

    Choice A correctly identifies the pulse rate. Choice B is the diastolic pressure reading. Choice C is the time the pressure was taken. Choice D is the systolic reading.

2. **Answer: (B) Hardwoods Only**

    Hardwoods Only has the lowest price at $210 (price plus shipping and handling). Choice A is much higher at $245. Choice C is also higher than Choice B at $250. Choice D is still higher than Choice B at $225.

3. **Answer: (B) 2**

    Choice B correctly identifies the number of times the woman would see the fountain on her trip. Choice A is not correct since the woman would see the fountain going and coming. Choices C and D are not correct, since the woman would not see the fountain any more than twice.

ReKap

Information can be compared using bar graphs or charts, line graphs, pie charts, and tables.

Advanced Paragraph and Passage Techniques

Imagine that you are seeing people coming out of a movie theater, and they are smiling and laughing. Based on this evidence, you might come to the conclusion that the movie was funny. You used the information at hand to draw a conclusion.

Common Uses in Health Care

- doctors' orders
- healthcare manuals
- patients' charts

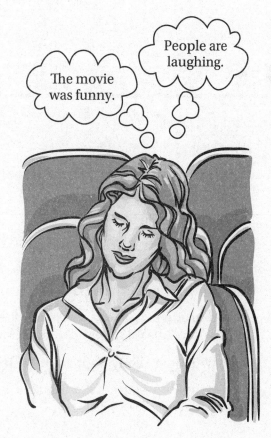

Key Terms/Formulas

- **bias** – prejudice in favor of or against one thing, person, or group

- **context** – information in a text that offers clues to help you understand the meaning of a word

- **historical and cultural context** – clues that help you understand the period when a text was written

- **inference** – a judgment made that is based on evidence that comes from the text

- **logical conclusion** – a theory based on the inferences in a text

- **prediction** – a logical inference about what might be true or occur in the future based on evidence in the text

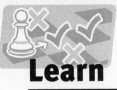

Learn

When you read, you need to put two and two together; that is, you need to be able to read between the lines. Sometimes authors tell you what they want you to know directly. Sometimes they hint at things. Figuring out what an author wants you to know is an ability that will help you make **logical inferences** and draw **conclusions** based on evidence that is in the text.

When you make an inference or draw a conclusion, you should be able to cite the evidence from the text that led you to your conclusion. This evidence will show that your conclusion is logical.

Making predictions is similar to drawing conclusions; you need to use the evidence in a text to make a prediction. This chart will clarify these three skills.

Skill	Process
Make an inference	Use reasoning to make a logical observation based on evidence
Draw a conclusion	Use reasoning to analyze evidence in order to come up with a theory
Make a prediction	Decide what may be true, or what may happen in the future, based on evidence

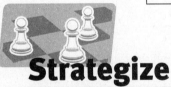

Strategize

Scan and Skim

What is the text mostly about?

Look through the text to identify the general theme or topic. Look for key words to help you figure it out.

Look for Evidence

Look to see if the author is suggesting or hinting at something. What evidence is there that this suggestion is logical?

Test the Conclusion's Logic

After you draw a conclusion, check to see that there is evidence to support your conclusion. Are you able to make inferences based on what you read?

What Will Most Likely Happen or Be True?

Based on what is written in a text, can you predict the author's viewpoint, or can you predict what the author may write next?

Apply

Read the following excerpt from a blog. Then answer the question.

Governor Pasquale's ratings are skyrocketing once again. He has the support of the people, and not just the people who voted him into office, but also the people who did not support him until he showed that he has what it takes to lead this state out of its many woes. Unemployment has never been lower, companies are hiring, and the public is buying cars and other high-end items. What more could we ask for?

A1. **What should the reader conclude about this excerpt?**

A) The author is a state politician.

B) The author works in the state house.

C) The author is a supporter of the governor.

D) The author dines frequently with the governor.

To answer this question, use the following strategies.

STEP 1: Scan and Skim

Ask yourself what the excerpt is mostly about.

Look for key words to help you figure it out. Is it about politics?

STEP 2: Look for Evidence

Look at what the author is saying about the governor. This is evidence you can use to form a conclusion.

STEP 3: Test the Conclusion's Logic

Check out each of the possible conclusions. Which one is supported by the evidence in the text? Eliminate the ones that are not supported by the text. Eliminate Choices A, B, and D. Choice C is the correct response.

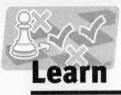

Learn

Many authors have a **bias** about the subject that they are writing about. Sometimes the bias is very noticeable; other times it is hidden. But even hidden bias may leave some clues for the reader to put together.

One way to check on an author's bias or prejudice regarding a topic is to look for statements that are opinions. As you learned in an earlier chapter, a statement based on an opinion reflects the speaker's personal feelings or viewpoint and cannot be proven.

It is important to find any opinions, hidden or overt, that the author may have, and to analyze them to see if they are strong enough to suggest a bias on the part of the author. Then, based on your evidence, you can make an inference about the author's bias.

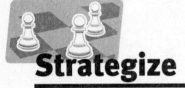

Strategize

Check for Opinions

What statements does the author make that are based on an opinion?

Try to determine what the author thinks of the subject. Does the author like the subject or dislike the subject? Look for hidden comments based on the author's opinion.

Apply

Read the following online advertisement. Then answer the question.

When Laurel Helmold began taking Isoprotempine last June, she was not optimistic. "I had tried every medication in the world for my migraines, but nothing helped. When I had one, I couldn't do anything. I was sick to my stomach and in terrible pain. And it lasted a long time before it went away."

All of that has changed since taking Isoprotempine. In a matter of weeks, Laurel noticed a dramatic change.

"I still had occasional migraines, but they didn't seem as bad. They lasted only a few hours and then just went away. I was so relieved."

Since that time, she has continued on her medication and now finds she is virtually free of terrible headaches.

It's the medication most people are reaching for.

For more information, visit isoprotempine.com

Click here for a full disclosure of side effects.

A2. What conclusion can the reader draw about the author's bias?

A) The author discovered the new drug.

B) The author thinks the medicine is ineffective.

C) The author has suffered from migraine headaches in the past.

D) The author is paid by the pharmaceutical company that makes the drug.

Now use some strategies to help you figure out the answer to the question.

STEP 1: Count

Ask yourself what the excerpt is mostly about.

Look for key words to help you determine what the excerpt is about. Is it about a new medicine?

STEP 2: Work Backwards

Which of the author's statements are based on opinion? Does the author show bias?

STEP 3: Predict and Match

Check out each of the possible conclusions. Which one is supported by the evidence in the text? Eliminate the ones that are not supported by the text. The advertisement includes statements about the benefits of the drug, but no first hand statements and nothing to indicate the author made the discovery. Eliminate Choices A, B, and C. The statement *didn't seem as bad* is an opinion. The statement *it's the medication that most people are reaching for* is not verified. It is likely the pharmaceutical company that makes the drug pays the author, Choice D.

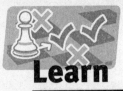

Learn

Context can help a reader figure out the meaning of unknown words or words that may have more than one meaning. **Context clues** are hints to a word's meaning and are found in the surrounding words, sentences, and paragraphs. The process of using context clues to figure out the meaning of a word is similar in process to drawing a conclusion.

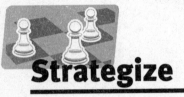

Strategize

Check for Hints

Look through the sentence or surrounding sentences for any hints or clues that help you understand the unknown word's meaning. These may include synonyms, antonyms, definitions, or examples. Use these clues to make a guess at the word's meaning and then find the answer choice that is closest in meaning to your guess.

 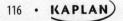

Apply

Read the following sentence. Then answer the question.

Instead of looking at each game's score separately, the judges add up all of the scores and judge a player on his or her <u>cumulative</u> record.

A3. Based on the context of the sentence above, what is the definition of the underlined word?

A) average

B) best

C) individual

D) total

STEP 1: Scan and Skim

Ask yourself what the excerpt is mostly about.

Look for key words to help you figure it out.

STEP 2: Check for Hints

What hints or clues are in the sentence that help you understand the meaning of the underlined word? Are there any synonyms, antonyms, definitions, or examples that can help you?

STEP 3: Test the Conclusion's Logic

Check out each of the possible answers. Which one is supported by the clues that you found in the text? The word *add* suggests that *cumulative* means the total of the scores. Choice D, total, is the correct response.

Learn

It is important to observe the historical and cultural context of what you read. For instance, someone writing hundreds of years ago would have beliefs and observations that might not apply in today's society. Someone who has grown up in a foreign culture might also have beliefs that are not accepted in America. Without the knowledge that the text was written long ago or was written by someone with a different cultural experience, you might have a misconception about the information. When you read a text that seems odd to you, look for context clues in the passage that will give you an idea of its historical or cultural background.

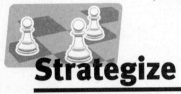

Strategize

Trust Your Instincts

When reading a text that you have no knowledge of, trust your instincts. Think about what the text makes you feel. Look to see if there is a citation about who wrote the text and when it was written. Consider this information when reading the text. Then you will be able to read the text in its proper historical or cultural context.

Apply

We learned to shoot with our bows and arrows when we were only three or four years old, and we were avid hunters. We went very early, making sure not to wake our elders, who knew nothing of our plans. We would walk quietly into the woods and lie await until we saw birds feeding on the ground. We were very careful not to make any noise, as that would drive them away. Then we would pull out arrows from our quivers and shoot the unsuspecting birds. We were ecstatic when we returned to camp and displayed our catch to the elders around the morning fire. They always forgave us for not asking their permission to hunt when they saw the large number of birds we brought home.

A4. Which statement best summarizes a cultural opinion held by the text's author?

A) Learning to hunt at a young age was a rarity for Native Americans.

B) Learning to hunt at a young age was a way of life for Native Americans.

C) Learning to hunt at a young age was extremely difficult for young Native Americans.

D) Learning to hunt at a young age was considered a way to teach Native American children obedience.

STEP 1: Scan and Skim

Ask yourself what the excerpt is mostly about.

Look for key words to help you figure it out. Is it about Native American children?

STEP 2: Check for Hints

What is different culturally about the text? In what ways are the actions of the children in the text different from the way children in today's society act?

STEP 3: Test the Conclusion's Logic

Consider each of the possible answers. Which one is supported by the clues that you found in the text? Choice B is supported by the details in the passage.

Guided Practice

1. Read the following text from a brochure. Then answer the question.

Clowns and Company will make you laugh, dance, and sing. You don't need to do anything. We do it all!

Clowns and Company is a professional entertainment company that will come to your home for parties. Our talent is unparalleled. There is no other entertainment group of our caliber in the city.

We have specially designed programs for the very young and for those adults who are young at heart.

Let us make that special day something memorable.

Call us at 684-8921 or go to our website at clownsandcompany.com.

You won't be sorry you did!

References available.

What can the reader conclude about this brochure?

A) Clowns and Company is competitively priced.

B) Clowns and Company has performed for people in the past.

C) Clowns and Company is sponsored by a not-for-profit group.

D) Clowns and Company is the only entertainment company in the city.

STEP 1: Skim and Scan

What is the passage mostly about?

_____

_____

STEP 2: Look for Evidence

What evidence can you find in the brochure?

_____

_____

STEP 3: What Will Most Likely Happen or Be True?

Based on the information in the brochure, what is most likely true of the entertainment company?

_____

_____

Look through the text to see what it is mostly about. Look for key words to help you figure it out.

2. Director Richard Moore has another blockbuster hit with *The Uranium Factor*. George Terry, played perfectly by Richard Burns, is a brilliant but somewhat eccentric (he sleeps in a Himalayan dome tent in his dorm room at MIT) college student. Bored with his courses, George designs and builds a time machine in the basement. On a cold, snowy January evening, he sets the time dial to 2150. With the push of a button, he is hurtled forward in time. Scenes rush by faster and faster until he passes out.

George wakens in a crater. Predictably, the dormitory is gone. He covers the time machine with a camouflage net. As he walks through the streets of Cambridge, there are destroyed buildings everywhere; there also don't seem to be any people. Rounding a corner, he sees a huge spaceship, guarded by armed robots over eight-feet tall. One fires at him and a laser beam blasts the pavement beneath him. George falls, only to be whisked away by a rider on a motorcycle, which can also fly.

I won't give the ending away, but the special effects are definitely award-winning. The camera work is stunning too, and the performance by Burns is first rate. This is his first role. The script, also by a newcomer, Alex Brandeis, is taut and suspenseful; however, the plot does seem to be a bit familiar. It's a story that occurs in the movies from time to time. Even so, this movie will leave you clutching your seat in excitement.

What can the reader predict about the author's bias?

A) The author knows the script writer.

B) The author thinks the film will be a flop.

C) The author enjoys watching science fiction films.

D) The author feels the actors were not experienced enough.

STEP 1: Skim and Scan

What is the text about? What is the author saying?

_____

_____

STEP 2: Check for Opinions

What opinions does the author have? Does he seem to have a bias?

_____

_____

STEP 3: Test the Conclusion's Logic

Which answer choice is supported by the evidence?

_____

_____

Guided Practice

3. Read the paragraph below. Then answer the question.

I have enclosed my ideas on the renovations you want done to your kitchen as well as a sketch of how it would look when completed. I have detailed the kinds of materials I would use in the project including the fixtures, refrigerator, cooktop, oven, and other equipment that would be needed and the cost of each. Finally, I have prepared a final <u>quote</u> for the work that I will do. If this is satisfactory to you, sign at the bottom and return with the agreed-upon down payment.

Based on the context of the paragraph above, what is the definition of the underlined word?

A) citation

B) design

C) price

D) process

STEP 1: Skim and Scan

What is the passage mostly about?

_____

_____

STEP 2: Look for Evidence

What context clues are there to help you understand the meaning of *quote?*

_____

_____

STEP 3: Test the Conclusion's Logic

What other word could replace the word *quote?*

_____

_____

Independent Practice

1. Use the graph below to answer the question.

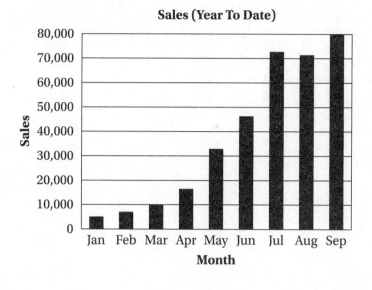

Sales (Year To Date)

This bar chart represents a new company's sales for the past year.

Based on the information in the bar chart, what can you predict about the company's future?

A) The company will have to downsize.

B) The company will hire more salespeople.

C) The company is planning to open a new location.

D) The company is likely to lose money in the future.

HINT *What trend does the bar chart show?*

2. Read the passage. Then answer the question.

When the poem was read, there was silence. It was not the kind of poetry that the audience was familiar with. Why weren't there any rhyming words? Why did it read like prose? These were the questions that lingered in the minds of those who witnessed this aberration, as one audience member called it.

The fact of the matter is that the so-called poem wasn't a poem at all, since it did not show any of the characteristics of, say, a sonnet or an ode. Rhyme and meter played no part in this text, which would be rejected by any intelligent person.

Here was someone experimenting with an art form that should not be tampered with. The audience was full of disdain. But then something happened. The author of the work walked down the aisle and took the podium. "This is the nature of art, to change," he said. "It is time to break the rules that have been suffocating so many so long."

There was a long silence. Then there was loud, thunderous applause.

Independent Practice

What specifically does the second paragraph suggest about the historical context of this text?

A) This was a period when people had ambitious goals for artists.

B) This was a time when free-thinking people were in great demand.

C) This was a time when people enjoyed experimenting with art forms.

D) This was a period in which people expected little deviation from the norm.

HINT   *What attitude is expressed in the second paragraph?*

3. What inference can you make about the poet?

A) He had little talent.

B) He wanted to please people.

C) He was passionate in his beliefs.

D) He was worried about his future.

HINT   *What kind of person would say what the poet said?*

4. Read the sentence. Then answer the question.

When other people act in an immoral and unprincipled way, it can be hard to maintain your <u>scruples</u>, especially when no one notices how hard you try to do the right thing.

Based on the context of the sentence above, what is the definition of the underlined word?

A) poor habits

B) even temper

C) moral principles

D) lack of discipline

HINT   *What clues are there in the sentence that can help you figure out the meaning of the underlined word?*

ReKap

In this lesson, you learned about the process for making logical conclusions and inferences. You also learned how to make predictions. You learned that any conclusion or prediction needs to be supported by evidence.

You learned how to recognize bias in a text and how to look for statements based on opinion.

You learned how to use context to figure out the meanings of words and how to recognize the historical and cultural contexts of passages that may seem odd to you when you first read them.

You learned strategies to help you answer test items. These strategies are:

- Scan and Skim
- Look for Evidence
- Test the Conclusion's Logic
- What Will Most Likely Happen or Be True?
- Check for Opinions
- Check for Hints
- Trust Your Instincts

? What are three skills that should be based on evidence?

_____

_____

_____

_____

Answers

Guided Practice

1. Step 1: The passage is about an entertainment company looking for work.

   Step 2: The company has references.

   Step 3: Likely, the company has performed before.

   Answer: (B) Clowns and Company has performed for people in the past.

2. Step 1: The text is a review of a movie. The author seems to like it.

   Step 2: The author says the movie will have you clutching at your seat. He says the plot seems familiar.

   Step 3: Choice C seems to be supported by the text.

   Answer: (C) The author enjoys watching science fiction films.

3. Step 1: The passage is a work proposal for a kitchen renovation.

   Step 2: The passage discusses the cost of materials for the renovation. It says the client needs to return a down payment if they agree to the terms.

   Step 3: The words *cost* and *price* could replace the word *quote*.

   Answer: (C) price

Independent Practice

1. **Answer: (B) The company will hire more salespeople.**

   The chart indicates that sales are continuously improving. The other answer choices are less likely to happen than Choice B. It does not seem likely that the company will have to downsize since it is doing very well, so Choice A is incorrect. Choice D is also not likely based on the company's past record. Choice C is a possibility; however, nothing in the graph suggests this option.

2. **Answer: (D) This was a period in which people expected little deviation from the norm.**

   Based on what is said in paragraph 2, this is the most logical conclusion. Choice A does not seem true, since the comments do not seem very ambitious. Choice B would be a very unlikely conclusion since the evidence in the paragraph does not support this. Choice C is not supported by the text either.

3. **Answer: (C) He was passionate in his beliefs.**

   Based on what the author says, he feels very strongly about his poetry and art. Choice A could be true, but that does not seem likely. Choice B does not seem to be true, since he is so outspoken. Choice D is also unlikely; this person does not seem to be worried about anything.

4. **Answer: (C) moral principles**

   Choice C, *moral principles*, makes sense when you substitute it for the underlined word. Choices A, B, and D do not.

ReKap

Making an inference, drawing a conclusion, and making a prediction are processes that should be based on evidence.

2 READING · LESSON 6
More Informational Techniques

Some of the passages and questions on the admissions test may take more thought than others. These detailed passages and questions will test your critical reading skills. Critical reading skills include the ability to analyze a passage and interpret the information in it. These skills differ from everyday comprehension because critical thinking includes judging the credibility of the information and analyzing the author's intention.

Common Uses in Health Care

- tables showing which medicines are indicated for certain diseases
- healthcare textbooks
- physicians' orders

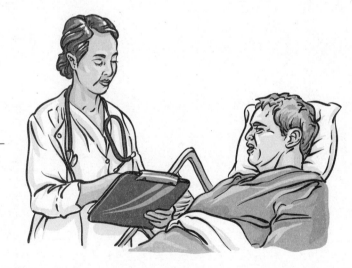

Key Terms/Formulas

- **appropriate source** – a source that can be trusted
- **critical reading skills** – skills that allow you to analyze and judge the credibility of a text and the author's intention
- **locating information** – the process of determining the most appropriate sources and finding specific information
- **recognizing bias** – analyzing whether an author has a prejudice in favor or against a thing, person, or group

Learn

You learned in an earlier lesson how to make inferences by putting two and two together and reading between the lines. You learned that sometimes authors tell you what they want you to know directly and that sometimes they hint at things. Other times, writing can reflect the opinions or biases of the writer, either by directly stating his or her thoughts, or through the language used, the information included, or the information the writer chooses to leave out.

You also learned how to make predictions based on the evidence in a text. When you make a prediction, you decide what may be true in the future based on the evidence in a text.

When you are working with more complex texts, you will have to use your **critical reading skills** to full capacity. That means that you must be able to understand and analyze what you read, make judgments about the information, and draw conclusions from the evidence in texts.

Here are the basic critical reading skills. These can be used as strategies to help you understand more complicated texts.

- Analysis
- Interpretation
- Citing evidence
- Making inferences
- Drawing conclusions
- Recognizing bias

These techniques can be applied to both technical and informational passages, and can even help you figure out the meaning of unknown words in a text.

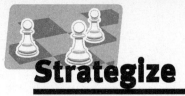

Strategize

Analyze

What kind of text is this? What is it mostly about?

Look through the text and determine its intent. Decide what it is mostly about.

Interpret

What is the text telling you between the lines?

Decide if there is something that the author is not telling you directly.

Cite Evidence

What evidence is found in the text?

Pinpoint the evidence that you need to draw a conclusion.

Make an Inference or Make a Prediction

What does the text suggest is true?

Make an inference or prediction based on the evidence in the text.

Sample Passage

Directive per Dr. Samuel Spears

Please make sure that the patient is comfortable at all times. Controlling the patient's body temperature is vital to the patient's treatment. Be sure to have warming blankets on the patient at all times.

Apply

Read the following text from a medical book.

In developed countries, a large proportion of all deaths are due to a disease called arteriosclerosis. Arteriosclerosis is a condition in which fatty material collects on the walls of the arteries, causing hardening of the arteries and possible blockage. Some of this hardening is caused by high cholesterol diets and by insufficient exercise; family history of the disease is a factor as well.

Exercise and a low-fat diet can help control the onset of the disease, and there are many procedures and medicines to help keep it under control should it develop.

Medical researchers believe that every man or woman, if he or she lives long enough, will inevitably suffer from arteriosclerosis. This is because arteriosclerosis is caused by the wear and tear resulting from the constant flow of blood through the arteries over the course of a lifetime.

A1. Which inference can the reader make based on this text?

A) Old age is caused by arteriosclerosis.

B) Exercise will prevent arteriosclerosis.

C) Old age and arteriosclerosis go hand in hand.

D) Clogged arteries can be cured with medication.

To answer this question, use the following strategies.

STEP 1: Analyze

Ask yourself what the excerpt is mostly about.

Look for key words to help you figure it out. Is it about an illness?

STEP 2: Cite Evidence

Look to see what the author is saying about arteriosclerosis. This is evidence you can use to form a conclusion.

STEP 3: Draw a Conclusion or Make a Prediction

Check out each of the possible conclusions. Which one is supported by the evidence in the text? Eliminate the ones that are not supported by the text. Choice C follows the text; the author states that arteriosclerosis is inevitable if a person lives long enough. Eliminate Choices A, B, and D for lack of supporting evidence. There is no mention that arteriosclerosis causes old age, that exercise cures arteriosclerosis, or that medication can eliminate clogged arteries.

Learn

The admissions test will ask you to figure out the meanings of unknown words or phrases by using context clues. As you learned in an earlier lesson, when you see a word or phrase that you do not know, read the sentence the word or phrase is in as well as the surrounding sentences. Many times the context of the passage will help you figure out the meaning of the phrase or word.

For example, what is the meaning of the phrase *greatest of diligence* in the following excerpt?

Before the accident, Angelina had been the most successful model in the country. Now the surgeons were struggling to reshape her nose to recapture her old beauty. The two surgeons worked with the greatest of diligence for many hours. If they could do their job successfully, Angelina's picture would continue to be on the cover of all the top magazines.

If you did not know the meaning of *greatest of diligence*, you could find the clues you need in the sentences around the sentence that the phrase is in. The excerpt says the surgeons worked for many hours and that if they were successful, Angelina would be a popular model again.

Think of a word or words that you could substitute for the phrase *greatest of diligence*, such as *terribly hard*. If you substitute that phrase for *greatest of diligence*, does the excerpt makes sense? If it does, you know you have the correct choice. This is a good way to determine the meaning of unknown words and phrases.

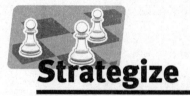

Strategize

Analyze the Text for Context Clues

Which words can help you determine the meaning of the unknown word or phrase?

Substitute the Word or Phrase for Another

What word could be substituted for the unknown word and make sense in the context of the sentence?

Apply

Read this excerpt from a medical report.

Although he performed several tests, the doctor was unable to <u>corroborate</u> any symptoms of heart palpitations even though they seemed evident to him. Therefore, he sent the patient to a specialist for further diagnosis.

A2. What is the meaning of the underlined word in the excerpt above?

A) answer

B) confirm

C) predict

D) solve

To answer this question, use the following strategies.

STEP 1: Analyze the Text for Context Clues

Which words can help you determine the meaning of the unknown word?

STEP 2: Substitute the Word for Another

Which word could be substituted for the unknown word and make sense in the context of the sentence?

STEP 3: Draw a Conclusion or Make a Prediction

Check out each of the possible answers. Which one fits into the context of the sentence? Context clues such as the doctor performing tests and then sending the patient to a specialist for further testing help the reader determine the meaning of the unknown word. Another clue is that the palpitations seemed to be present, but the tests did not show them. Choice B, *confirm*, is the meaning of the word corroborate.

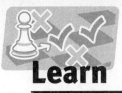

Learn

You will need to learn how to locate information and to make sure that it is from an appropriate source. An appropriate source is one that is reliable. Today, the Internet is used constantly as a means to locate information, but the problem with the Internet is that everyone has access to it and can post information that is inaccurate or unreliable.

But how do you recognize whether a source is reliable? You need to check its references in the same way you would check the references of someone you were hiring for a job. You need to know where the information is coming from and if the source is recognized as being credible.

Reliable sources include websites of well-known agencies, the government, and nonprofit groups dedicated to education. Textbooks also make good sources.

When you locate information, you will need to make sure that it is the exact information you are looking for and not just something loosely related to the topic.

You should also analyze the information to see if there is any bias in the text. You will need to analyze any prejudice that an author may have in order to check the credibility of the text.

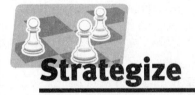

Strategize

Check for Appropriateness

Can this source be trusted? Is this the best source?

Check to see if the source is appropriate. Check to see if the source will supply exact information.

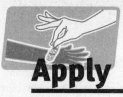

A3. A runner wants to learn ways to warm up before setting off on a jog. Which of the following would be an appropriate source for providing this information?

A) *The Happy Jogger*, a novel

B) "Jogger Supplies," a retail website

C) *Stretching Before You Jog*, a nonfiction book

D) "Common Jogging Injuries," an article about jogging injuries

To answer this question, use the following strategies.

STEP 1: Analyze

What does the question ask you? What are the possible answers?

STEP 2: Check for Appropriateness

Which source would be most appropriate for the runner to use? Which would most likely give the information that the runner is seeking?

STEP 3: Draw a Conclusion or Make a Prediction

Check out each of the possible answers. Which one is directly related to what the runner wants to find out? While all sources seem to be reliable, only one of them addresses the information that the runner wants; the runner wants to know what to do to warm up. The title of the nonfiction book (Choice C) suggests it would cover this information, so this is the best answer.

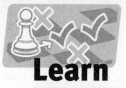
Learn

Some questions on the admissions test may ask about the information in a table or the information in the yellow pages. Other questions could ask you to comprehend the information in a communication such as an invitation or memo.

Tables are useful graphics. Complicated information can be presented in a visual form, making it easier to read and to compare products or services.

One way a table can be useful is to determine which product is the most desirable, at the best price, to meet a person's needs.

For example, this table compares the prices of flowers.

Type of Flower	Price
Roses	$19.99 per dozen or $1.75 each
Tulips	$14.99 per dozen or $1.50 each
Daffodils	$11.99 per dozen or $1.20 each.

This table organizes information about three different types of flowers and how much they cost, per dozen and for each one. If this information were presented in a sentence or a paragraph, it would be more difficult to analyze the cost of each type of flower. That is why a table is useful. It is a visual representation of information.

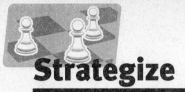
Determine the Purpose of a Text

What does the text do? Does it compare things? Does it tell you what to do? Does it help you find what you need?

Decide What Is Being Compared

Look through the table and see what information is in it. What is being compared?

Sample Texts

The first sample text is an excerpt from the yellow pages listing entries related to oil: oil change and lube, oils for fuel and heating, lubricating oil, petroleum oil, and waste and used oil. The second sample text has information related to a work anniversary party.

Oil Change & Lube -(Cont'd)	Oils Petroleum
Valvoline Instant Oil Change 8200 Market St Wilm . . . . . .**681-0244** **Valvoline Instant Oil Change** 4417 S 17th St Wilm **392-7279**	**Amerada Hess Corp** . . . .**763-8147** **Amerada Hess Corp** 1312 S Front St Wilm . . . . .**763-5122** **Apex Oil Co** River Rd . . . . . .**799-0030** **Colonial Oil Industries Inc** 4002 S Front St Wilm . . . . .**762-1747** **Dearybury Oil Inc** 1929 Sandwedge Pt Wilm . .**256-2450** **Dearybury Oil Inc** 1929 Sandwedge Pt Wilm . .**256-5766**
Oils Fuel & Heating	
Atlantic Coast Fuel & Lubes 3607 Lynn An Cstl Hayne . . .**623-4559** **Damar Oil Co** 13025 Castle Hayne Rd . . . .**762-0312** **Great Lakes Petroleum** Toll Free "1" & then . . . **800-686-3455** **Springer Burbank** 123 Shipyard Blvd Wilm . .**343-1991** *See Display Ad This Page* **Springer Burbank** 10 S Cardinal Dr Wilm **790-0284**	**VOPAK OIL RECOVERY LLC** **BULK CHEMICAL STORAGE** WWW.VOPAK.COM 1710 Woodhouse St . . .**763-0104**
Oils Lubricating	**Oils Waste & Used**
Amsoil Direct Jobber 103 Broadview Ln Hampstead **270-7776** **Brewer-Hendley Oil Co Inc** Toll Free "1" & then **800-613-8465** **SHELL LUBRICANTS** A complete line of auto, truck, and industrial oils, greases and coolants. • Rotella® T • Pennzoil® • Rimula® • Quaker State® • Tellus® **DILMAR OIL CO** **1325 Castle Hayne Rd Wilmington** Toll Free "1" & then . . **800-489-4626**	**BFP OIL RECOVERY LLC** **★ NO JOB TOO SMALL ★** ✓ Residential & Commercial ✓ Totes & Drums Provided ✓ Waste Oil-Filters-Diesel-Gas-Antifreeze ✓ Sludge - Solid Waste & Mixed Water www.BFPoilRecovery.com . . . .**259-0389** **P & W Waste Oil Service Inc 392-9760** **SR & R ENVIRONMENTAL INC** 4520 US Hwy 421 N Wilmington **763-6274**

Memo

To: All Employees

Re: Anniversary Celebration

Please be advised that the office will close early on Friday afternoon at 3:30 pm so that we can enjoy our five-year anniversary celebration. This will be a potluck party, although management will provide a mean chili dish and a delicious cake. We are asking everyone to bring a favorite dish to share. Non-alcoholic drinks will also be provided. Please contact Pete in HR to sign up for a specific dish. He is coordinating the effort so we don't have ten potato salads or eight franks and beans. If you prefer not to bring a dish, contact Eileen in room 121 who will collect a monetary contribution in lieu of food. She will be purchasing additional foods with the funds she collects. The party will run until 6 pm. If you cannot join us, please let Kate in room 204 know so we can plan accordingly.

Congratulations to all of you for a job well done!

Apply

A4. A student in California wants to buy a textbook called *This World of Biology*. She went online and found this table.

Stores/Prices for *This World of Biology*

Store	Location	Price	Shipping and Handling
Books Are Us	Chicago, IL	$90	Free shipping and handling
Education Texts	Chicago, IL	$85	$15 (free on purchases of $50 or more)
Technical Textbooks	San Francisco, CA	$80	$20
Tons of Texts	San Francisco, CA	$90	$20 (free in state)

From which store should the student purchase the book in order to get the best price?

A) Books Are Us

B) Education Texts

C) Technical Textbooks

D) Tons of Texts

STEP 1: Determine the Purpose of a Text

What does the table show? Does it compare things?

STEP 2: Decide What Is Being Compared

Look through the table and see what information is in it. What is being compared?

STEP 3: Interpret

Determine which book would be the least expensive based on the details in the question and the table. Some stores offer the book at a cheaper price, but the shipping and handling has to be figured into the cost. Overall, *Education Texts*, Choice B, provides the books at the best price.

TIP: Do not jump to conclusions about the data, but factor in the details found in the question and the table.

Guided Practice

1. The human eye is a very sensitive organ since so much of it is exposed to the environment. Luckily the facial structure around the eye is designed to protect the exposed parts of the eye from harm, or at least keep harm to a minimum. The brow shields the eye from the top while the nose and cheekbones guard it at the sides and below.

   There are other aspects of the eye that help protect the organ from threats, including the tear glands and the eyelid. Tear ducts perform an important role because they provide the fluids that keep the eye moist, which is necessary to the well-being of the organ. The eyelid is equally essential since it shuts over the eye, protecting it from dust or other airborne materials that could irritate the eye.

   What inference could be made based on the evidence in the passage?

   A) The eye is the most protected part of the human body.

   B) Parts of the design of the human body are helpful to the body's safety.

   C) The eye is just one of many parts of the body that are constantly at risk.

   D) Accident prevention is the main focus of the design of the human body.

   STEP 1: Analyze

   What is this passage mostly about?

   _____

   _____

   STEP 2: Cite Evidence

   How does the design of the body protect the eye?

   _____

   _____

   STEP 3: Draw a Conclusion

   Which answer choice is supported by the evidence?

   _____

   _____

2. I've been through every file in my file cabinet and I cannot find the information about how much I paid for the improvements to my house. I guess I will have to <u>start from scratch</u> and go through it all again.

What is the meaning of the underlined phrase?

A) begin again

B) start at the end

C) review the information

D) come up with a new figure

STEP 1: Analyze the Text for Context Clues

Which words help you determine the meaning of the unknown word or words?

_____

_____

STEP 2: Substitute One Word or Words For Another

Which word or words would make sense in the context of the sentence?

_____

_____

STEP 3: Draw a Conclusion

Which answer choice is closest to your substitute words?

_____

_____

Guided Practice

Store	Unit Price: 1 to 10 cases	Unit Price: 11 or more cases	Shipping and Handling
Tech Time	$10	$9	$30 total fee for any order
Super Savings	$12	$10	$20 total fee for any order
Work Tech	$11	$9	$25 for orders under $100; free on purchases of $100 or more
Supplies and More	$10	$8	$2 per case

3. A company in Massachusetts wants to buy 12 cases of oil. Which store will provide the best total order price?

A) Tech Time

B) Super Savings

C) Work Tech

D) Supplies and More

STEP 1: Determine the Purpose of a Text

What does the table do?

_____

_____

STEP 2: Decide What Is Being Compared

What is the cost of the oil and shipping and handling?

_____

_____

STEP 3: Interpret

How much would each option cost?

_____

_____

Independent Practice

1. Memo
To: Employees
Re: Weekend Workshop

We are organizing our weekend workshop and wanted to update everyone on the schedule. We plan to have four major sessions on Saturday and three on Sunday. The weekend will commence with a dinner on Friday evening at 6 pm. Saturday's sessions will run from 8:30 am to 4:30 pm. There will be two sessions in the morning and two in the afternoon. During the evening there will be a casual get-together after dinner to discuss the day's activities. Sunday will run from 1 to 4 pm with two sessions.

Transportation is being arranged as follows: People whose last name begins with a letter A through D should contact Jim Thorne about a ride to the workshop. Those whose last name begins with a letter from E through L should contact Ellen Avena for information about transportation. Those whose last name begins with a letter from M to P should call John Marlin. All others should call Mitzi Ladner.

We are looking forward to this workshop and feel it will go far to increase productivity and morale. More specifics about the different sessions will follow.

Peggy Ruiz wants to find out about her transportation to the workshop. Who should she contact?

A) Jim Thorne

B) Ellen Avena

C) John Marlin

D) Mitzi Ladner

HINT *What letter does Peggy's last name begin with?*

2. Not all blind people use dogs as guides. A growing number of people who are sightless are turning to miniature horses to ensure their safety and ability to move about. These tiny animals are equally able to keep a master out of harm's way and because of certain attributes, a small horse may be more desirable than a seeing-eye dog.

Miniature horses are no strangers to hard work. Many of their ancestors worked in the coal mines in England and Wales. They have been used for mining in this country as well. Some of these animals never saw the light of day, living their entire lives underground. The obvious reason for miniature horses working in a mine is their height. They measure 35 inches at their withers. But there were other reasons as well. These little horses are very obedient, easy-going, and able to work long hours. All of these traits make them excellent candidates as guide animals.

They also have other valuable assets. They are hypoallergenic, so people with allergies may prefer them over dogs. They live longer than traditional guides, up to 40 years, so people may only have to have one guide animal in their lifetime. They also don't mind spending their down time out of doors, though they can be housetrained.

There's another factor to consider as well. Many people are nervous around dogs, but feel more comfortable with a small horse. These horses are never aggressive, but they are strong enough to help individuals with physical disabilities, including helping a handler rise from a chair if that is a difficult thing to do. Another good point, say owners, is that dogs are often seen as pets and it takes some explaining to allow them to act as guides. Little horses, however, are recognized quickly as guide animals. Also, horses are very clean and, unlike dogs, don't get fleas. Plus they are incredibly sweet and willing to take care of their charge.

Independent Practice

They are also very adaptable. One sightless person flew with his miniature horse from the farm where she was trained to his home. The horse's name was Cuddles, and she slept beside her master for most of the flight. The two of them also took a trip to New York City, where locals were impressed by this animal and how she was even able to navigate the subway!

Of course dogs and horses are not the exclusive animals that have served as service animals. Pigs are also trained from time to time as guide animals, and monkeys have proved useful to those with serious physical handicaps. Therefore, the saying should probably be changed to "It's not just a dog that is man's best friend."

Based on the passage, who do you predict is most likely to choose a miniature horse rather than a dog as a service animal?

A) a person who grew up on a farm

B) a person who likes to live in a city

C) a person who has never owned a dog

D) a person who is afraid of being bitten

HINT   *What would motivate each person?*

---

3. A person wants to find out how much keeping his house warm in the winter will cost him. Which heading would he look under in the yellow pages?

A) Oils Petroleum

B) Oils Lubricating

C) Oil Fuel & Heating

D) Oils Waste & Used

Oil Change & Lube -(Cont'd)

Valvoline Instant Oil Change
8200 Market St Wilm **681-0244**
Valvoline Instant Oil Change
4417 S 17th St Wilm **392-7279**

Oils Fuel & Heating

Atlantic Coast Fuel & Lubes
3607 Lynn An Cstl Hayne ... **623-4559**
Damar Oil Co
13025 Castle Hayne Rd **762-0312**
Great Lakes Petroleum
Toll Free "1" & then ... **800-686-3455**
Springer Burbank
123 Shipyard Blvd Wilm ...**343-1991**
See Display Ad This Page
Springer Burbank
10 S Cardinal Dr Wilm **790-0284**

Oils Lubricating

Amsoil Direct Jobber
103 Broadview Ln Hampstead **270-7776**
Brewer-Hendley Oil Co Inc
Toll Free "1" & then **800-613-8465**
SHELL LUBRICANTS ─────
   A complete line of auto, truck, and
   industrial oils, greases and coolants.

   • Rotella® T • Pennzoil® • Rimula®
       • Quaker State® • Tellus®
DILMAR OIL CO
1325 Castle Hayne Rd Wilmington
Toll Free "1" & then .. **800-489-4626**

Oils Petroleum

Amerada Hess Corp **763-8147**
Amerada Hess Corp
1312 S Front St Wilm **763-5122**
Apex Oil Co River Rd **799-0030**
Colonial Oil Industries Inc
4002 S Front St Wilm **762-1747**
Dearybury Oil Inc
1929 Sandwedge Pt Wilm .. **256-2450**
Dearybury Oil Inc
1929 Sandwedge Pt Wilm .. **256-5766**
VOPAK OIL RECOVERY LLC ─────
   BULK CHEMICAL STORAGE
      WWW.VOPAK.COM
   1710 Woodhouse St ... **763-0104**

Oils Waste & Used

BFP OIL RECOVERY LLC ─────
   ★ NO JOB TOO SMALL ★
   ✓ Residential & Commercial
      ✓ Totes & Drums Provided
   ✓ Waste Oil-Filters-Diesel-Gas-Antifreeze
   ✓ Sludge - Solid Waste & Mixed Water
      www.BFPoilRecovery.com
   .... **259-0389**
P & W Waste Oil Service Inc **392-9760**
SR & R ENVIRONMENTAL INC
4520 US Hwy 421 N Wilmington
   .... **763-6274**

ReKap

In this lesson, you learned about the process for making logical conclusions and inferences. You also learned how to make predictions. You learned that any conclusion or prediction needs to be supported by evidence.

You learned how to use context to figure out the meanings of words and phrases.

You learned how to locate information and to check to see if it is appropriate and reliable. You also learned to check for an author's bias or prejudice in a text.

You learned strategies to help you answer test items. These strategies are:

- Analyze

- Interpret

- Cite Evidence

- Make an Inference or Make a Prediction

- Analyze the Text for Context Clues

- Substitute the Word or Phrase For Another

- Check for Appropriateness

- Determine the Purpose of a Text

- Decide What Is Being Compared

? What critical reading skills require using evidence in a text?

_____

_____

_____

_____

Answers

Guided Practice

1. Step 1: The passage is about how the eye is protected by the design of the body.

    Step 2: The brow and cheekbones shield the eye. The tear glands and eyelid protect it.

    Step 3: The evidence of the passage support Choice B.

Answer: (B) Parts of the design of the human body are helpful to the body's safety.

2. Step 1: The words *go through it all again* give clues about the meaning of the unknown word.

    Step 2: In the context of the sentence, the words *start over* would make sense.

    Step 3: Choice A, *begin again*, is closest to the substituted words.

Answer: (A) begin again

3. Step 1: The table compares buying cases of oil.

    Step 2: The cost of the oil and shipping and handling are all different.

    Step 3: The cost for Tech Time is $138 ($9 × 12 + $30); Super Savings, $140 ($10 × 12 + $20); Work Tech, $108 ($9 × 12 + free shipping); Supplies and More, $120 ($8 × 12 + $2 × 12). $108 is the least cost listed.

Answer: (C) Work Tech

Independent Practice

1. **Answer: (D) Mitzi Ladner**

    The memo indicates the individual that people should contact regarding transportation by listing the names of people and telling employees that the person to contact depends on the first letter of their last name. The name of the person who wants to find out about transportation begins with the letter R, so Choices A, B, and C can all be eliminated. While the memo does not actually tell the first letters that are assigned to Mitzi Ladner, the reader can figure out that she gets the names beginning with the letters after P.

2. **Answer: (D) a person who is afraid of being bitten**

    Based on what is said in paragraph 4, Choice D is the most logical prediction. Choice A could be a possibility, but there is no direct evidence to support it. Choice B could be possible, but again there is no real evidence that this person would pick a miniature horse as a guide. Choice C is possible, but it is not supported by the text.

3. **Answer: (C) Oil Fuel & Heating**

    The question asks about someone who wants to know how much it will cost to keep his house warm in the winter. This question is about heating his house. There is only one heading that deals with oil heating, so Choice C is the correct answer. The other headings deal with different aspects of oil.

ReKap

Each of the critical thinking skills – analysis, interpretation, citing evidence, making inferences, drawing conclusions, and recognizing bias – requires using evidence in a text.

UNIT 3 Math

3

MATH · LESSON 1
Numbers

Have you ever had to deal with temperatures so cold that the thermometer drops into the negative? Have you worked with square roots lately? Remember that the questions you will tackle on the test are meant to be answered without a calculator. Fortunately, this just means they are simple enough to be solved with a pencil and paper!

Some of the most basic number concepts—negative numbers, absolute values and square roots—may seem abstract at first, but relating them to a number line helps to visualize and make sense of them. Let's take a look at them now!

Common Uses in Health Care

- working with changes in temperature
- calculating deficits and shortages
- measuring increases or decreases in medication doses

Key Terms/Formulas

- **absolute value** – the distance, in units, of a number from zero on a number line
- **negative number** – a number less than zero
- **number line** – a line with numbers marked as units
- **square root** – a number that, when multiplied by itself, yields a given value

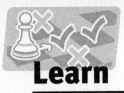

Learn

Comparing Numbers

Let's begin by talking about positive and negative numbers. We'll see how to order and compare them. Refer to a number line to compare numbers.

$$\xleftarrow{\hspace{3cm}}\underset{\substack{-10 \quad -8 \quad -6 \quad -4 \quad -2 \quad\; 0 \quad\; 2 \quad\; 4 \quad\; 6 \quad\; 8 \quad\; 10}}{\overline{|\,|\,|\,|\,|\,|\,|\,|\,|\,|\,|\,|\,|\,|\,|\,|\,|\,|\,|\,|\,|}}\xrightarrow{\hspace{3cm}}$$

If you ignore negative signs, the numbers on the number line are counted up from 0 in both directions. They are not really counted up from 0 when it comes to negative numbers, though. The key to comparing numbers on a number line is this:

You know that 8 is greater than 1, and you can see that it is farther to the right of 0 than 1 (seven units to the right, to be exact!).

We also say that –2 is greater than –5 for the same reason. On the number line, –2 is three units to the right of –5. Likewise, –6 is less than –3 because it is several units to the left of –3 on the number line.

You can also use the number line to think about addition and subtraction.

- To add a positive number, move that many units to the right on the number line.
- To add a negative number, move that many units to the left on the number line.
- To subtract a positive number, move that many units to the left on the number line.
- To subtract a negative number, move that many units to the right on the number line.

The rules for the finding the sign of the products and quotients with signed numbers are below.

Rules for Multiplying Signed Numbers	Rules for Dividing Signed Numbers
positive × positive = positive	positive ÷ positive = positive
negative × positive = negative	negative ÷ positive = negative
positive × negative = negative	positive ÷ negative = negative
negative × negative = positive	negative ÷ negative = positive

For both multiplication and division, the result is positive when the signs are the same. The result is negative when the signs are different.

You can also use a number line to compare fractions as points on a number line between the whole numbers.

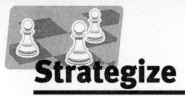

Strategize

Visualize

To compare or order numbers, especially negative numbers, plot them on a number line.

To draw a number line:

- Remember to count positive numbers up from zero, from left to right.

- Count negative numbers (–1, –2, –3) away from 0 from right to left.

- Remember that as you count the negative numbers left from 0, their value decreases.

Plot the numbers on the number line and compare their positions. The number on the right is the greater number.

The X Method for Comparing Fractions

To compare fractions on a number line, you can estimate where each should be placed. If you are dealing with fractions with different numerators and denominators, though, placing them in relative positions can be difficult. There is another strategy that is helpful for comparing fractions.

To compare two positive fractions:

- Draw lines between the denominator of the one and the numerator of the other to form an X.

- Multiply *denominator* × *numerator* for each line and record the result above each fraction.

$$5\times2=10 \qquad 3\times4=12$$

$$\frac{2}{3}\diagdown\diagup\frac{4}{5}$$

The fraction beneath the greater product is the greater fraction. For instance, because 12 > 10 in the example above.

$$\frac{4}{5}>\frac{2}{3}$$

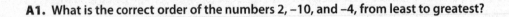
Let's take a look at some examples.

A1. **What is the correct order of the numbers 2, –10, and –4, from least to greatest?**

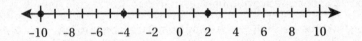

STEP 1: Plan

Plot each number on the number line.

STEP 2: Follow through

I see that –10 is to the left of –4, and –4 is to the left of 2. So, –4 is greater than –10, and 2 is greater than –4.

STEP 3: Solve

The order from least to greatest is –10, –4, 2.

A2. **Which temperature is colder, –8°C or –3°C?**

STEP 1: Plan

Since higher (warmer) temperatures are represented by greater numbers, the colder temperature has a lower value. Think: I should plot the numbers of degrees on a number line and look for the lesser value.

STEP 2: Follow through

The number –8 is to the left of –3 on the number line.

STEP 3: Solve

So, –8°C is colder than –3°C.

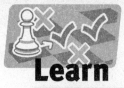

Learn

Absolute Value

If the temperature in a freezer is –5°C, how many degrees below zero is the temperature? The answer is 5. If you got that, you already grasp the idea of *absolute value*. A temperature of –5°C is five units away from 0°C on a thermometer.

The absolute value of a number is its distance from zero on a number line. So, the absolute values of –5 and 5 are same. Both are five units from 0, just in opposite directions. Each number has an absolute value of 5.

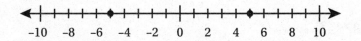

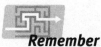
Remember

The absolute value of a number (even a negative one) is positive.

To symbolize absolute values, we place a vertical line on each side of a number or expression, like brackets.

The expression |–5| stands for the absolute value of 5: |–5| = 5.

The expression |4 – 5| stands for the absolute value of 4 – 5. Since 4 – 5 = –1, |4 – 5| = |–1| = 1.

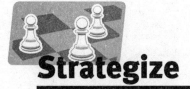

Strategize

Count!

For basic questions involving absolute value, just count units from zero. Remember that the direction does not matter.

Ask yourself:

- Where do I count from on the number line?

- How do I go about simplifying absolute value expressions?

For more complicated arithmetic questions involving absolute value, be sure to apply the absolute value operations at the right point in your calculations.

For an expression like |4 – 8|, find the value of the expression inside the lines. Then, find the absolute value of that number.

Apply

A3. What is $|{-8}| - |{-3}|$?

STEP 1: Plan

This involves two absolute value expressions. Find each absolute value and then subtract.

STEP 2: Follow through

Since −8 is 8 units to the left of zero, $|{-8}| = 8$; −3 is 3 units to the left of zero, so $|{-3}| = 3$.

STEP 3: Solve

$|{-8}| - |{-3}| = 8 - 3 = 5$

A4. What is $|{-9} + 4|$?

STEP 1: Plan

Although the expression has two numbers, both are inside the lines. Think: I have to find the sum of the numbers inside, and then find the absolute value of the numbers.

STEP 2: Follow through

$-9 + 4 = -5$, $|{-9} + 4| = |{-5}| = 5$

STEP 3: Solve

$|{-5}| = 5$

Learn

Square Roots

The square of a number is the product of the number and itself. Since $5 \times 5 = 25$, the square of 5 is 25. Since $-6 \times -6 = 36$ (note that the product of two negative numbers is always positive), the square of -6 is 36.

Think of square roots as involving the opposite relationship. Since $5 \times 5 = 25$, a square root of 25 is 5. To get the square root of a given number, you have to find what number you have to square to get the given number.

Every positive number actually has two square roots. One is its positive square root, and the other is the negative of that root. We've already said that 5 is a root of 25, but so is -5, because $-5 \times -5 = 25$.

We use the sign $\sqrt{}$ (*a radical sign*), with a number inside, to represent the positive square of a number. So, $\sqrt{25} = 5$ and $\sqrt{36} = 6$. An expression like $\sqrt{25}$ is called a radical.

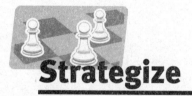

Strategize

Estimate and Adjust

You might know some square roots by heart; many people will remember offhand that a square root of 9 is 3. But do you know the positive square root of 289 offhand?

If not, you can begin by making a guess. Is 19 the square root? Try it!

$20 \times 20 = 400 \rightarrow$ Too high!

Go a little lower. What about 15?

$15 \times 15 = 225 \rightarrow$ Too low!

Try a number in the middle

$17 \times 17 = 289 \rightarrow$ Perfect!

Sometimes you have to play a bit of a *high-low* game, adjusting higher or lower if you do not hit the target.

Apply

A5. A square bandage has an area of 64 square centimeters. What is the length of each side of the bandage?

STEP 1. Plan.

The area of a square is the product of its length and width, which are the same. So, the side length is the square root of 64, the area.

STEP 2. Follow through.

Estimate. Could the side length be 12?

$12 \times 12 = 144 \rightarrow$ Too high, go lower

$6 \times 6 = 36 \rightarrow$ Too low, go higher

$8 \times 8 = 64 \rightarrow$ The square root is 8

STEP 3. Solve.

So, the correct answer is 8 centimeters.

A6. The square root of 200 is between which two whole numbers?

STEP 1. Plan.

You don't have to calculate the actual square root of 200 to answer this question. Instead, find two whole numbers with squares nearest to 200, with one less than 200 and one greater.

STEP 2. Follow through.

Try squaring different numbers, based on estimates.

$13 \times 13 = 169 \rightarrow$ Close?

$14 \times 14 = 196 \rightarrow$ Very close!

$15 \times 15 = 225 \rightarrow$ Greater than 200!

STEP 3. Solve.

Because the square of 14 is less than 200 and the square of 15 is greater, the square root of 200 is between 14 and 15.

Guided Practice

Let's work through a few examples together. Look back at the lesson content as often as necessary to help you apply the concepts and strategies you learned.

1. Which number is less than −10 and greater than −15?

   A) −18

   B) −12

   C) 13

   D) 16

   STEP 1: Visualize

   _____

   _____

   STEP 2: Plot

   _____

   _____

   STEP 3: Compare

   _____

   _____

2. Which number is closest to the value of $\sqrt{90}$?

   A) 7

   B) 8

   C) 9

   D) 10

   STEP 1: Estimate

   The number 90 is not a perfect square, and you don't need to find the exact square root. However, you can estimate based on the positive square roots of numbers that are close to 90.

   $\sqrt{81} =$

   $\sqrt{100} =$

   _____

   _____

Guided Practice

STEP 2: Test

Let's see what happens when we split the difference. The number 9.5 is midway between 9 and 10, so let's square it.

_____

_____

STEP 3: Compare

Consider how does the square root of 90 compare to the answer options.

_____

_____

3. What is the value of $|-9 - 4| - |4 - 18|$?

   A) −9

   B) −1

   C) 1

   D) 9

STEP 1: Work inside the lines

Start on the inside, and work your way out.

_____

_____

STEP 2: Calculate absolute values

_____

_____

STEP 3: Simplify

_____

_____

Independent Practice

1. Which of the following inequalities is correct?

A) $-25 > -18$

B) $-24 < -15$

C) $-23 > -21$

D) $-22 < -26$

HINT > *One negative number is less than a second negative number if it is closer to 0 on the number line.*

2. What is the value of $\sqrt{144}$?

A) 12

B) 16

C) 32

D) 72

HINT > *What number can be multiplied by itself to get 144?*

3. What is the sum of $|-5|$ and $|9|$?

A) -14

B) -4

C) 4

D) 14

HINT > *Remember to find the absolute values before adding.*

4. Which of the following orders the fractions $\dfrac{3}{8}$, $\dfrac{2}{5}$, and $\dfrac{1}{4}$, from least to greatest?

A) $\dfrac{1}{4}, \dfrac{2}{5}, \dfrac{3}{8}$

B) $\dfrac{1}{4}, \dfrac{3}{8}, \dfrac{2}{5}$

C) $\dfrac{3}{8}, \dfrac{1}{4}, \dfrac{2}{5}$

D) $1\dfrac{3}{8}, \dfrac{2}{5}, \dfrac{1}{4}$

HINT > *How does each pair of fractions compare, based on the X Method?*

ReKap

In this lesson, you learned how to compare and order signed numbers, how to work with square roots, and how to work with absolute values. Remember the following techniques:

- Plot numbers on a number line to compare them.

- Use the X Method to compare fractions.

- Think of absolute value as distance from 0 on a number line.

> **?** **Suppose a falls to the right of b on a number line and $|a| = |b| = 7$. Use what you learned to find the values of a and b.**
>
> _____
>
> _____
>
> _____

Answers

Guided Practice

1. Step 1: Draw a number line. For example,

   Step 2: Mark the two numbers on the line.

   Step 3: Realize that −10 is to the right of −15. A number that is greater than −15 will be to the right of it, and a number less than −10 will be to the left of −10. So, a number that is less than −10 and greater than −15 must be between those numbers on the number line. Only Choice B fits between the two points.

   Answer: (B) −12

2. Step 1: $\sqrt{81} = 9$

   $\sqrt{100} = 10$

   So, the positive square root of 90 must be between 9 and 10.

   Step 2: $9.5^2 = 9.5 \times 9.5 = 90.25$

   Step 3: 9 is closer than 10 to the square root of 90.

   TIP: Don't be tempted to say that it's closer to 10 just because it's greater than 9.

   Answer: (C) 9

3. Step 1: Start on the inside, and work your way out.

   $|-9 - 4| - |4 - 18|$

   $-9 - 4 = -13$

   $4 - 18 = -14$

   So, $|-13| - |-14|$

   Step 2: $|-13| - |-14| = 13 - 14$

   Step 3: $13 - 14 = -1$.

   TIP: Don't rule out the negative answers just because the expression involves absolute values.

   Answer: (B) −1

Independent Practice

1. **Answer: (B) −24 < −15**

   Sketch a number line. Use the values in the answer choices to determine the starting and ending value on the number line. You only need to show values between −26 and −15. Plot the numbers in the answer choices. Compare the positions of each pair of numbers on the line. Remember, the farther left, the lesser the number. −24 is to the left of −15, so −24 < −15.

Answers

2. **Answer: (A) 12**

   If you know that 10 is the square root of 100, which is not that far from 144, you can work your way up from there.

   $11 \times 11 = 121 \rightarrow$ too low, go higher

   $12 \times 12 = 144$

3. **Answer: (D) 14**

   The absolute values of $|-5|$ and $|9|$ are 5 and 9, respectively. The sum of 5 and 9 is 14.

4. **Answer: (B)** $\dfrac{1}{4}, \dfrac{3}{8}, \dfrac{2}{5}$

   To order the fractions, compare them in pairs using the X Method.

   Compare $\dfrac{3}{8}$ and $\dfrac{2}{5}$, we get $3 \times 5 = 15$ and $2 \times 8 = 8$. So $\dfrac{2}{5} > \dfrac{3}{8}$

   Compare $\dfrac{3}{8}$ and $\dfrac{1}{4}$, we get $3 \times 4 = 12$ and $1 \times 8 = 8$. So $\dfrac{3}{8} > \dfrac{1}{4}$

   This is enough to conclude that the correct order from least to greatest is $\dfrac{1}{4}, \dfrac{3}{8}, \dfrac{2}{5}$

MATH • LESSON 2

Evaluating Numerical Expressions

Suppose you have to fill a complicated order of medical supplies. What would be the simplest way to calculate the number of packs of gauze being shipped in several cases of different sizes? That could require both addition and multiplication. How do you handle both at once? In this lesson, you'll learn to work through combinations of basic calculations smoothly.

Common Uses in Health Care

- Making calculations with dosages
- Working with vital signs

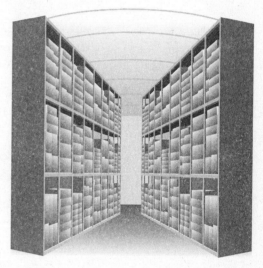

Key Terms/Formulas

- **difference** – the result of subtracting one number from another

- **evaluating** – the process of finding the value of an expression by carrying out different operations

- **expression** – a combination of numbers with symbols for operations [such as 2 + 2, 5 × (8 − 3)]

- **operations** – any calculation you use to combine two numbers

- **order of operations** – the rules for the order in which to apply the operations while evaluating an expression

- **powers** – an expression where a number is multiplied by itself a given number of times

- **product** – the result of multiplying two numbers

- **quotient** – the result of dividing one number from another

- **regrouping** – the process of rearranging numbers in an addition or subtraction problem

- **sum** – the result of adding two numbers

Learn

Order of Operations

The key to evaluating any expression is the Order of Operations. Use the made-up word *PEMDAS* to remember the order in which to perform the operations in an expression. PEMDAS stands for:

- Parentheses
- Exponents
- Multiplication and Division (from left to right)
- Addition and Subtraction (from left to right)

Be sure to memorize this term and what the letters stand for.

Let's take a look at each part of PEMDAS in more detail.

- Always deal with operations in parentheses first. For instance, if an addition operation is in parentheses, you would take care of it before you carry out multiplication:

$$3 \times (4 + 5) \times 6 = 3 \times 9 \times 6$$

- Next in the ordering is exponents. An exponent is the small number in the power. For instance, the exponent in the power 6^3 is 3. We call the big number, 6, the *base* of the power. A power is written: $(\text{base})^{(\text{exponent})}$.

A power is just shorthand for repeated multiplication. To evaluate a power, multiply the base by itself as many times as the exponent tells you to. Look at the multiplication expressions that represent the powers in the chart below.

Power	Equivalent Multiplication Expression	Value
2^3	$2 \times 2 \times 2$	$2^3 = 8$
3^4	$3 \times 3 \times 3 \times 3$	$3^4 = 81$
5^2	5×5	$5^2 = 25$

- Once you have dealt with any operations in parentheses and with exponents, you move to multiplication/division, going from left to right.
- Finally, perform addition and subtraction, going from left to right.

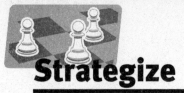

Strategize

Use PEMDAS

Remember the sentence "Please Excuse My Dear Aunt Sally." You can abbreviate that as PEMDAS, so it's a helpful device for remembering the order of operations.

To apply this as you evaluate an expression, ask these questions:

- Are there parentheses or other grouping symbols?
- Are there exponents?
- Are these numbers to multiply or divide?
- Are these numbers to add or subtract?

Always target one operation at a time. Carry out the operation and rewrite the expression with the new result.

If you carry out operations in the wrong order, there is a very good chance you will get an incorrect value. The value of $2 + 3 \times 4$ is 14 (the sum of 2 and the product of 3 and 4). If you add first, you would wind up multiplying 5 (the sum of 2 and 3) by 4, for a product of 20.

Take it Step-by-Step

To keep things orderly, write out your calculations step by step, following PEMDAS to guide you. Perform each operation one at a time, and then simplify before you move on.

$\boxed{(3+4)} \times 2 - 5^2 + 6$ Start with parentheses.

$7 \quad \times 2 - 5^2 + 6$ Simplify.

$7 \times 2 - \boxed{5^2} + 6$ Now apply the exponent.

$7 \times 2 - 25 + 6$ Simplify.

$\boxed{7 \times 2} - 25 + 6$ Next, multiply.

$14 \quad - 25 + 6$ Simplify.

$\boxed{14 - 25} + 6$ Add/subtract, starting on the left.

$-11 + 6$ Simplify.

-5 Add.

Remember, the time you take to write things out, rather than doing the math in your head, will pay off when you get the right answer!

Apply

Let's take a look at an example.

A1. What is the value of $4 + 6 \times (7 - 2)$?

STEP 1: Identify the Operations

I see that the expression has addition, multiplication, and subtraction in a set of parentheses.

STEP 2: Plan

Use PEMDAS to determine the order in which to perform the operations.

- Parentheses
- Multiplication
- Addition

STEP 3: Solve

The expression in parentheses, $7 - 2$, has a value of 5. So,

$4 + 6 \times \underline{(7 - 2)} = 4 + 6 \times \underline{5}$

The product of 6 and 5 is 30, so

$4 + \underline{6 \times 5} = 4 + \underline{30}$

And the sum of 4 and 30 is 34.

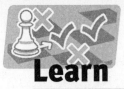

Learn

Addition and Subtraction

When adding and subtracting with numbers with several digits, you might need to regroup.

Take the sum of 56 and 23. You could add those numbers by adding the digits in the two columns:

$$\begin{array}{r} 56 \\ +23 \\ \hline 79 \end{array}$$

Always start with the right-most digits and work your way left, one column at a time, while adding vertically. Here, start by adding down the ones column: $6 + 3 = 9$. Then add down the tens column: $5 + 2 = 7$.

▶Let's take a look at another example, 56 + 48. Set the problem up vertically.

$$\begin{array}{r} 56 \\ +28 \\ \hline - \end{array}$$

Start by adding down the ones column to find the ones digit in the result: $6 + 8 = 14$. We are only allowed to record one digit per place value at a time in the result. But 14 has two digits, so it won't fit! You should *regroup* when you get a two-digit sum for a column, as we did here. The ones digit in 14 is 4; put that in the ones column of the result. The tens digit in 14 is 1; record that digit above the next column to the left, in the tens column.

$$\begin{array}{r} {}^{1}\\ 56 \\ +28 \\ \hline 4 \end{array}$$

This is called *carrying* the 1 because you are *carrying* it to the top of the next column to the left. We've taken care of the ones column. Now add down the tens column to find the tens digit in the result. Make sure you include the *carried* 1 in this sum: $1 + 5 + 2 = 8$.

$$\begin{array}{r} {}^{1}\\ 56 \\ +28 \\ \hline 84 \end{array}$$

▶Now let's talk about subtraction, starting with 67 – 25. Again, record subtraction problems vertically.

$$\begin{array}{r} 67 \\ -25 \\ \hline 42 \end{array}$$

Again, just as in adding, our rules are to start with the right-most column. Place only one digit at a time in the result. Subtract 5 from 7 in the ones column to get 2. Subtract 2 from 6 in the tens column to get 4. Putting those results together, we get $67 - 25 = 42$.

▶ **Let's take a look at another difference, 67 – 29. Take a look at the ones column.**

$$\begin{array}{r} 67 \\ -29 \\ \hline \end{array}$$

Note that 9 > 7, so we can't subtract and get a positive result. To handle this, we regroup with subtraction. You can *borrow* a *1* from the tens column and bring it over to the ones column. We use a little 1 to show that the one is borrowed.

$$\begin{array}{r} 6\,{}^{1}7 \\ -2\ 9 \\ \hline \end{array}$$

Now, to account for 1 we borrowed, we must deduct 1 from the tens column. Cross out 6, and take away 1 to write 5 in the tens column.

$$\begin{array}{r} {}^{5}\!\!\!\not{6}\,{}^{1}7 \\ -2\ 9 \\ \hline \end{array}$$

Now we are set up to subtract down each column and get one positive digit at a time in the result. Subtract 17 – 9 to get 8 in the ones column and 5 – 2 to get 3 in the tens column.

$$\begin{array}{r} {}^{5}\!\!\!\not{6}\,{}^{1}7 \\ -2\ 9 \\ \hline 3\ 8 \end{array}$$

So, 67 – 29 = 38.

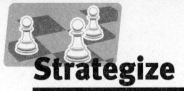

Strategize

Rearranging Numbers

Always look for opportunities to group sums into pairs that are easy to combine mentally. The most helpful rearrangements give you zeroes (through subtraction) or multiples of ten. Such numbers are easier to combine with others.

Take the expression 67 + 79 + 33. Before you start evaluating it, look to see whether any pairs of numbers might be added to get a nice round number. You might notice that 67 and 33 end with digits that add up to 10, so that might be a nice fit. Indeed, 67 and 33 have a sum of 100. When you see that, you can add more easily:

$$67 + 79 + 33 = (67 + 33) + 79$$
$$= 100 + 79$$

Sure, it requires a bit of extra thought and planning, but someone is more likely to make a mistake when adding 67 and 79, and then adding 33 to the sum.

Avoid rearranging numbers in an expression that involves a combination of different operations.

Estimating by Rounding

If the answer options on a test question aren't very close together, you might be able to get by with estimation. A common way of estimating involves rounding.

Rather than adding 92 and 59, you could round 92 down to 90 and 59 up to 60. The sum of 90 and 60 is 150, so 92 + 59 must be close to 150.

Original Sum: 92 + 59
Round: ↓   ↓
                90   60
Estimate: 150

The actual sum of 92 and 59 is 151, so we were only off by one! If you were given answer options of 141, 151, 161, and 171, you could pick 151 as the correct answer without making a precise calculation.

Apply

Let's take a look at an example.

A2. What is the value of 98 + 19 + 32 + 35 + 11?

STEP 1: Examine

I see that 98 and 32 end in digits with a sum of 10, Also, 19 and 11 end with digits with a sum of 10.

STEP 2: Plan

These numbers could be rearranged to make my work easier.

STEP 3: Solve

With this in mind, rearrange and group the numbers:

$$98 + 19 + 32 + 35 + 11 = (98 + 32) + (19 + 11) + 35$$
$$= \quad 130 \quad + \quad 30 \quad + 35$$
$$= \qquad\qquad 195$$

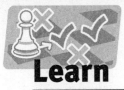

Learn

Multiplication and Division

Multiplying multi-digit numbers

When you multiply, you have to keep track of the position of numbers, and be sure to carry numbers as well.

Take the product of 52 and 38. Set it up vertically, lining up corresponding digits in columns:

$$\begin{array}{r} 52 \\ \times\, 38 \\ \hline \end{array}$$

Start with the ones column of the number on the bottom. Multiply this digit by the ones column of the top number: $8 \times 2 = 16$. We can only record one digit at a time in the result, so we must carry the 1 in 16 to the next column to the left. Record 6 as the ones digit in the result and record the small, *carried* 1 above the tens column.

$$\begin{array}{r} {}^{1}\,52 \\ \times\, 38 \\ \hline 6 \end{array}$$

Now, multiply 8 by the tens digit in 52, 5: $8 \times 5 = 40$. Remember your carried 1 here. You must add this 1 to the product: $40 + 1 = 41$. Again, record the ones digit, 1, as the next digit in your result, and carry the tens digit, 4, in the next column to the left, the hundreds column.

$$\begin{array}{r} {}^{4\,1}\,52 \\ \times\, 38 \\ \hline 16 \end{array}$$

There is no hundreds digit to multiply by in the top number, so we simply record the carried 4 in the result.

$$\begin{array}{r} {}^{4\,1}\,52 \\ \times\, 38 \\ \hline 416 \end{array}$$

We are finished multiplying 52 by the ones digit in 38, 8. Now we will multiply 52 by the tens digit in 38, 3, and record the product below what we already have. We have to show that we are really multiplying 52 by 30, since 3 is in the tens place. To do that, we multiply put a zero in the ones place of the new product.

$$\begin{array}{r} 52 \\ \times\, 38 \\ \hline 416 \\ 0 \end{array}$$

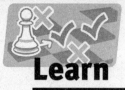

Use the same process we used before, multiplying 3 this time by each digit in 52. The product of 52 and 3 is 156. Put that on the line in front of the zero.

$$
\begin{array}{r}
52 \\
\times\,38 \\
\hline
416 \\
1560
\end{array}
$$

Finally, add the two products to get a final result.

$$
\begin{array}{r}
52 \\
\times\,38 \\
\hline
416 \\
+1560 \\
\hline
1976
\end{array}
$$

Long division

To divide multi-digit numbers, you might have to rely on long division. Take the following steps to divide 550 ÷ 25 using long division.

STEP 1:

Start by looking at the left-most digit of the number you are dividing into, 550. Does 25 go into 5? It does not, so record a 0 above the first 5 in 550.

$$
\begin{array}{r}
0 \\
25\overline{)550}
\end{array}
$$

STEP 2:

We recorded a 0 as the first digit in the result, so we can move on to the next digit to the right in 550. Does 25 go into 55? Yes, it goes twice because $2 \times 25 = 50$, which is less than 55. Record a 2 in the result above the second 5 in 55.

$$
\begin{array}{r}
02 \\
25\overline{)550}
\end{array}
$$

STEP 3:

Multiply the 2 we just recorded by 25 and record the result below 55. Subtract 50 from 55 to get 5.

$$
\begin{array}{r}
02 \\
25\overline{)550} \\
-50 \\
\hline
5
\end{array}
$$

STEP 4:

We are ready to move on to the next digit in 550, the 0. Bring the 0 down next to the difference we just found, 5.

```
      02
25 ) 550
    −50 ↓
      50
```

Does 25 go into 50? Yes, it goes twice. Record a 2 in the result above the 0 in 550.

```
      022
25 ) 550
    −50↓
      50
```

STEP 5:

Multiply the 2 we just recorded by 25 and record the result below 50. Subtract 50 from 50 to get 0.

```
      022
25 ) 550
    −50↓
      50
    −50
       0
```

Once you subtract and get a difference of zero, you're done.
Our result is 550 ÷ 25 = 22.

Rearranging

Just as with addition and subtraction, you can group with multiplication and division. Grouping a pair of numbers like 2 and 5 for multiplication might be helpful. That would give you a product of 10, which might be easy to handle.

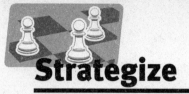

Strategize

Estimate by rounding

As with addition and subtraction, you can estimate products and quotients with rounding.

When multiplying 38 by 23, for instance, you could round those numbers to the nearest ten and find the product:

$$38 \times 23$$

$$\downarrow \times \downarrow$$

Round: 40   20

Estimate: 800

The actual product of 38 and 23 is 874.

When dividing 238 by 26, you could round in the same manner.

$$238 \div 26$$

$$\downarrow \quad \downarrow$$

Round: $240 \div 30$

Estimate: 8

Even if you need to carry out multiplication or division to get a precise result, you can still use estimation to check whether your product or quotient is reasonable. If your estimate of a product is 800, but you got 6,430 when carried out the whole calculation, you'll know to retry it.

Apply

Let's take a look at an example.

A3. What is the value of 492 ÷ 12 × 36?

STEP 1. Examine

I see that the expression involves one division operation and one multiplication operation.

STEP 2. Plan

According to PEMDAS, I should take these steps in order:

- do the division, since it appears first
- multiply the result of the division by 36

STEP 3. Solve

Use long division to divide 492 by 12:

$$
\begin{array}{r}
41 \\
12\overline{)492} \\
\underline{48} \\
12 \\
\underline{12} \\
0
\end{array}
$$

Now, multiply that quotient by 36:

$$
\begin{array}{r}
41 \\
\times\,36 \\
\hline
246 \\
\underline{1230} \\
1476
\end{array}
$$

So, 492 ÷ 12 × 36 = 1,476

Guided Practice

1. What is the value of (61 − 40) × (36 − 18)?

   A) 189

   B) 378

   C) 641

   D) 738

STEP 1: Examine

What operations are performed first?

_____

_____

STEP 2: Plan

What are the values of the expressions in parentheses?

_____

_____

STEP 3: Solve

What is the product of the values?

_____

_____

2. What is the value of $16 + 8^2 + 144 \div 16$?

A) 14

B) 29

C) 89

D) 585

STEP 1: Examine

Which operation comes first?

_____

_____

_____

STEP 2: Plan

Does addition or division come next?

_____

_____

STEP 3: Solve

What is the final value?

_____

_____

Guided Practice

3. What is the value of $8^2 + (2 + 5)^2 + 6^2 - 3^2$

A) 118

B) 125

C) 140

D) 152

STEP 1: Examine

Which operation comes first?

_____

_____

STEP 2: Plan

What is the next operation?

_____

_____

STEP 3: Solve

What is the final value?

_____

_____

Independent Practice

1. **What is the value of $56 + 36 \div (3^2 - 5)$?**

   A) 20

   B) 23

   C) 60

   D) 65

   HINT *Remember to divide before adding.*

2. **What is the value of $453 + 677 - 53 - 17$?**

   A) 1,040

   B) 1,050

   C) 1,060

   D) 1,070

   HINT *Rearranging the numbers will make this expression easier to evaluate.*

3. **What is the value of $81 + 324 \div 27 - 18 + 17 \times 12$?**

   A) 143

   B) 195

   C) 201

   D) 279

   HINT *Since there are no powers or parentheses, take care of division and multiplication first.*

ReKap

Remember these key points about evaluating expressions:

- If an expression has more than one operation, you should carry them out in a particular order:

- Perform operations inside parentheses first.

- Find the values of powers next. Powers are really just a kind of multiplication operation, where a number is multiplied by itself a given number of times.

- Perform any multiplication and division operations.

- Finally, perform any addition and subtraction operations.

Remember these key points about addition and subtraction operations:

- You can narrow down answer choices by estimating with rounding.

- Regrouping makes it possible to add and subtract more multi-digit numbers in columns.

- Rearranging numbers can make it easier to evaluate long expressions.

Remember these key points about multiplication and division operations:

- You can narrow down answer choices by estimating with rounding.

- Rearranging numbers can make it easier to evaluate long expressions.

? **What is the value of $5 + 6 \times (5^2 + 2^3)$?**

_____

_____

Answers

Guided Practice

1. Examine: multiplication and subtraction within parentheses

    Plan: (61 - 40) × (36 - 18)
           (61 - 40) = 21; (36 - 18) = 18

    Solve: 21 × 18 = 378

Answer: (B) 378

2. Examine: The first operation, according to PEMDAS, is the exponent (since no parentheses are involved here). This means we have to find the product of 8 and 8 (we "square" 8).

    Plan: Division comes next, according to PEMDAS. Addition comes last in the order of operations.

    Solve: 16 + **64** + 144 / 16 =
            16 + 64 + **9** =
            89

Answer: (C) 89

   * Trap: You might get 585 if you added before evaluating the power.

3. Examine: The addition operation in parentheses comes before anything else (remember PEMDAS)

    Plan: Exponents come next in PEMDAS. Apply the exponents, going from left to right.

    Solve: $8^2 + (2 + 5)^2 + 6^2 - 3^2 =$
            $8^2 + (7)^2 + 6^2 - 3^2 =$
            $64 + 49 + 36 - 9 =$
            140

Answer: (C) 140

Independent Practice

1. **Answer: (D) 65**

    Solve: $56 + 36 / (3^2 - 5) =$
                $56 + 36 / (9 - 5) =$
                $56 + 36 / (4) =$
                $56 + 9 =$
                65

   * Tip: Although the parentheses come before powers, here the power is within the parentheses. When there is more than one operation in parentheses, use the order of operations to simplify within the parentheses.

2. **Answer: (C) 1060**

    Solve: $452 + 677 - 53 - 17$
                1060

Answers

3. **Answer: (D) 279**

Solve: $81 + 324 / 27 - 18 + 17 \times 12$
$81 + 12 - 18 + 204$
$93 - 18 + 204$
279

ReKap Question

$5 + 6 \times (5^2 + 2^3) =$
$5 + 6 \times \mathbf{(25 + 8)} =$
$5 + 6 \times \mathbf{(33)} =$
$5 + \mathbf{198} =$
203

MATH · LESSON 3

Operations with Fractions and Decimals

Medication must be administered in precise dosages. What if you need to calculate multiple dosages? If some directions use fractions and others use decimals, how would you combine them? This lesson reviews operations with fractions and decimals, as well as conversions among them.

Common Uses in Health Care

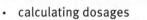

- calculating dosages
- converting prescription information
- working with vital measurements in different forms

Key Terms/Formulas

- **common denominator** – a denominator shared by a number of given fractions
- **denominator** – the lower part of a fraction
- **least common multiple (LCM)** – the smallest number that is a multiple of two given numbers
- **mixed number** – a fraction greater than one that is written as a combination of a whole number and a fraction
- **numerator** – the upper part of a fraction
- **place value** – the values expressed by a given decimal place; for instance, the first decimal place represents tenths, and the second represents hundredths
- **quotient** – the number that results from dividing one number by another
- **reciprocal** – a fraction that results from switching the numerator and denominator of a given fraction
- **simplest form** – a fraction is in simplest form when the numerator and denominator have no common factors other than 1
- **whole numbers** – a set of numbers that contains the numbers you count with and zero (0, 1, 2, 3, 4, ...)

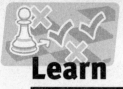

Learn

Operations with Fractions

It is easy to add or subtract fractions that have the same denominator. Just add or subtract the numerators and use the common denominator for the result.

$$\frac{3}{7} + \frac{2}{7} = \frac{3+2}{7} = \frac{5}{7}$$

If the denominators are not the same, then you must find a common denominator. To find a common denominator, find the least common multiple (LCM) of the given denominators. For each fraction, multiply the numerator by the same number you multiply the denominator by to get the new common denominator.

For example, the common denominator of $\frac{1}{3}$ and $\frac{1}{4}$ is 12 (the LCM of 3 and 4). To get 12 in the denominator of $\frac{1}{3}$, you have to multiply 3 by 4. To get 12 in the denominator of $\frac{1}{4}$, you have to multiply 4 by 3. Make sure you multiply by the same number in the top and bottom of the fraction you are writing with a new denominator.

$$\frac{1\times 4}{3\times 4} = \frac{4}{12} \qquad \frac{1\times 3}{4\times 3} = \frac{3}{12}$$

Each fraction has been written as an equivalent fraction with a denominator of 12. Now that the fractions have common denominators, you can combine them with addition or subtraction.

To multiply fractions, multiply the numerators straight across, and then multiply the denominators straight across.

$$\frac{2}{5} \times \frac{2}{3} = \frac{2\times 2}{5\times 3} = \frac{4}{15}$$

To divide fractions, multiply the first by the reciprocal of the second.

$$\frac{1}{8} \div \frac{3}{4} = \frac{1}{8} \times \frac{4}{3} = \frac{1\times 4}{8\times 3} = \frac{4}{24}$$

In an expression that involves fractions and either a whole number or a mixed number, it may be helpful to convert the other numbers to fractions. To convert a whole number to a fraction, write the whole number as the numerator and 1 as the denominator. For instance, $2 = \frac{2}{1}$.

To convert a mixed number, $2\frac{1}{4}$ for instance, to a fraction:

- Multiply the whole number part by the denominator of the fraction part: 2×4.

- Add this product to the numerator of the fraction part: $(2 \times 4) + 1$.

- Record this result as the numerator: $\frac{(2\times 4)+1}{}$.

- Keep the denominator the same as in the fraction part: $\frac{(2\times 4)+1}{4}$.

Simplify to write the fraction: $2\frac{1}{4} = \frac{(2\times 4)+1}{4} = \frac{8+1}{4} = \frac{9}{4}$.

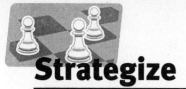

Strategize

Using Common Denominators

Consider the problem $\frac{2}{3} - \frac{1}{4}$. To subtract, you must first get a common denominator. Identify the LCM of 3 and 4. List the first few multiples of each until you find a number that appears in both lists.

Multiples of 4: 4, 8, 12, etc.

Multiples of 3: 3, 6, 9, 12, etc.

The least number in both sets of multiples is 12. Write both fractions with a denominator of 12.

To convert $\frac{2}{3}$ to a fraction with a denominator of 12, you must multiply the denominator 3 by 4 to get 12. Remember to multiply the top of the fraction by 4 as well. $\frac{2}{3} = \frac{2 \times 4}{3 \times 4} = \frac{8}{12}$

Write $\frac{1}{4}$ also as a fraction with a denominator of 12. Multiply the denominator 4 by 3. To make sure the resulting fraction is equivalent to $\frac{1}{4}$, you must multiply the numerator by the same number. $\frac{1}{4} = \frac{1 \times 3}{4 \times 3} = \frac{3}{12}$

Now you can subtract: $\frac{8}{12} - \frac{3}{12} = \frac{8 - 3}{12} = \frac{5}{12}$

Working with Mixed Numbers

To add $4\frac{5}{8}$ and $1\frac{3}{4}$, you will first need to convert these mixed numbers to fractions. Find the numerator by multiplying 4 by 8, and then adding this product to 5. Leave the denominator, 8, untouched:

$$4\frac{5}{8} = \frac{4 \times 8 + 5}{8} = \frac{32 + 5}{8} = \frac{37}{8}$$

Next, convert $1\frac{3}{4}$ to a fraction. Multiply 1 by 4 and add the product to 3 to find the numerator. Leave the denominator the same:

$$1\frac{3}{4} = \frac{4 \times 1 + 3}{4} = \frac{4 + 3}{4} = \frac{7}{4}$$

To add $\frac{37}{8}$ and $\frac{7}{4}$, get common denominators. The LCM of 8 and 4 is 8, so you only need to convert $\frac{7}{4}$.

$$\frac{7}{4} = \frac{7 \times 2}{4 \times 2} = \frac{14}{8}$$

Finally, $\frac{37}{8} + \frac{14}{8} = \frac{51}{8}$

That sum can be converted to $6\frac{3}{8}$, since 51 divided by 8 is 6, with a remainder of 3.

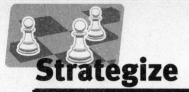

Strategize

Writing in Simplest Form

When fractions appear as answer choices on test questions, they are likely to be in simplest form, which may be different from the fraction you get after adding, subtracting, etc. To get a fraction in simplest form, find a common factor, and divide both parts by it. Keep doing this until there are no more common factors.

To simplify $\frac{4}{12}$, note that 4 is a factor of both 4 and 12. Divide both parts of the fraction by 4.

$$\frac{4}{12} = \frac{4 \div 4}{12 \div 4} = \frac{1}{3}$$

So, $\frac{4}{12}$ is $\frac{1}{3}$ in its simplest form.

Apply

A1. What is $5\frac{2}{5} - 1\frac{2}{3}$, written in simplest form?

STEP 1: Plan

To carry out this subtraction, you'll have to convert the mixed numbers to fractions, and then to fractions with common denominators. If you get an improper fraction after subtracting, you'll have to convert the resulting fraction back to a mixed number.

STEP 2: Follow Through

$5\frac{2}{5} = \frac{5 \times 5 + 2}{5} = \frac{27}{5}$ and $1\frac{2}{3} = \frac{1 \times 3 + 2}{3} = \frac{5}{3}$. Remember that you multiply the whole number by the denominator, and add the product to the numerator.

Find common denominators. The LCM of 5 and 3 is 15.

$$\frac{27}{5} = \frac{27 \times 3}{5 \times 3} = \frac{81}{15} \qquad \frac{5}{3} = \frac{5 \times 5}{3 \times 5} = \frac{25}{15}$$

Now subtract: $\frac{81}{15} - \frac{25}{15} = \frac{56}{15}$

*Tip: Identify the LCM (least common multiple) of the denominators, 5 and 3, using the following method: List the first few multiples of 5 (5, 10, 15, 20, 25, 30, . . .) and 3 (3, 6, 9, 12, 15, 18, . . .).

Circle the least number that appears in both lists, 15.

STEP 3: Solve

Now that you have subtracted, convert the improper fraction $\frac{56}{15}$ to a mixed number.

Note that 56 divided by 15 is 3 with a remainder of 11. So $\frac{56}{15} = 3\frac{11}{15}$.

The fraction part of the mixed number, $\frac{11}{15}$, is in its simplest form since there are no common multiples. Three is a factor of 9 and 15, so we can divide both parts of the fraction.

Therefore, the correct answer is $3\frac{11}{15}$.

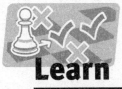

Learn

Operations with Decimals

The key to operating with decimals is keeping track of decimal places. The first decimal place is the *tenths* place, the second is the *hundredths* place, and so on. So, we read 0.5 as "five tenths," 0.05 as "five hundredths," and so on.

When you add or subtract decimals, you must be sure to line up the decimal places. When adding 0.4 to 0.25, for instance, use a vertical format with the decimal points recorded one directly above the other.

$$\begin{array}{r} \downarrow \\ 0.4 \\ -0.25 \\ \hline \end{array}$$

When you multiply decimals, you can start by ignoring the decimal places and multiply whole numbers. Then, add the numbers of decimals places of the numbers you multiplied. The sum is the number of decimal places of the product.

For instance, to multiply 0.4 by 0.75, ignore the decimal places in the first step. Multiply 4 by 75 to get 300. Count the number of digits to the right of a decimal point in the original decimals, 0.4 and 0.75. Since 0.4 has one decimal place and 0.75 has two, the product of 0.4 and 0.75 has 3 decimal places (1 + 2 = 3).

So, 0.4 × 0.75 = 0.300. You can abbreviate 0.300 as 0.3.

Division also requires careful attention to decimal places. We'll go over that below.

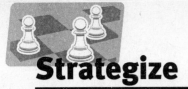

Strategize

Line Up Decimal Points

When adding or subtracting decimals, arrange the numbers so that the decimal points are lined up. To subtract 0.4 from 0.85, start with this.

$$
\begin{array}{r}
0.85 \\
-\ \ 0.4 \\
\hline
\end{array}
$$

You can always put zeroes after the last digit in a decimal, so that the decimals have the same number of places.

$$
\begin{array}{r}
0.85 \\
-\ \ 0.40 \\
\hline
\end{array}
$$

Next, bring the decimal point down.

$$
\begin{array}{r}
0.85 \\
-\ \ 0.40 \\
\hline
\end{array}
$$

Finally, you can subtract, as if you are subtracting 40 from 85.

$$
\begin{array}{r}
0.85 \\
-\ \ 0.40 \\
\hline
0.45
\end{array}
$$

Keep Track of Decimal Places

When multiplying decimals, keep track of the original decimal places. When multiplying 0.13 by 0.02, you can begin by multiplying as if you are multiplying whole numbers with the given digits (here, 13 and 2):

$$
\begin{array}{r}
13 \\
\times 2 \\
\hline
26
\end{array}
$$

The product of 0.13 and 0.02 is not 26, though; we have to account for our decimals. Identify the number of digits to the right of the decimal point in each decimal. An easy way to do this is to put your pencil at the end of the number and scoop under the digits one by one until you get to the decimal point.

$$
\underset{2\ \ 1}{0.0\ 2} \qquad \underset{2\ \ 1}{0.\ 1\ 3}
$$

There are 2 digits to the right of the decimal point in 0.13 and 2 in 0.02. So, there are 2 + 2, or 4 digits to the right of the decimal point altogether in the product, 0.0026.

$$
\underset{4\ 3\ 2\ 1}{0.\ 00\ 2\ 6}
$$

Write the product without decimals accounted for, 26, and scoop 4 spots from the last digit to locate the position of the decimal point. Use 0's to hold the places of any scoops that don't already contain a digit.

The product of 0.13 and 0.02 is 0.0026.

Use Long Division

The first steps of long division involving decimals work the same way as long division with whole numbers. You just have to account for the decimal points as a last step. For instance, to divide 5.5 by 25, you would start by positioning a decimal point:

$$25\overline{)5.50}$$

Then work around the decimal as you divide:

$$
\begin{array}{r}
0.22 \\
25\overline{)5.50} \\
\underline{50} \\
50 \\
\underline{50} \\
0
\end{array}
$$

If you are dividing by a decimal, shift the decimal point in the quotient one digit to the right for each decimal place in the number you are dividing by. To divide 5.5 by 2.5 instead of 25, you would take 0.22 and move the decimal point one digit to the right, to wind up with 2.2 (meaning that 5.5 divided by 2.5 is 2.2!).

Apply

A2. What is 0.43 + (0.36 ÷ 0.45)?

STEP 1: Plan

This question requires two operations: division and addition. Always do the operation in parentheses first (remember the PEMDAS strategy from Lesson 2). That will involve long division. You can then add the result of that division to 0.43.

STEP 2: Divide

You can't divide 3 or 36 by 45, but you can divide 360 by 45 to get 8. Add a zero to the end of 0.36 so you can divide.

$$
\begin{array}{r}
0.008 \\
45\overline{)0.360} \\
\underline{360} \\
0
\end{array}
$$

Remember that you are dividing by 0.45, not 45. This means that we need to adjust the decimal point. Since 0.45 has two decimal places, we move the decimal point in 0.008 two places to the right. The result is 0.8.

Apply

STEP 3: Add

Add 0.43 and 0.8 by lining up the decimal points. Put an extra zero in the second number so you can proceed as if you were adding two 2-digit numbers.

$$\begin{array}{r} 0.43 \\ +\quad 0.80 \\ \hline 1.23 \end{array}$$

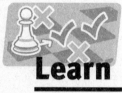

Learn

Converting Fractions and Decimals

You can work with decimal places to convert fractions to decimals.

The first decimal place is known as the tenths place. The digit there represents a number of tenths. So, 0.6 is six-tenths, or $\frac{6}{10}$.

Add a zero to the denominator to find the fraction represented by each place value to the right of a given decimal place. The decimal 0.06, for instance, is equal to the fraction $\frac{6}{100}$. The next one is the thousandths place, and so on. The decimal 0.006 is equal to the fraction $\frac{6}{1000}$, and so on.

Likewise, you can convert any fraction with 10 or a power of 10 (100, 1,000, 10,000, and so on) into a decimal in one step. The fraction $\frac{8}{10}$ is equivalent to the decimal with an 8 in the tenths place, 0.8. Here are some other conversions:

$$\frac{7}{100} = 0.07, \quad \frac{9}{1,000} = 0.009.$$

For fraction denominators that are not powers of 10, you can use division. The decimal equivalent of a fraction is the result of dividing the numerator by the denominator.

The fraction $\frac{1}{4}$ is equivalent to 0.25, since $1 \div 4 = 0.25$.

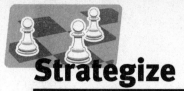

Strategize

Identify Decimal Places

Identify place value of right-most digit. Count the number of decimal places to find what denominator to use when you convert a decimal to a fraction. For instance, consider the fraction 0.0807. This decimal has four decimal places, to the ten-thousandths place. So, the equivalent fraction should have 10,000 in the denominator.

You can begin to fill in the fraction with the denominator. In this case, that would be $\dfrac{}{10,000}$.

Once you've found that denominator, you can just use the digits behind the decimal point in the numerator. For instance, the decimal 0.0807, which runs to the ten-thousandths place, is equivalent to $\dfrac{807}{10,000}$.

Use Powers of Ten

To convert a fraction to a decimal, divide the numerator by the denominator.

Since dividing by 10 or a power of 100 just involves moving the decimal place to the left, it is easy to convert fractions with such denominators.

$$\frac{3}{10} = 0.3 \qquad \frac{2}{100} = 0.02 \qquad \frac{14}{1,000} = 0.014$$

Apply

A3. **What is the mixed number equivalent of 3.213?**

STEP 1: Plan

You will need to convert the part of this number behind the decimal (0.213), to a fraction. Remember that any such decimal can be converted to a fraction with a denominator that is a power of 10.

Once you've converted, you can combine the fraction with the number in front of the decimal point, 3, to get your mixed number.

STEP 2: Follow Through

Since the decimal goes to the thousandths place, the fraction has a denominator of 1,000. Use the part of the number behind the decimal point, 213, as the numerator.

$$0.213 = \frac{213}{1,000}$$

STEP 3: Solve

Combine this fraction with the number in front of the decimal.

$$3.213 = 3 + 0.213 = 3 + \frac{213}{1,000} = 3\frac{213}{1,000}$$

Guided Practice

1. What is the sum of $1\frac{5}{8}$ and $\frac{7}{12}$?

   A) $2\frac{1}{24}$

   B) $2\frac{5}{24}$

   C) $2\frac{7}{24}$

   D) $2\frac{11}{24}$

   STEP 1

   What is the fraction equivalent of the mixed number?

   _____

   _____

   STEP 2

   What is the sum of the fractions?

   _____

   _____

   STEP 3

   What is the mixed number equivalent of the improper fraction?

   _____

   _____

2. Which decimal is equivalent to $1\frac{1}{2} \div 2\frac{2}{5}$?

   A) 0.125

   B) 0.375

   C) 0.625

   D) 0.875

   STEP 1

   What are the fraction equivalents of the mixed numbers?

   _____

   _____

STEP 2

How should you apply the rule for writing a quotient of a fraction as a product?

_____

_____

STEP 3

Which technique should you use to convert your answer to a decimal?

_____

_____

3. Which fraction is the product of 0.03 and 0.25?

A) $\dfrac{75}{100,000}$

B) $\dfrac{75}{10,000}$

C) $\dfrac{75}{1,000}$

D) $\dfrac{75}{100}$

STEP 1

What is the product of related whole numbers?

_____

_____

STEP 2

How do you rewrite this product as a decimal?

_____

_____

STEP 3

What fraction is equivalent to this decimal?

_____

_____

Independent Practice

1. What is the value of $\frac{1}{2} \times \left(\frac{7}{12} - \frac{3}{8} \right)$?

   A) $\frac{3}{12}$

   B) $\frac{5}{48}$

   C) $\frac{3}{24}$

   D) $\frac{5}{12}$

   HINT *What is a common denominator of the two fractions in the parentheses?*

2. What is the product of 0.32 and $\frac{10}{21}$?

   A) $\frac{8}{105}$

   B) $\frac{16}{105}$

   C) $\frac{32}{105}$

   D) $\frac{64}{105}$

   HINT *Look at the answer choices. Do you need to find a decimal or a fraction? You could be asked for either, but should know which way you will need to go with your calculations before starting!*

3. Which of the following results from dividing 0.2 by 0.08?

   A) $\frac{1}{4}$

   B) $\frac{9}{20}$

   C) $2\frac{1}{2}$

   D) $4\frac{1}{4}$

   HINT *What are the fraction equivalents of 0.2 and 0.08?*

ReKap

Remember these key points about adding, subtracting, multiplying, and dividing with fractions:

- You must find common denominators to add and subtract fractions.

- To multiply, you can write the product of the numerators over the product of the denominators.

- To divide by a fraction, multiply by the reciprocal of the fraction.

Remember these key points about adding, subtracting, multiplying, and dividing with decimals:

- To add and subtract decimals, use a vertical format. Make sure to line up the decimal points, one directly above the other.

- Use the rules for shifting the decimal point in the answer to multiplication and division problems with decimals.

To convert between fractions and decimals:

- Use place values (tenths, hundredths, thousandths, etc.) to convert decimals to fractions.

- Use long division to convert fractions to decimals.

? **What is $2\frac{3}{4} \div 1\frac{1}{3}$, written as a decimal?**

_____

_____

Answers

Guided Practice

1. Step 1: Convert $1\frac{5}{8}$ to a fraction:

$$1\frac{5}{8} = \frac{(1 \times 8) + 5}{8} = \frac{8 + 5}{8} = \frac{13}{8}$$

Step 2: Find a common denominator for $\frac{13}{8}$ and $\frac{7}{12}$. The LCM of 8 and 12 is 24. Once you have converted each fraction, you can add.

$$\frac{13}{8} + \frac{7}{12} = \frac{13 \times 3}{8 \times 3} + \frac{7 \times 2}{12 \times 2} = \frac{39}{24} + \frac{14}{24} = \frac{53}{24}$$

Step 3: Now convert $\frac{53}{24}$ to a mixed number. When we divide 53 by 24, we get 2 with a remainder of 5. That remainder becomes the numerator in the fraction part of the mixed number. So, $\frac{53}{24} = 2\frac{5}{24}$.

Answer: (B) $2\frac{5}{24}$

2. Step 1: $1\frac{1}{2} = \frac{(1 \times 2) + 1}{2} = \frac{2 + 1}{2} = \frac{3}{2}$

$$2\frac{2}{5} = \frac{(2 \times 5) + 2}{2} = \frac{10 + 2}{5} = \frac{12}{5}$$

Step 2: To divide $\frac{3}{2}$ by $\frac{12}{5}$, multiply $\frac{3}{2}$ by the reciprocal of $\frac{12}{5}, \frac{5}{12}$:

The product $\frac{15}{24}$ can be reduced to $\frac{5}{8}$ by dividing the numerator and denominator each by the same number, 3.

$$\frac{15}{24} = \frac{15 \div 3}{24 \div 3} = \frac{5}{8}$$

Step 3: To convert $\frac{5}{8}$ to a decimal, divide the numerator by the denominator.

$$\frac{5}{8} = 5 \div 8 = 0.625$$

Answer: (C) 0.625

3. Step 1: Putting aside the decimals, we get 75 as the product of 3 and 25.

Step 2: Since 0.03 and 0.25 have two decimal places each, we add two and two to get four places in the product. The 5 in 75 has the fourth place (the ten-thousandths place) and the 7 has the third place (the thousandths place). So, the product is 0.0075.

Step 3: The decimal 0.0075 is seven thousands and five ten-thousandths, for a total of 75 ten-thousandths.

Answer: (B) $\frac{75}{10,000}$

Independent Practice

1. **Answer: (B)** $\dfrac{5}{48}$

    Use PEMDAS to determine how to approach this problem. There is an operation in parentheses and multiplication in this expression. Start by finding the difference in parentheses. The LCM of 12 and 8 is 24, and the fractions inside the parentheses are equivalent to $\dfrac{14}{24}$ and $\dfrac{9}{24}$, respectively.

    The difference between them is $\dfrac{5}{24}$. Now multiply: $\dfrac{1}{24} \times \dfrac{5}{24} = \dfrac{1 \times 5}{2 \times 24} = \dfrac{5}{48}$

2. **Answer: (B)** $\dfrac{16}{105}$

    The decimal goes to the hundredths place with a digit in the tenths place as well. So, the digit 3 represents $\dfrac{1}{10}$ or $\dfrac{30}{100}$ and the digit 2 represents $\dfrac{2}{100}$

    $$\dfrac{30}{100} + \dfrac{2}{100} = \dfrac{32}{100}$$

    Multiply $\dfrac{32}{100}$ by $\dfrac{10}{21}$ by multiplying the numerators and denominators: $\dfrac{32}{100} \times \dfrac{10}{21} = \dfrac{320}{2100}$

    Simplify this fraction by dividing both parts by a common factor: 20

    $$\dfrac{320}{2100} = \dfrac{320 / 20}{2,100 / 20} = \dfrac{16}{105}$$

3. **Answer: (C)** $2\dfrac{1}{2}$

    Since 0.2 is greater than 0.08, the result of dividing should be greater than 1. Remember that any fraction where the numerator is greater than the denominator is greater than 1.

    Divide, being mindful of the decimal points:

    $$
    \begin{array}{r}
    2.5 \\
    0.08\overline{)0.20} \\
    16 \\
    \hline
    40 \\
    40 \\
    \hline
    0
    \end{array}
    $$

    The decimal 0.5 is equivalent to $\dfrac{5}{10}$, which you can simplify to $\dfrac{1}{2}$. So, 2.5 is $2\dfrac{1}{2}$, the sum of 2 and $\dfrac{1}{2}$

Answers

ReKap

- Convert the fractions to mixed numbers:

$$2\frac{3}{4} = \frac{(2\times4)+3}{4} = \frac{8+3}{4} = \frac{11}{4}$$

$$1\frac{1}{3} = \frac{(1\times3)+1}{3} = \frac{4+1}{3} = \frac{4}{3}$$

- Divide by multiplying $\frac{11}{4}$ by the reciprocal of $\frac{4}{3}$:

$$\frac{11}{4} \div \frac{4}{3} = \frac{11}{4} \times \frac{3}{4} = \frac{33}{16}$$

- Divide 33 by 16 to convert this number to a decimal. The result is 2.0625.

MATH · LESSON 4
Ratios and Proportions

You may already know that high density lipoprotein (HDL) is the *good* cholesterol and low density lipoprotein (LDL) is the *bad* cholesterol. A patient's HDL, LDL, and total cholesterol levels are important to help guide healthcare and lifestyle choices. However, the patient's ratio of total cholesterol to good cholesterol is also important. In fact, ratios play an important role in a number of health care applications.

Common Uses in Health Care

- calculating cholesterol ratio
- determining medication dosages
- reporting quantities of substances present in blood

Key Terms/Formulas

- **cross-multiply** – multiply the numerator of one ratio in a proportion by the denominator of the other ratio

- **proportion** – a mathematical statement equating two ratios

- **rate** – a comparison of two quantities with different units

- **ratio** – a comparison of two quantities

- **unit rate** – the number of units of the first quantity in a rate that correspond to one unit of the second quantity

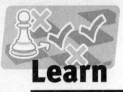

A ratio is a comparison of two quantities. It can compare a part to a part, a part to a whole, or a whole to a part. For example, if a patient has an HDL level of 40 mg/dL and an LDL level of 100 mg/dL, the ratio of HDL to LDL is 40 to 100, and the ratio of HDL to total cholesterol is 40 to 140.

A ratio can be written with the word *to*, with a colon, or as a fraction. The two numbers in a ratio are called the *terms*.

40 to 100   40:100 $\dfrac{40}{100}$

A ratio can be simplified much like a fraction. To simplify a ratio, divide each term by the greatest common factor of the terms. For instance, the ratio on the left below is simplified by dividing each term by 20 to get the ratio on the right.

40:100 = 2:5

A rate is a special ratio in which the numerator and denominator have different units. A unit rate tells the number of units of the first quantity that correspond to one unit of the second quantity. In the example above, the HDL level of 40 mg/dL is a unit rate of 40 mg of HDL per 1 dL of blood.

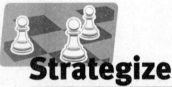

Strategize

Identify Parts and Wholes

The first step in approaching a ratio problem is to identify the quantities that you must compare. A ratio problem may ask you to compare a part to a part or a part to a whole, so determine which type of ratio you are asked for.

Once you have identified the quantities that you will compare, go back and read the question again to determine whether those quantities are provided. If you are asked to compare a part to a whole, but are provided with two parts, you will need to add the parts together to find the whole. On the other hand, if you are asked to compare a part to a part, but are provided with one part and the whole, you will need to subtract the given part from the whole to find the other part.

Ask Yourself

1. What quantities do I need to compare?

2. What quantities am I given?

Find the Unit Rate

A unit rate problem will typically ask you to find the number of units of one quantity *per* one unit of a second quantity.

To find a unit rate, divide the first quantity by the number of units of the second quantity.

Ask Yourself

Which unit should the rate be in terms of?

Apply

A1. There are 35 staff members at a meeting. Fifteen of the staff members are nurses. The rest of the staff members are doctors. What is the ratio of doctors to nurses?

Identify Parts and Wholes

The *whole* is the number of staff members, 35.

One *part* is the number of nurses, 15.

The other *part* is the number of doctors, 35 – 15 = 20.

Part: Nurses	Part: Doctors
Whole: Staff Members	

The ratio of doctors to nurses is 20:15.

- Make sure you are writing the ratio that is asked for.

- Write the numbers in the order in which the ratio was described

A2. If it takes Hannah 36 minutes to run 4 miles, how long does it take her to run 1 mile?

Find the Unit Rate

It takes Hannah 36 minutes per 4 miles.

Find the number of minutes that correspond to 1 mile.

Divide each quantity by the number of units of the second quantity, 4 miles.

$$\frac{36 \text{ minutes}}{4 \text{ miles}} = \frac{36 \div 4}{4 \div 4} = \frac{9 \text{ minutes}}{1 \text{ mile}}$$

- Be sure to write the unit rate in terms of the correct unit.

- The unit rate can be the answer, or a strategy for finding the answer.

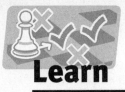
A proportion is a statement that two ratios are equal. In a proportion, the ratios are generally written as fractions.

$$\frac{2}{4} = \frac{4}{8}$$

In a proportion, the numerators describe the same quantities and the denominators describe the same quantities. In other words, the units in the numerators on either side of the equal sign match and the units in the denominators on either side of the equal sign match. For example, the proportion below describes salt solutions. Each numerator represents a mass of salt, and each denominator represents a volume of water.

$$\frac{12 \text{ mg}}{2 \text{ dL}} = \frac{18 \text{ mg}}{3 \text{ dL}}$$

If you know one of the ratios in a proportion and either the numerator or the denominator of the other ratio, you can solve for the unknown quantity.

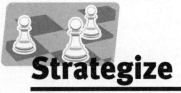

Strategize

Set Up a Proportion with a Variable

Since a proportion states that two ratios are equivalent, you can use the relationships among the known quantities to determine an unknown quantity. Write the proportion using a variable for the unknown quantity.

For example, given that the ratio of green apples to red apples in a display case is 2:3 and there are 15 red apples, you can set up a proportion to find the number of green apples.

Let g be the number of green apples.

Write the ratio of green apples to red apples in the display: $\dfrac{\text{green}}{\text{red}} = \dfrac{g}{15}$

Write a proportion: $\dfrac{2}{3} = \dfrac{g}{15}$

Ask Yourself

1. Does the problem give a ratio of two quantities and ask a question related to one of the quantities?

2. What quantity is unknown?

Cross-Multiply to Solve a Proportion

You can use cross-products to solve a proportion. A cross-product is equal to the numerator times the denominator on opposite sides of the equal sign. For instance, the cross-products in the proportion below are 1×4 and 2×2. You can draw an X over the equal signs in a proportion to identify cross-products.

$$\frac{1}{2} \times \frac{2}{4}$$

 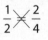

There is a special relationship among the quantities in a proportion: the cross-products are equal.

Look at the proportion below.

$$\frac{1}{2} = \frac{2}{4}$$

Multiply the numerator of the first ratio by the denominator of the second ratio to get the first cross-product: $1 \times 4 = 4$

Multiply the denominator of the first ratio by the numerator of the first ratio to get the second cross-product: $2 \times 2 = 4$

The cross-products of any proportion are equal. Therefore, if you have a proportion with a variable, you can use the cross-products of a proportion to write and solve an equation to find the value of the variable:

$$\frac{2}{3} = \frac{g}{15}$$

$2 \times 15 = 3g$ Set the cross-products equal.

$30 = 3g$ Simplify.

$\dfrac{30}{3} = \dfrac{3g}{3}$ Divide by 3 on both sides.

$10 = g$ Simplify.

Use a Unit Rate

You can also use unit rates to solve a problem with proportions. Given a rate, find the unit rate, and then multiply by the number of units of the second quantity to find the number of units of the first quantity. You can use the information provided in a problem to determine if you can use a unit rate to solve it.

Ask Yourself

1. Does the problem involve a pair of units that are compared to each other?

2. Does the problem ask for the number of units of one quantity that correspond to a given number of units of a second quantity?

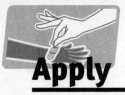

Apply

A3. Solve the proportion.

$$\frac{x}{15} = \frac{16}{20}$$

Cross-Multiply

$20 \times x = 15 \times 16$ Multiply each numerator by the denominator of the other ratio.

$20x = 240$ Simplify.

$\dfrac{20x}{20} = \dfrac{240}{20}$ Divide each side by the x-coefficient, 20.

$x = 12$ Simplify.

- Be careful to multiply the correct quantities. Do not multiply the numerators together and the denominators together.

A4. Marcus paid \$3.75 to make 25 photo prints. How much will 40 photo prints cost?

Set Up a Proportion with a Variable

Let c represent the cost of 40 prints.

Write a proportion with the numbers of prints in the same position and the costs in the same position.

$$\frac{3.75}{25} = \frac{c}{40}$$

Cross-Multiply

$$\frac{3.75}{25} = \frac{c}{40}$$

$25 \times c = 3.75 \times 40$

$25c = 150$

$c = 6$

Forty prints will cost \$6.00.

- Set up the proportion with the same units in the numerators and the same units in the denominators.

- Cross-multiply numerators by denominators.

Guided Practice

Let's work through a few examples together. Look back at the lesson content as often as necessary to help you apply the concepts and strategies you learn.

---

1. There are 24 half-inch nails and 18 one-inch nails in a toolbox. What is the simplified ratio of the number of half-inch nails to the total number of nails in the toolbox?

A) 3:4

B) 4:3

C) 3:7

D) 4:7

STEP 1

What are the parts and the wholes?

_____

_____

STEP 2

What is the unsimplified ratio?

_____

_____

STEP 3

What is the simplified ratio?

_____

Guided Practice

2. The ratio of men to women on a committee is 2:3. There are 12 women on the committee. How many men are on the committee?

   A)   8

   B)   11

   C)   18

   D)   20

STEP 1

What are the parts and wholes?

_____

_____

_____

STEP 2

What proportion represents the relationship?

_____

_____

STEP 3

What is the number of men?

_____

_____

3. Suppose you can complete 12 math problems in 16 minutes. How many problems will you be able to complete in 40 minutes?

   A) 20

   B) 24

   C) 30

   D) 45

STEP 1

How do you know this problem involves a proportion?

_____

STEP 2

How can you use a proportion to solve for the number of problems?

_____

_____

STEP 3

How can you use a unit rate to check the answer?

_____

_____

Independent Practice

You are ready to show what you know! Answer the questions below without looking back at the lesson content. Use the Hints to help you.

1. There are 12 cats and 21 dogs at a shelter. Write the ratio of cats to dogs in simplest terms.

   A) 4:7

   B) 7:4

   C) 4:11

   D) 12:21

   HINT ▷ *Write the ratio using the numbers given in the problem. Then divide the terms by the greatest common factor to simplify the ratio.*

2. Casey walked 6 miles and ran 9 miles. What is the ratio of the number of miles Casey walked to the total number of miles he traveled?

   A) 2:3

   B) 2:5

   C) 3:5

   D) 5:2

   HINT ▷ *Read the question carefully. What quantities should the ratio compare?*

3. Find the value of x.
   $$\frac{5}{x} = \frac{30}{15}$$

   A) 2.5

   B) 4

   C) .5

   D) 0

   HINT ▷ *Remember to cross-multiply.*

4. The ratio of blue pens to black pens in a variety pack is 3:4. There are 12 black pens. How many blue pens are there?

A) 8

B) 9

C) 11

D) 16

HINT *Set up a proportion using a variable. What color pen goes in the numerator?*

5. A serving of 12 crackers has 132 calories. Brent ate 16 crackers. How many calories did he consume?

A) 84

B) 148

C) 176

D) 192

HINT *You can use a proportion or a unit rate to solve this problem.*

ReKap

Remember that a ratio is a comparison of two quantities. It can be written in one of three ways:

4:3   4 to 3 $\dfrac{4}{3}$

A proportion is a statement that two ratios are equal. For instance, $\dfrac{4}{3} = \dfrac{8}{6}$.

If two ratios are equal, you can use a proportion to find an unknown quantity. Use a variable to represent the unknown quantity and cross-multiply.

A rate compares two quantities with different units. Examples of rates are: 64 miles in 4 hours; $5.00 for 2 pounds.

A unit rate tells the number of units of the first quantity that correspond to the second quantity. For instance, if 64 miles are traveled in 4 hours, the unit rate is 64 ÷ 4, or 16 miles per hour.

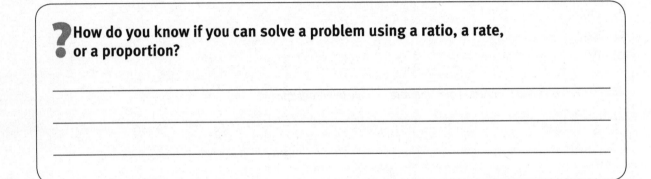

? **How do you know if you can solve a problem using a ratio, a rate, or a proportion?**

_____

_____

_____

Answers

Guided Practice

1. Step 1: The parts are the number of half-inch nails (24) and the number of one-inch nails (18).

   The whole is the total number of nails: 24 + 18 = 42

   Step 2: half-inch nails : total nails (24:42)

   Step 3: 24:42 = 4:7.

   * You divide each term in the ratio by the greatest common factor (GCF) of the terms to simplify the ratio.

Answer: (D) 4:7

2. Step 1: The first part is the number of men.

   The second part is the number of women.

   men:women = 2:3

   Step 2: Let m be the number of men

   $$\frac{2}{3} = \frac{m}{12}$$

   Step 3: $\dfrac{2}{3} = \dfrac{m}{12}$

   $3 \times m = 2 \times 12$

   $3m = 24$

   $$\frac{3m}{3} = \frac{24}{3}$$

   $m = 8$

Answer: (A) 8

3. Step 1: It provides a rate and asks for an unknown quantity related to that rate.

   Step 2: $\dfrac{12}{16} = \dfrac{p}{40}$

   $16 \times p = 12 \times 40$

   $16p = 480$

   $$\frac{16p}{16} = \frac{480}{16}$$

   $p = 30$

   Step 3: If you solve 12 problems in 16 minutes, you solve $\dfrac{12}{16} = 0.75$ problems per minute.

   $40 \text{ minutes} \times \dfrac{0.75 \text{ problems}}{1 \text{ minute}} = 30 \text{ problems}$

Answer: (C) 30

Answers

1. **Answer: (A) 4:7**

    The problem asks for the ratio of cats to dogs. Both of those quantities are provided in the problem.

    The ratio of cats to dogs is 12:21.

    The factors of 12 are 1, 2, 3, 4, 6, and 12.

    The factors of 21 are 1, 3, 7, and 21.

    The greatest common factor of 12 and 21 is 3. Divide each number by 3.

    The ratio of cats to dogs is 4:7.

2. **Answer: (B) 2:5**

    Identify the parts and wholes.

    The problem asks for the ratio of number of miles walked (part) to the total number of miles (whole).

    The whole is not provided, so add the number of miles walked to the number of miles run to find the total number of miles: $6 + 9 = 15$

    The ratio of number of miles walked to total number of miles is 6:15.

    To simplify the ratio, divide each number by the greatest common factor of 6 and 15, which is 3. So, the simplified ratio is 2:5.

3. **Answer (A) 2.5**

    The cross-products of a proportion are equal. Multiply numerator by opposite denominator to find the cross-products: $30 \times x = 5 \times 15$, or $5 \times 15 = 30 \times x$.

    Solve the equation for x:

    $30x = 75$

    $$\frac{30x}{30} = \frac{75}{30}$$

    $x = 2.5$

4. **Answer: (B) 9**

    Pay close attention to the information in the problem. In the ratio, the number of blue pens is the first number, but the number of black pens (the second number in the ratio) is provided. Set up a proportion. Let b represent the number of blue pens.

    $$\frac{3}{4} = \frac{b}{12}$$

    Cross-multiply and solve for b.

    $4 \times b = 3 \times 12$

    $4b = 36$

    $$\frac{4b}{4} = \frac{36}{9}$$

    $b = 9$

5. Answer: (C) 176

The two quantities compared are crackers and calories. The units are different, which makes this a rate. You can use a proportion to solve this problem or you can use the unit rate.

To use a proportion, choose a variable and then set up the proportion. Let c be the number of calories. Check that the numerators and the denominators have the same units.

$$\frac{12 \text{ crackers}}{132 \text{ calories}} = \frac{16 \text{ crackers}}{c \text{ calories}}$$

Cross multiply and solve for c

$$\frac{12}{132} = \frac{16}{c}$$

$$12 \times c = 132 \times 16$$

$$12c = 2112$$

$$\frac{12c}{12} = \frac{2112}{12}$$

$$c = 176$$

ReKap

For example, if a problem compares two quantities or asks you to compare two quantities, you can probably use a rate, a ratio, or a proportion to solve it.

MATH · LESSON 5
Applications of Percents

Consider two patients who each lost 20 pounds by following their doctors' advice to exercise more and make healthier eating choices. Although their absolute weight losses were equal, their relative weight losses might differ, depending on their starting weights. In many medical situations, it is important to consider not only the absolute change, but also the percent change.

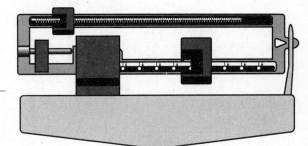

Common Uses in Health Care

- calculating correct dosages of medicines

- determining quantities of substances in the bloodstream

- computing a relative (percent) change in a patient's weight

Key Terms/Formulas

- **percent change equation** –

  % change = $\dfrac{\text{amount of change}}{\text{original amount}} \times 100$, where amount of change = |original – final|

- **percent decrease** – percent change from the initial quantity to the final quantity, where the final quantity is less than the initial quantity

- **percent equation** – percent · whole = part

- **percent increase** – percent change from the initial quantity to the final quantity, where the final quantity is greater than the initial quantity

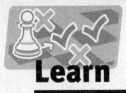

A percent is a part of 100. For example, 40% is 40 parts out of 100. You can also think of a percent as a part-to-whole ratio in which 100 is the whole.

The percent equation relates the percent, the whole, and the part:

$$\text{percent} \cdot \text{whole} = \text{part}$$

You can use the percent equation to solve a variety of problems:

- Given a whole and a percent, you can find a percent of a number

- Given a part and a percent, you can find the whole

- Given a part and a whole, you can find the percent

You can relate a percent to a fraction by translating the symbol % or the phrase *percent* as a fraction over 100.

- The percent 20% is equivalent to the fraction $\frac{20}{100}$, which simplifies to $\frac{1}{5}$.

- The phrase 3 *percent* refers to the fraction $\frac{3}{100}$.

You can relate a percent to a decimal by moving the decimal point in the percent 2 places to the left.

- The percent 15%, which is the same as 15.0%, is equivalent to the decimal 0.15.
  15% = 0.1 5
        ‿‿
        2 1

- The percent 2%, which is the same as 2.0%, is equivalent to the decimal 0.02.
  2% = 0.0 2
       ‿‿
       2 1

To convert a decimal to a percent, move the decimal point in the decimal 2 places in the opposite direction, to the right.

- The decimal 0.56 is equivalent to the percent 56%.
  0. 5 6 = 56%
     ‿ ‿
     1 2

- The decimal 1.8 is equivalent to the percent 180%.
  1. 8 0 = 180%
     ‿ ‿
     1 2

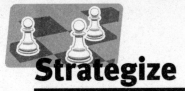
Strategize

Write Percents as Decimals to Make Calculations

To perform calculations with percents, first write the percent as a decimal. Remember to move the decimal point two places to the left.

$$32\% = 0.32$$

$$8\% = 0.08$$

$$175\% = 1.75$$

Some percent problems ask for a percent as the answer. If your computations result in a decimal, move the decimal point two places to the right to write the decimal as a percent.

$$0.65 = 65\%$$

$$0.032 = 3.2\%$$

$$2.9 = 290\%$$

Notice that percents greater than 100% correspond to decimals greater than 1, and percents less than 1% correspond to decimals less than 0.1. By thinking about the relative sizes of the decimals and percents in the problem, you can provide a check for whether you have converted quantities correctly.

Use the Percent Equation

For a problem dealing with percents, identify the *whole*, the *part*, and the *percent*, and then substitute the quantities into the percent equation.

$$\text{percent} \cdot \text{whole} = \text{part}$$

Use a variable for the unknown quantity.

For example, percent problems commonly ask about interest and tips. The table below demonstrates how the percent equation can be set up to solve different types of problems involving interest and tips.

	Interest	Tips
	rate · principle = interest	**percent tip · bill = tip amount**
Unknown Whole	Given the interest rate and the amount of interest earned, find the principle, x. rate $\cdot$ x = interest	Given the percent tip and the amount of the tip, find the amount of the restaurant bill, x. percent $\cdot$ x = tip
Unknown Part	Given the interest rate and the principle, find the interest earned, x. rate $\cdot$ principle = x	Given the percent tip and the amount of the restaurant bill, find the amount of the tip x. percent $\cdot$ amount of bill = x
Unknown Percent	Given the amount of interest earned and the principle, find the interest rate, x. x $\cdot$ principle = interest	Given the amount of the tip and the amount of the restaurant bill, find the percent tip x. x $\cdot$ amount of bill = tip

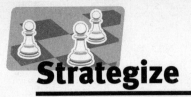

Strategize

Translate from Words to Equations

Some percent problems are purely mathematical and do not involve real-world situations. While you can use the percent equation to solve these problems, in some cases it is easier to translate the problem directly into its own equation.

For example, what percent of 40 is 12?

What is an unknown quantity that can be represented with a variable.

Percent tells you that the unknown quantity is a percent.

Of means to multiply.

Is means equals.

So, "What percent of 40 is 12" can be written as $x \cdot 40 = 12$, where x is a percent.

Apply

A1. Juan deposited $500 in a savings account. One year later, he had earned $9 in interest. What interest rate did the savings account pay?

Identify the whole, part, and percent.

- The principle (whole) is $500.

- The interest (part) is $9.

- The interest rate (percent) is unknown.

Use the percent equation.

percent · whole = part

interest rate · principle = interest

Use a variable for the missing piece of the equation.

The problem tells you to find the interest rate (percent). Let x be the interest rate. Substitute the whole, part, and percent into an equation you can solve for x.

$$x \cdot 500 = 9$$

$$\frac{500x}{500} = \frac{9}{500}$$

$$x = 0.018$$

Write the decimal as a percent: $0.018 \cdot 100 = 1.8\%$.

The savings account paid 1.8% interest.

To summarize our approach:

- Determine whether the whole, the part, or the percent is unknown and identify the known quantities.

- Substitute the values into the percent equation.

- Write the decimal as a percent.

A2. Caroline took her parents out to dinner to celebrate their wedding anniversary. Before tax, the restaurant bill came to $72.80. Caroline wants to leave a 15% tip. How much should Caroline leave as a tip?

Identify the whole, part, and percent.

- The restaurant bill (whole) is $72.80.

- The percent tip is 15% (percent).

- The tip amount (part) is unknown.

Write percents as decimals before calculating.

$15\% = 0.15$

Use the percent equation.

percent · whole = part

percent tip · restaurant bill = tip amount

Use a variable for the missing piece of the equation.

The problem tells you to find the tip amount (part). Let x be the tip amount. Substitute the whole, part, and percent into an equation you can solve for x.

$0.15 \cdot 72.80 = x$

$\qquad 10.92 = x$

Caroline should leave a tip of $10.92.

To summarize our approach:

- Determine whether the whole, the part, or the percent is unknown and identify the known quantities.

- Write the percent as a decimal.

- Substitute the values into the percent equation.

- Round to the nearest cent, if necessary.

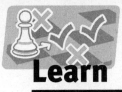

Learn

Percent problems commonly ask for the percent of change. These types of problems will typically ask you to find the percent increase or percent decrease in a quantity. For example, you may be asked to find the percent increase in population over an interval of time, or the percent decrease in price of an item on sale.

Percent change is the ratio of the change to the original amount.

$$\% \text{ change} = \frac{\text{amount of change}}{\text{original amount}} \times 100$$

For a percent increase, the original amount is less than the final amount.

For a percent decrease, the original amount is greater than the final amount.

ASK YOURSELF

Am I looking for a percent increase or a percent decrease?

What is the original amount?

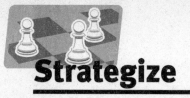

Strategize

Organize

Read the question carefully to determine whether the question is asking for a percent increase or a percent decrease. Identify the original amount and the amount of change.

If the problem does not provide the amount of change, it will likely provide the original amount and the final amount. Subtract to find the amount of change:

amount of change = final amount − original amount

If the amount of change is positive, it is a percent increase. If it is negative, it is a percent decrease.

ASK YOURSELF

What is the direction of change? Is it an increase or a decrease?

Is the amount of change provided, or do I need to compute it?

Use the Percent Change Equation

Once you have identified the amount of change and the original amount, substitute those values into the percent change equation:

$$\% \text{ change} = \frac{\text{amount of change}}{\text{original amount}} \times 100$$

Apply

A3. Natalie bought a painting for $450. Ten years later, the value of the painting had increased by $54. What was the percent increase in the value of the painting?

> **Organize.**
>
> The original value was $450.
>
> The amount of change was $54.
>
> **Use the percent change equation.**
>
> $$\% \text{ change} = \frac{\text{amount of change}}{\text{original amount}} \times 100$$
>
> $$= \frac{54}{450} \times 100 \qquad \text{Substitute.}$$
>
> $$= \frac{54 \times 100}{450}$$
>
> $$= \frac{540\cancel{0}}{45\cancel{0}} \qquad \text{Cancel 0's.}$$
>
> $$= \frac{540}{45}$$
>
> $$= 12 \qquad \text{Use long division to find } 540 \div 45.$$

The value of the painting increased by 12%.

To summarize our approach:

- Identify the amount of change.

- Identify the original amount.

- Substitute the values into the percent change equation.

Apply

A4. Bryce and Isobel bought a house for $225,000. Five years later, they sold the house for $215,000. What was the percent change in the value of the house?

Organize.

The original value was $225,000.

The final value was $215,000.

The final value was less than the original value, so the change was a decrease.

Subtract to find the change in the value of the house: $215,000 - 225,000 = -10,000$.

Use the percent change equation.

$$\% \text{ change} = \frac{\text{amount of change}}{\text{original amount}} \times 100$$

$$= \frac{10,000}{225,000} \times 100 \qquad \text{Substitute.}$$

$$= \frac{10,000 \times 100}{225,000}$$

$$= \frac{1,000,000}{225,000} \qquad \text{Cancel 0's.}$$

$$\approx 4.4 \qquad \text{Use long division to divide } 1000 \div 225.$$

The value of the home decreased by 4.4%.

Remember

The amount of change was negative because the value decreased. You do not need to use the negative sign in your further computations.]

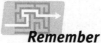

Remember

Unless otherwise directed, round the answer to the nearest tenth of a percent

Guided Practice

Let's work through a few examples together. Look back at the lesson content as often as necessary to help you apply the concepts and strategies you learned.

---

1. What is 20% of 56?

    A) 2.8

    B) 7.6

    C) 11.2

    D) 35.7

STEP 1

What are the whole, the part, and the percent?

_____

_____

STEP 2

What is the percent equation for this problem?

_____

_____

STEP 3

What is 20% of 56?

_____

_____

Guided Practice

2. Joanna bought a sweater for $23.27, including 6% sales tax. What was the price of the sweater before tax?

A) $13.96

B) $21.95

C) $23.45

D) $24.72

STEP 1

What is the whole? Is it less than or greater than the part?

_____

_____

STEP 2

How can you find the percent?

_____

_____

STEP 3

What is the percent equation for this problem?

_____

_____

3. Jamal was driving at a rate of 55 miles per hour. As he approached a curve in the road, his speed was 48 miles per hour. What was the percent change in Jamal's speed?

A) 12.7% decrease

B) 12.7% increase

C) 14.6% decrease

D) 14.6% increase

STEP 1

Did Jamal's speed increase or decrease?

_____

_____

STEP 2

What was the amount of change?

_____

_____

STEP 3

What was the percent of change?

_____

_____

Independent Practice

You are ready to show what you know! Answer the questions below without looking back at the lesson content. Use the Hints to help you.

---

1. **40 is 32% of what number?**

   A) 12.8

   B) 24.6

   C) 80

   D) 125

   HINT *Translate the question into an equation.*

2. **Alexa had lunch at a restaurant with her friends. The bill came to $74.80. Since they formed a large party, they decided to leave an 18% tip. How much did Alexa and her friends leave as a tip?**

   A) $4.16

   B) $13.46

   C) $17.24

   D) $24.06

   HINT *The restaurant bill is the whole. The tip is the part.*

3. **Marcus bought a certificate of deposit (CD) that paid 2.8% interest over one year. At the end of the year, his investment was worth $257. How much did Marcus invest?**

   A) $200

   B) $245

   C) $250

   D) $265

   HINT *The initial investment is the whole. Is the percent greater or less than 100%?*

4. Last year, 85 people attended a lecture series. This year, 98 people attended the same lecture series. By what percent did the number of attendees increase?

A) 15.3%

B) 13.3%

C) 9.2%

D) 8.7%

HINT *You will need to find the amount of change before you can determine the percent change.*

5. The population of Smithville in 2000 was 22,071. In 2010, the population was 21,446. What was the percent decrease in the population of Smithville from 2000 to 2010?

A) 0.28%

B) 0.29%

C) 2.8%

D) 2.9%

HINT *Be careful when changing the decimal to a percent.*

ReKap

Remember that a percent is a part of 100. You can also think of a percent as a part-to-whole ratio in which 100 is the whole.

The percent equation relates the percent, the whole, and the part:

$$\text{percent} \cdot \text{whole} = \text{part}$$

You can use the percent equation to solve a variety of problems:

- Given a whole and a percent, you can find a percent of a number
- Given a part and a percent, you can find the whole
- Given a part and a whole, you can find the percent

If you are asked to find the percent of increase or decrease in a quantity, you can use the percent change equation:

$$\% \text{ change} = \frac{\text{amount of change}}{\text{original amount}} \times 100$$

- For a percent increase, the original amount is less than the final amount.
- For a percent decrease, the original amount is greater than the final amount.

? **How can you determine whether you should use the percent equation or the percent change equation?**

_____

_____

Answers

Guided Practice

1. Step 1: The whole is 56, the percent is 20%, and the part is unknown.

    Step 2: $0.20 \times 56 = x$

    Step 3: $0.20 \times 56 = 11.2$

Answer: (C) 11.2

2. Step 1: The whole is the original price, and it is less than the part.

    Step 2: The original price of the sweater is 100% of the price. The amount of the tax is 6%. So, the price with tax is 106% of the price of the sweater.

    Step 3: $1.06 \times x = 23.27$

Answer: (B) $21.95

3. Step 1: Jamal's speed decreases

    Step 2: $55 - 48 = 7$ miles per hour

    Step 3: $\% \text{ change} = \dfrac{\text{amount of change}}{\text{original amount}} \times 100$

    $$= \dfrac{7}{55} \times 100$$

    $$= \dfrac{700}{55}$$

    $$\sim 12.7$$

Answer: (A) 12.7% decrease

Independent Practice

1. **Answer: (D) 125**

    The whole is unknown. The part is 40. The percent is 32%, or 0.32.
    The question translates to $40 = 0.32 \times x$.
    Dividing each side of the equation by 0.32 gives $x = 125$.
    Check the answer by finding 32% of 125. The answer should be 40.

2. **Answer: (B) $13.46**

    Write 18% as a decimal: 0.18.
    Substitute $74.80 for the whole, 0.18 for the percent, and x for the part, which is the tip.
    $0.18 \times 74.80 = x$
    $x = 13.46$
    They left a tip of $13.46.
    Is the answer reasonable? The bill was about $70. The tip was about 20%. Find 20% of 70 to check: $0.20 \times 70 = 14$.

3. **Answer: (C) $250**

    The whole is the initial investment. The part is $257. Since the value of the investment at the end of the year is equal to the initial investment plus the interest, the value of the investment at the end of the year is

Answers

100% + 2.8%, or 102.8%, of the original investment. So, the percent is 102.8%, or 1.028.
c. Set up the percent equation: $1.028 \times x = \$257$.
Divide each side of the equation by 1.028 to get $x = \$250$.

4. **Answer: (A) 15.3%**

The original number is 85. The final number is 98.
Subtract to find the amount of change: $98 - 85 = 13$.
Use the percent change equation:

$$\% \, \text{change} = \frac{\text{amount of change}}{\text{original amount}} \times 100$$

$$= \frac{13}{85} \times 100$$

$$= \frac{1300}{85}$$

$$\sim 15.3$$

5. **Answer: (C) 2.8%**

The original population is 22,071. The final population is 21,446.
Subtract to find the amount of change: $21,446 - 22,071 = -625$.
Use the percent change equation:

$$\% \, \text{change} = \frac{\text{amount of change}}{\text{original amount}} \times 100$$

$$= \frac{625}{21,466} \times 100$$

$$= \frac{62,300}{21,466}$$

$$\sim 2.8$$

ReKap

The percent equation is used to find the percent, the whole, or the part of a given number. The percent change equation is used when one is asked to find the percent of increase or decrease in a quantity.

MATH · LESSON 6
Measurement Conversions

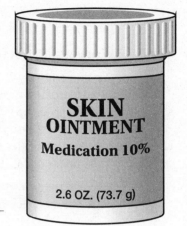

Suppose you are asked to administer 0.01 grams of medication to a patient, but your scale measures weight in milligrams. How would you know when you have measured the right amount?

Common Uses in Health Care

- converting from customary units to metric
- converting measurements in prescriptions

Key Terms/Formulas

- **conversion rate** – an equation that compares a measurement into two different units

- **conversion ratio** – an expression that presents a conversion rate in the form of a fraction; you can multiply a measurement by a conversion ratio to convert it into a measurement with a different unit

- **customary system** – the measurement system used mainly in the United States, which uses units such as feet, miles, pounds, and gallons

- **dimensional analysis** – a process used to guide the steps of converting from one unit to another

- **metric system** – a measurement system used in most parts of the world (and by scientists in the United States), based on the decimal system; it uses units such as centimeters, kilograms, and liters

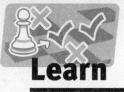

Conversions

The three kinds of measurements you will need to work with are length, weight, and volume. Volume may be less familiar to you than length (how long something is) and weight (how heavy something is). Volume is a measurement of how much space an object takes up. Volume is often used as a measure of an amount of liquid. When you buy a gallon of milk or a liter bottle of water, you are buying a measured volume.

Conversion Rates in Customary Measurement System

You are probably very familiar with the customary system of measurement. It is the system used to make everyday measurements in the U.S. Several examples of customary units are: inches, miles, cups, gallons, pounds, tons. The table below shows the conversion rates for some common customary units. You will be given conversion rates between customary units in the wording of the questions on the test, but you should familiarize yourself with the rates ahead of time in order to prepare yourself for the types of calculations you will use on test day.

Customary Measurement System		
Selected conversion rates		
Weight	**Volume**	**Length**
1 pound (lb) = 16 ounces (oz) 1 ton (T) = 2,000 pounds (lb)	1 cup (c) = 8 fluid ounces (fl oz) 1 pint (pt) = 2 cups (c) 1 quart (qt) = 2 pints (pt) 1 gallon (g) = 4 quarts (qt)	1 foot (ft) = 12 inches (in.) 1 yard (yd) = 3 feet (ft) 1 mile (mi) = 5,280 feet (ft)

Conversion Rates in Metric Measurement System

Many Americans rarely use the metric system, but scientists, nurses, and doctors use it all the time. The basic units in the metric system are gram (for weight), liter (for volume), and meter (for length). These units are often abbreviated. Gram has the abbreviation *g*, liter has the abbreviation *L*, and meter has the abbreviation *m*.

Converting within the metric system is easier than the customary system because metric unit conversions always involve powers of ten (10, 100, 1000, etc.). You will not be given the conversion rates within the wording of the question in order to make conversions within the metric system, so you should memorize the meanings of these prefixes before test day.

Common Metric System Prefixes		
Selected conversion rates		
Prefix	**Meaning**	**Example**
Kilo (k)	Thousand	1 **kilo**meter = 1,000 meters
Hecto (h)	Hundred	1 **hecto**gram = 100 grams
Deka (da)	Ten	1 **deka**liter = 10 liters
Deci (d)	One tenth	1 **deci**gram = $\frac{1}{10}$ gram = 0.1 gram
Centi (c)	One hundredth	1 **centi**meter = $\frac{1}{100}$ meter = 0.1 meter
Milli (m)	One thousandth	1 **milli**liter = $\frac{1}{1,000}$ liter = 0.001 liter

Units based off of grams, liters, and meters are abbreviated by combining the abbreviations of prefixes (shown in parentheses in the first column of the table above) with the basic abbreviations. So, milligram can be abbreviated as *mg*, kiloliter as *kL*, and centimeter as *cm*.

The table below shows the conversion rates for some common metric units. You can use the prefix table to find any other conversion rate in the metric system.

Metric System		
Selected conversion rates		
Weight	**Volume**	**Length**
1 gram = 100 centigrams 1 kilogram = 1,000 grams	1 liter = 1,000 milliliters 1 kiloliter = 1,000 liters	1 meter = 1,000 millimeters 1 hectometer = 100 meters

Conversion Rates Between Systems

Sometimes, you may have to convert between units in the two different systems. The table below shows the most common conversion rates you would use. You will be given the relevant rates in the wording of the questions on the test, so you do not have to memorize them. However, you should familiarize yourself with the rates before test day.

Conversions Between Systems		
Selected conversion rates		
Weight	**Volume**	**Length**
1 kilogram ≈ 2.2 pounds 1 ounce ≈ 28 grams	1 liter ≈ 1.06 quarts 1 fluid ounce ≈ 30 milliliters 1 teaspoon ≈ 5 milliliters 1 gallon ≈ 3.785 liters	1 inch ≈ 2.54 centimeters 1 meter ≈ 39.37 inches 1 mile ≈ 1,609 meters 1 meter ≈ 1.094 yards

Converting

To convert from one unit to another you must multiply the given measurement by the appropriate conversion ratio. A conversion ratio is a ratio of two equivalent measurements. The result will be an equivalent measurement with a different unit.

Use dimensional analysis to set up the math to make a conversion. For instance, say you must convert a measurement given in gallons to an equivalent measurement in liters. Let's look only at the units in play for this type of problem, leaving aside numbers. To convert, you would multiply the original unit, gallons, by a conversion ratio that relates gallons and liters. The original unit, gallons, should be in the denominator of the conversion ratio:

$$\text{gallons} \times \frac{\text{liters}}{\text{gallons}}$$

Simplify this expression in the same way that you would simplify if the factors were numbers instead of units. The expression fits the same pattern as the product of a whole number and a fraction. Just as you would multiply the whole number by the numerator of the fraction, multiply gallons by liters in the top of the fraction.

$$\text{gallons} \times \frac{\text{liters}}{\text{gallons}} = \frac{\text{gallons} \times \text{liters}}{\text{gallons}}$$

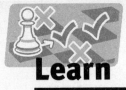

To simplify that result, you would *cancel* the common factor, gallons, from the numerator and denominator:

$$\text{gallons} \times \frac{\text{liters}}{\text{gallons}} = \frac{\text{gallons} \times \text{liters}}{\text{gallons}} = \frac{\cancel{\text{gallons}} \times \text{liters}}{\cancel{\text{gallons}}} = \text{liters}$$

The product has the units you want to convert to, liters.

To solve a test problem, you will have to work also with numbers attached to units. To do so, you will use conversion ratios. For example, to convert 5 centimeters to inches you would work with the ratio $\frac{1 \text{ inch}}{2.54 \text{ cm}}$. If you look on the chart, you find that that 1 inch is equal to 2.54 cm. So, multiplying by $\frac{1 \text{ inch}}{2.54 \text{ cm}}$ is the same as multiplying by a form of 1.

Multiply the original measurement, 5 centimeters, by the conversion ratio to convert from centimeters (cm) to inches (in).

When you multiply by a conversion ratio, you can cancel units common to the numerator and denominator, in the same way that you would cancel numbers that are common to the numerator and denominator in a fraction. Take a look below for an example.

$5 \,\text{cm} = 5 \text{ cm} \times \dfrac{1 \text{ in.}}{2.54 \text{ cm}}$ Multiply by the conversion ratio.

$= \dfrac{5 \cancel{\text{ cm}} \times 1 \text{ in.}}{2.54 \cancel{\text{ cm}}}$ Cancel the common unit, cm.

$= \dfrac{5 \times 1}{2.54} \text{ in.}$ Write the remaining factors with the remaining units, inches.

$\approx 1.97 \text{ in.}$ Calculate.

This shows that 5 centimeters is approximately equal to 1.97 inches.

We'll talk more about this conversion process, and how to identify the appropriate conversion ratio, in the Strategize section below.

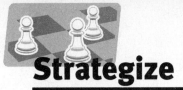

Strategize

Use Dimensional Analysis to Convert

To convert from one unit to another, you should use *dimensional analysis*. The following are the four steps you should use to convert a measurement from one unit to another using dimensional analysis:

Step 1: Use the units given in the problem to identify the appropriate conversion ratio.

Step 2: Multiply the original measurement by the conversion ratio, written as a fraction.

Step 3: Cancel common units.

Step 4: Record the result with the unit that did not cancel and simplify the numerical expression to find the answer.

Use the saying *U M*ust *C*onvert *S*uccessfully, or *UMCS* to remember this process:

U—Use the **Units** in the problem to identify the correct conversion ratio.

M—**Multiply** the given measurement by the conversion ratio.

C—**Cancel** the common units.

S—**Simplify** to find the answer.

Let's take a look at these steps in action by converting 6 kilograms (kg) to pounds (lb).

Conversion ratio: $\dfrac{2.2 \text{ lb}}{1 \text{ kg}}$ **Step 1: U**se units to identify conversion ratio.

$6 \text{ kg} = 6 \text{ kg} \times \dfrac{2.2 \text{ lb}}{1 \text{ kg}}$ **Step 2: M**ultiply by conversion ratio.

$= \dfrac{6 \ \cancel{\text{kg}} \times 2.2 \text{ lb}}{1 \ \cancel{\text{kg}}}$ **Step 3: C**ancel common units.

$= \dfrac{6 \times 2.2 \text{ lb}}{1}$ **Step 4: S**impliy.

$= 13.2 \text{ lb}$

Look back at the steps as you read more about each below.

More on Step 1:

The conversion rate for pounds to kilograms is 1 kilogram ≈ 2.2 pounds. How do you know to interpret the corresponding conversion ratio as $\dfrac{2.2 \text{ lb}}{1 \text{ kg}}$ and not $\dfrac{1 \text{ kg}}{2.2 \text{ lb}}$?

Well, the denominator of the appropriate conversion ratio must have the same unit as the measurement you are converting *from*. This is so that the common units will cancel, leaving you with the unit you set out to convert to. Because our original measurement is in kilograms, we use the conversion ratio with kilograms on the bottom: $\dfrac{2.2 \text{ lb}}{1 \text{ kg}}$.

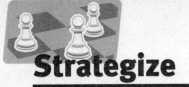

More on Step 2:

Once you have identified the appropriate conversion ratio, multiply the original measurement by it: $6 \text{ kg} \times \dfrac{2.2 \text{ lb}}{1 \text{ kg}}$.

Perform the multiplication in the same way that you would multiply a non-fractional number by a fraction. For instance, look at $8 \times \dfrac{2}{3} = \dfrac{8 \times 2}{3}$. Just as the non-fractional number gets multiplied into the numerator of the fraction in this example, 6 kg gets multiplied into the numerator in Step 2 of the conversion: $6 \text{ kg} \times \dfrac{2.2 \text{ lb}}{1 \text{ kg}} = \dfrac{6 \text{ kg} \times 2.2 \text{ lb}}{1 \text{ kg}}$.

More on Step 3

Remember that we selected a conversion ratio so that we could cancel kilograms on the top with kilograms on the bottom. Since the unit *kg* appears in both the numerator and denominator, it cancels: $\dfrac{6 \text{ kg} \times 2.2 \text{ lb}}{1 \text{ kg}} = \dfrac{6 \cancel{\text{ kg}} \times 2.2 \text{ lb}}{1 \cancel{\text{ kg}}}$.

More on Step 4:

Note that pounds is the only unit not crossed out after cancelling common units; that is the unit to attach to your result. Record the unit and simplify the numerical expression to finish up:

$$\frac{6 \cancel{\text{ kg}} \times 2.2 \text{ lb}}{1 \cancel{\text{ kg}}} = \frac{6 \times 2.2 \text{ lb}}{1} = \left(\frac{6 \times 2.2}{1}\right) \text{lb} = 13.2 \text{ lb}$$

Use Multiple Conversion Ratios

You might encounter a conversion problem that does not give a conversion rate from the given unit to the unit you have to reach. Instead, you might have to work with two different rates at once.

Suppose you are asked to convert a length in meters to a length in inches. You might not have the conversion rate to go directly from meters to inches, but if you know that 1 meter = 100 centimeters and 1 inch ≈ 2.54 centimeters, you can convert in two steps. Go from meters to centimeters to inches.

- Use 1 meter = 100 centimeters to go from meters to centimeters. Write the conversion ratio so that the original unit, meters, will cancel with the unit in the denominator of the conversion ratio: $\dfrac{100 \text{ cm}}{1 \text{ m}}$. Take away the numbers to think about what will happen with the units when you multiply meters by this conversion factor: $\text{m} \times \dfrac{\text{cm}}{\text{m}} = \dfrac{\cancel{\text{m}} \times \text{cm}}{\cancel{\text{m}}} = \text{cm}$. The result will be in centimeters.

- Now use 1 inch ≈ 2.54 centimeters to go from centimeters to inches. Your original unit is now centimeters. Write the conversion ratio with centimeters in the denominator: $\dfrac{1 \text{ in.}}{2.54 \text{ cm}}$. Again, take away the numbers to think about what will happen with the units when you multiply centimeters by this conversion factor: $\text{cm} \times \dfrac{\text{in.}}{\text{cm}} = \dfrac{\cancel{\text{cm}} \times \text{in.}}{\cancel{\text{cm}}} = \text{in.}$. The result will be in inches, which is what we want.

Let's apply the UMCS steps with two conversion ratios in play this time in order to convert 4 meters (m) to inches (in.).

Conversion ratios: $\dfrac{100 \text{ cm}}{1 \text{ m}}$ and $\dfrac{1 \text{ in.}}{2.54 \text{ cm}}$ Step 1: **U**se units to identify conversion ratios.

$$4 \text{ m} = 4 \text{ m} \times \frac{100 \text{ cm}}{1 \text{ m}} \times \frac{1 \text{ in.}}{2.54 \text{ cm}}$$ Step 2: **M**ultiply by conversion ratios.

$$= \frac{4 \text{ m} \times 100 \text{ cm} \times 1 \text{ in.}}{1 \text{ m} \times 2.54 \text{ cm}}$$ Step 3: **C**ancel common units.

$$= \frac{4 \times 100 \times 1 \text{ in.}}{1 \times 2.54}$$ Step 4: **S**impliy.

$$\approx 157 \text{ in.}$$

So, 4 meters is equivalent to approximately 157 inches.

Apply

Let's take a look at a couple of examples.

A1. What is the volume of a 15-gallon fuel tank in liters?

Remember: **U M**ust **C**onvert **S**uccessfully. Identify **Units** and then **Multiply** by the conversion ratio. Then **Cancel** units and **Simplify**.

Step 1: Use the Units

Use the units given in the problem to identify the appropriate conversion ratio. This is a volume conversion from gallons to liters. The conversion tables indicate that 1 gallon (gal) ≈ 3.785 liters (L).

The original unit is gallons. Write the conversion ratio with gallons in the bottom, so the unit *gallons* will cancel: $\dfrac{3.785 \text{ L}}{1 \text{ gal}}$.

Step 2: Multiply

Multiply the original measurement, in gallons, by the conversion ratio:

$$15 \text{ gal} \times \frac{3.785 \text{ L}}{1 \text{ gal}} \ .$$

Step 3: Cancel the Common Units

Next, cancel the unit gallons and record the remaining factors and unit.

$$15 \text{ gal} \times \frac{3.785 \text{ L}}{1 \text{ gal}} = \frac{15 \text{ gal} \times 3.785 \text{ L}}{1 \text{ gal}} = \frac{15 \text{ gal} \times 3.785 \text{ L}}{1 \text{ gal}} = \frac{15 \times 3.785 \text{ L}}{1}$$

Step 4: Simplify

Simplify the numerical expression and attach the remaining unit, L, to the result.

$$\frac{15 \times 3.785\,\text{L}}{1} = \left(\frac{15 \times 3.785}{1}\right)\text{L} = 56.775\,\text{L}$$

So, 15 gallons is equal to approximately 56.775 liters.

A2. **What is the length of a 24-centimeter rod in meters?**

Step 1: Use the Units

This is a length conversion from centimeters to meters.

Based on the conversion tables, you will apply the rate 1 meter (m) ≈ 100 centimeters (cm).

This means that the centimeter unit will have to be in the denominator of the ratio:

$$\frac{1\,\text{m}}{100\,\text{cm}}$$

Step 2: Multiply

Multiply the given measurement by that the appropriate conversion ratio:

$$24\,\text{cm} \times \frac{1\,\text{m}}{100\,\text{cm}}$$

Step 3: Cancel the Common Units

Next, cancel the centimeter units:

$$24\,\text{cm} \times \frac{1\,\text{m}}{100\,\text{cm}} = \frac{24\,\text{cm} \times 1\,\text{m}}{100\,\text{cm}} = \frac{24\,\cancel{\text{cm}} \times 1\,\text{m}}{100\,\cancel{\text{cm}}} = \frac{24 \times 1\,\text{m}}{100}$$

Step 4: Simplify

Simplify the numerical expression and attach the remaining unit, m, to the result.

$$\frac{24 \times 1\,\text{m}}{100} = \left(\frac{24 \times 1}{100}\,\text{m}\right) = 0.24\,\text{m}$$

So, 24 centimeters is equal to 0.24 m.

Guided Practice

1. **What is the length of a 12.6 foot piece of rope in yards? (Note: 1 yard = 3 feet.)**

   A) 4.2

   B) 6.3

   C) 25.2

   D) 37.8

   STEP 1: What conversion rate applies?

   _____

   _____

   STEP 2: What ratio should be used, and what unit should be in the denominator of that ratio?

   _____

   _____

   STEP 3: What is the converted length?

   _____

   _____

Guided Practice

2. Which distance is closest to 2.1 miles? (Note: 1 kilometer ≈ 1,000 meters and 1 mile ≈ 1,609 meters.)

  A) 476 km

  B) 766 km

  C) 1,302 m

  D) 3,379 m

STEP 1: What conversion rates apply?

_____

_____

STEP 2: How do the rates apply?

_____

_____

STEP 3: What are the converted lengths?

_____

_____

3. **What is the approximate volume of 15 fluid ounces of liquid in liters? (1 fluid ounce ≈ 30 milliliters and 1 liter = 1,000 milliliters.)**

   A) 0.045

   B) 0.05

   C) 0.45

   D) 0.5

   STEP 1: How do I set up the conversion?

   _____

   _____

   _____

   STEP 2: What conversion ratios apply?

   _____

   _____

   STEP 3: What is the converted volume?

   _____

   _____

Independent Practice

1. What is the approximate volume of 6 gallons of water in liters? (Note: 1 gallon ≈ 3.785 liters.)

   A) 1.5

   B) 4.5

   C) 11.25

   D) 22.71

   HINT *Use a conversion ratio that cancels out the gallons unit.*

2. Which distance is equivalent to 500 millimeters? (Note: 1,000 meters = 1 kilometer, 1 meter = 1,000 millimeters, 1 meter = 10 decimeters, 1 meter = 100 centimeters.)

   A) 5 meters

   B) 5 kilometers

   C) 5 decimeters

   D) 5 centimeters

   HINT *Find the unit that is equivalent to 100 millimeters.*

3. Approximately how many ounces are there in 3.3 kilograms? (Note: 1 kilogram ≈ 2.2 pounds and 1 pound = 16 ounces.)

   A) 24

   B) 53

   C) 116

   D) 158

   HINT *Set up two separate conversion ratios.*

ReKap

Remember these key points about converting measurements:

- Always work with unit rates.

- When working with a unit rate, multiply to convert from a larger unit to a smaller one.

- When working with a unit rate, divide to convert from a smaller unit to larger one.

- Conversions between customary and metric units are always approximate.

? **What is the equivalent of 0.1 liters in teaspoons?**

_____

_____

Answers

Guided Practice

1. Step 1: Since the conversion is from feet to yards, use the rate 1 yard = 3 feet.

   Step 2: Since the original measurement is given in feet, that unit should go in the denominator of the ratio. So, multiply $\dfrac{1\,\text{yard}}{3\,\text{feet}}$

   Step 3: 4.2 yards

   Answer: (A) 4.2

2. Step 1: Since 1 mile ≈ 1,609 meters and 1 kilometer ≈ 1,000 meters, you can work with the rates
   $$\frac{1,609\,\text{meters}}{1\,\text{mile}} \quad \text{and} \quad \frac{1\,\text{kilometer}}{1,000\,\text{miles}}$$

   Step 2: You can use the first ratio to convert from miles to meters. If you need to go further, you could use the second ratio to convert from meters to kilometers.

   Step 3: 3,378.9 meters and 3.3789 kilometers.
   Apply the *Multiply, Cancel, and Simplify* steps:

   $$2.1\,\cancel{\text{miles}} \times \frac{1,609\,\text{meters}}{1\,\cancel{\text{mile}}} = 3,378.9\,\text{meters}$$

   You can use that converted measurement to find the distance in kilometers.

   $$3,378.9\,\cancel{\text{meters}} \times \frac{1\,\text{kilometer}}{1,000\,\cancel{\text{meters}}} = 3.3789\,\text{kilometers}$$

   Answer: (D) 3,379 m

3. Step 1: Since the conversion tables given in this lesson do not give a direction conversion rate between fluid ounces and liters, you have to combine two conversion ratios with multiplication, and convert in two steps.

   TIP: U—Use the Units in the problem to identify the correct conversion ratio.

   Step 2: Since 1 fluid ounce ≈ 30 milliliters and 1 liter = 1,000 milliliters, use the ratios
   $$\frac{30\,\text{milliliters}}{1\,\text{fluid ounce}} \quad \text{and} \quad \frac{1\,\text{liter}}{1,000\,\text{milliliters}}$$

   The units fluid ounces and milliliters will cancel out, leaving the liter unit in the final result of multiplication.

   Step 3: 0.45 liters
   Carry out the remaining three steps:
   M—Multiply the given measurement by the conversion ratio.
   C—Cancel the common units.
   S—Simplify to find the answer.

   $$15\,\cancel{\text{fluid ounces}} \times \frac{30\,\cancel{\text{milliliters}}}{1\,\cancel{\text{fluid ounces}}} \times \frac{1\,\text{liter}}{1,000\,\cancel{\text{milliliters}}} = 0.45\,\text{liters}$$

   Answer: (C) 0.45

Independent Practice

1. Answer: (D) 22.71

Since 1 gallon ≈ 3.785 liters, multiply 6 gallons by the conversion ratio.

$$6 \text{ gallons} \times \frac{3.785 \text{ liters}}{1 \text{ gallon}} = 22.71 \text{ liters}$$

2. Answer: (C) 5 decimeters

Because each answer option involves a different unit, you might apply different conversions to rule out answer options in a process of elimination. If you get the units in meters first, you can easily convert to the other units in the answer choices.

Since 1 meter = 1,000 millimeters,

$$500 \text{ millimeters} \times \frac{1 \text{ meter}}{1000 \text{ millimeters}} = 0.5 \text{ meters}.$$

This rules out choice A.

Since 1 kilometer = 1,000 meters,

$$500 \text{ millimeters} \times \frac{1 \text{ meter}}{1000 \text{ millimeters}} \times \frac{1 \text{ kilometer}}{1000 \text{ millimeters}} = 0.0005 \text{ kilometers}$$

That rules out choice B.

Since 1 meter = 10 decimeters,

$$500 \text{ millimeters} \times \frac{1 \text{ meter}}{1000 \text{ millimeters}} \times \frac{10 \text{ decimeter}}{1 \text{ meter}} = 5 \text{ decimeters}$$

Choice C is correct.

3. Answer: (C) 116

Since 1 kilogram ≈ 2.2 pounds and 1 pound = 16 ounces, you can set up conversion ratios so units will cancel out.

$$3.5 \text{ kilograms} \times \frac{2.2 \text{ pounds}}{1 \text{ kilogram}} \times \frac{16 \text{ ounces}}{1 \text{ pound}} = 116.16 \text{ ounces}$$

The product of 3.3 and 2.2 is 7.26.

The product of 7.26 and 16 is 116.16.

So 7.26 is about 116.16 ounces, which is close to 116 ounces.

ReKap

1 liter = 1,000 milliliters, and 1 teaspoon = 5 milliliters.

Combine the ratios $\frac{1,000 \text{ milliliters}}{1 \text{ liter}}$ and $\frac{1 \text{ teaspoon}}{5 \text{ milliliters}}$

$$0.1 \text{ liters} \times \frac{1,000 \text{ milliliters}}{1 \text{ liter}} \times \frac{1 \text{ teaspoon}}{5 \text{ milliliters}} = 20 \text{ teaspoons}$$

So 100 milliliters is about 20 teaspoons.

3 MATH · LESSON 7
Operations with Polynomials

Imagine you take an oral dose of medication. As the medication dissolves in the gastrointestinal tract and is released into the bloodstream, the level of the drug in the blood slowly increases until it reaches a peak. Then, as the drug is metabolized by the body, the level of the drug decreases. If you were to graph the level of drug over time, the curve would resemble an upside-down U. This shape curve is typical of a quadratic relationship, which can be modeled with a polynomial.

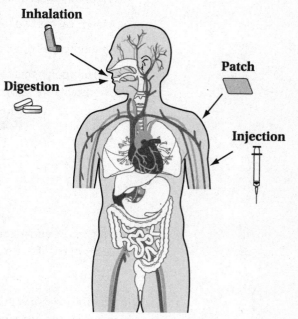

Common Uses in Health Care

- modeling levels of substances in the blood over time

Key Terms/Formulas

- **binomial** – a polynomial with two terms

- **coefficient** – a number that is multiplied by a variable

- **constant** – a quantity that is not a variable

- **exponent** – the number that shows how many times a base is multiplied by itself in a power, shown as a superscript

- **like terms** – terms that have the same variable raised to the same power

- **monomial** – a polynomial with one term

- **polynomial** – a mathematical expression made up of terms that are variables, constants, or the product of variables and constants

- **term** – a variable, constant, or product of variables and constants

- **variable** – a quantity that changes, usually represented by a letter like *x* or *y*

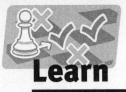
A polynomial is a mathematical expression that is a sum of terms. The terms can be numbers (constants), variables, or the products of constants and variables. When a constant is multiplied by a variable, the constant is called the coefficient of the variable.

For example, look at the polynomial below.

$$4x + 3$$

The polynomial is the sum of two terms, $4x$ and 3.

- The first term is the product of a constant, 4, and a variable x. So, the coefficient of the variable x is 4.

- The second term is the constant 3.

A polynomial can be named according to the number of terms it has.

- A monomial has one term, for example, $5p$ or y.

- A binomial has two terms, for example, $3n - 6$.

- A trinomial has three terms, for example, $x^2 + 2x + 7$.

The terms of a polynomial are called *like* terms if they have the same variable raised to the same power. Constants are also considered like terms.

Like Terms	Not Like Terms
$4x$ and $8x$	$4x$ and $4y$
$\dfrac{x}{2}$ and $\dfrac{x}{3}$	$\dfrac{x}{2}$ and $\dfrac{y}{2}$
x^2 and $-x^2$	x and x^2
25 and 0.8	x and xy

Like terms can be added together to simplify a polynomial. To add the like terms, add the coefficients of the like terms and keep the variable part the same.

$$6y^2 + 2y^2 = (6 + 2)y^2 = 8y^2$$

Remember, a variable with no coefficient can be written with a coefficient of 1. For instance, x is written as 1x in the equation below.

$$5x + x = 5x + 1x = (5 + 1)x = 6x$$

Before you combine like terms, make sure you convert all subtraction signs in the polynomial into addition signs. Then follow the rules for adding signed integers to combine coefficients.

$$-3x^2 - 8x^2 = -3x^2 + (-8x^2) = (-3 + (-8))x^2 = -11x^2$$

$$6y - 9y = 6y + (-9y) = (6 + (-9))y = -3y$$

When multiplying or dividing polynomials, you may need to multiply or divide variable terms.

When you multiply terms with the same variable, add the exponents together. Remember, a variable with no exponent can be written with an exponent of 1.

$$(x^2)(x) = (x^2)(x^1) = x^{2+1} = x^3$$

When you divide terms with the same variable, subtract the exponent of the divisor from the exponent of the dividend. In fraction form, subtract the exponent of the denominator from the exponent of the numerator.

Division sign form: $m^3 \div m^2 = m^{3-2} = m^1 = m$

Fraction form: $\dfrac{y^5}{y^2} = y^{5-2} = y^3$

If the variables have coefficients, multiply or divide the coefficients, and multiply or divide the variables.

$$(2x^2)(4x^3) = (2 \cdot 4)(x^2 \cdot x^3) = 8x^{2+3} = 8x^5$$

$$\frac{15y^3}{3y} = \frac{15}{3} \cdot \frac{y^3}{y^1} = 5y^{3-1} = 5y^2$$

You will need to apply the rules of integer multiplication in order to multiply or divide positive and negative constants or coefficients.

- If two integers have the same sign, the product or quotient is positive: $(-5)(-2x) = 10x$.

- If two integers have different signs, the product or quotient is negative: $\dfrac{12x}{-3} = -4x$.

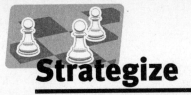

Strategize

Group Like Terms

When you add or subtract polynomials, you will need to combine like terms to find the simplified answer. When you combine like terms, you add or subtract the coefficients of terms that have the same variable raised to the same power.

You can rearrange the terms of a polynomial without changing its value, and your calculations will be easier if like terms are next to each other.

For example, add $(3x^2 - x + 5) + (2x^2 + 4x - 7)$

$(3x^2 - x + 5) + (2x^2 + 4x - 7)$	Copy the original expression.
$(3x^2 + (-x) + 5) + (2x^2 + 4x + (-7))$	Rewrite subtraction as addition.
$3x^2 + (-x) + 5 + 2x^2 + 4x + (-7)$	Remove the parentheses.
$3x^2 + 2x^2 + (-x) + 4x + 5 + (-7)$	Group like terms.
$(3 + 2)x^2 + (-1 + 4)x + (5 + (-7))$	Rewrite to add coefficients.
$5x^2 + 3x - 2$	Combine like terms.

Multiplying or dividing polynomials may also result in a product or quotient polynomial that has like terms. Rewrite the product or quotient polynomial to group like terms, and then add or subtract the coefficients of like terms.

Distribute the Factor

When you multiply a polynomial by a monomial, you need to multiply each term in the polynomial by the monomial. Make sure you follow the rules for multiplying coefficients with the same signs and with opposite signs, and remember to add the exponents when you multiply terms with the same variable.

For example, multiply $2x(x^2 + 4x - 6)$.

$2x(x^2 + 4x - 6)$	Copy the original expression.
$2x(x^2 + 4x + (-6))$	Rewrite subtraction as addition.
$2x(x^2) + 2x(4x) + 2x(-6)$	Distribute the factor.
$2(x \cdot x^2) + (2 \cdot 4)(x \cdot x) + (2 \cdot -6)x$	Multiply coefficients and variables.
$2x^{1+2} + 8x^{1+1} + (-12)x$	Add exponents to multiply variables.
$2x^3 + 8x^2 - 12x$	Simplify.

Use FOIL

When you multiply a binomial by a binomial, you must multiply each term in the first polynomial by each term in the second polynomial. That is four products! Follow these steps to make sure you find all four products correctly:

1. Multiply the first terms in each polynomial.

2. Multiply the outside terms in each polynomial.

3. Multiply the inside terms in each polynomial.

4. Multiply the last terms in each polynomial.

Use the mnemonic FOIL to help you remember: **F**irst, **O**utside, **I**nside, **L**ast.

For example, multiply $(5x + 1)(2x - 3)$

$(5x)(2x)$	$+$	$(5x)(-3)$	$+$	$(1)(2x)$	$+$	$(1)(-3)$
Product of the First Terms		Product of the Outside Terms		Product of the Inside Terms		Product of the Last Terms

$(5x + 1)(2x - 3)$	Copy the original expression.
$(5x)(2x) + (5x)(-3) + (1)(2x) + (1)(-3)$	Use FOIL.
$10x^2 - 15x + 2x - 3$	Multiply.
$10x^2 - 13x - 3$	Combine like terms.

Break Apart the Numerator

When you divide a polynomial by a monomial, divide each term in the polynomial by the monomial. Then, in each part, divide the coefficients and the variables. Remember, to divide variables, subtract the exponents.

For example, divide $(12x^3 + 8x^2 - 4x) \div 2x$

$\dfrac{12x^3 + 8x^2 - 4x}{2x}$	Write the problem as a fraction.
$\dfrac{12x^3}{2x} + \dfrac{8x^2}{2x} + \dfrac{-4x}{2x}$	Break apart the numerator.
$\dfrac{12}{2}x^{3-1} + \dfrac{8}{2}x^{2-1} + \dfrac{-4}{2}x^{1-1}$	Divide coefficients and variables.
$6x^2 + 4x - 2$	Simplify.

Apply

A1. Subtract.

$$(3x^2 - 5x + 2) - (7x^2 + 9)$$

Step 1: Write Subtraction as Addition of the Opposite

$$(3x^2 - 5x + 2) - (7x^2 + 9) = (3x^2 + (-5x) + 2) + (-1)(7x^2 + 9)$$

Step 2: Distribute the Factor

Multiply each term in the second polynomial by -1.

$$(3x^2 + (-5x) + 2) + (-1)(7x^2 + 9)$$

$$= (3x^2 + (-5x) + 2) + (-1)(7x^2) + (-1)(9)$$

$$= (3x^2 + (-5x) + 2) + (-7x^2) + (-9)$$

Step 3: Group and Combine Like Terms

Rewrite the polynomial so that like terms are next to each other. Remember that it does not matter what order you add in, so the parentheses around the first three terms can be removed.

$$(3x^2 + (-5x) + 2) + (-7x^2) + (-9)$$

$$= 3x^2 + (-7x^2) + (-5x) + 2 + (-9)$$

Now you can combine the like terms by adding coefficients.

$$3x^2 + (-7x^2) + (-5x) + 2 + (-9)$$

$$= (3 + (-7))x^2 + (-5x) + (2 + (-9))$$

$$= -4x^2 + (-5x) + (-7)$$

$$= -4x^2 - 5x - 7$$

A2. Multiply.

$$(x + 4)(2x^2 - 3x)$$

Step 1: Write Subtraction as Addition of the Opposite

$$(x + 4)(2x^2 - 3x) = (x + 4)(2x^2 + (-3x))$$

Step 2: Use FOIL

Multiply the first terms: $(x)(2x^2)$

Multiply the outside terms: $(x)(-3x)$

Multiply the inside terms: $(4)(2x^2)$

Multiply the last terms: $(4)(-3x)$

$(x + 4)(2x^2 + (-3x))$

$= (x)(2x^2) + (x)(-3x) + (4)(2x^2) + (4)(-3x)$

$= (2x^{2+1}) + (-3x^{1+1}) + (4 \times 2)x^2 + (4 \times -3)x$

$= 2x^3 + (-3x^2) + 8x^2 + (-12x)$

Step 3: Combine Like Terms

$2x^3 + (-3x^2) + 8x^2 + (-12x)$

$= 2x^3 + (-3 + 8)x^2 + (-12x)$

$= 2x^3 + 5x^2 - 12x$

Guided Practice

Let's work through a few examples together. Look back at the lesson content as often as necessary to help you apply the concepts and strategies you learned.

1. **Find the sum.**

   $$(3x^2 + 8x - 9) + (x^2 - 10x + 5)$$

   A) $2x^2 - 2x - 14$

   B) $2x^2 + 18x - 14$

   C) $4x^2 - 2x - 4$

   D) $4x^2 + 2x + 4$

   STEP 1

   What are the like terms?

   _____

   STEP 2

   How can you combine like terms?

   _____

   STEP 3

   What is the sum?

   _____

2. Multiply.

$$2x(5x^2 - 3x + 7)$$

A) $7x^2 - 6x + 14$

B) $10x^2 - 6x^2 + 14x$

C) $7x^3 + 6x^2 + 14x$

D) $10x^3 - 6x^2 + 14x$

STEP 1

How can you multiply a trinomial by a monomial?

_____

STEP 2

How do you multiply terms with coefficients and variables?

_____

STEP 3

How do you determine the exponent in the product of two like variables?

_____

Guided Practice

3. Simplify.

$$\frac{3x(6x+4)}{2x}$$

A) $\dfrac{9x+7}{2}$

B) $9x+\dfrac{2}{x}$

C) $9x+6$

D) $9x^3+6x^2$

STEP 1

What is the product of the monomial and the trinomial in the numerator?

_____

STEP 2

How can you break apart the numerator?

_____

STEP 3

How can you divide coefficients and variables?

_____

Independent Practice

You are ready to show what you know! Answer the questions below without looking back at the lesson content. Use the Hints to help you.

---

1. Add.

$$(4y^2 - 6y + 12) + (-5y^2 + 3y - 8)$$

A) $-y^2 - 3y + 4$

B) $-y^2 - 9y - 4$

C) $9y^2 - 3y + 4$

D) $9y^2 + 3y - 4$

> **HINT** *Write like terms next to each other, then add the coefficients to combine like terms.*

2. Multiply.

$$3x^2(2x^2 - x + 5)$$

A) $5x^3 - 3x^2 + 8x$

B) $5x^4 - 3x^3 + 8x^2$

C) $6x^3 - 3x^2 + 15x$

D) $6x^4 - 3x^3 + 15x^2$

> **HINT** *Multiply each term in the trinomial by $3x^2$.*

3. Simplify.

$$\frac{(x^2 + 6x) + (5x^2 - 4x)}{2x}$$

A) $6x^2 + 2x$

B) $3x + 5$

C) $3x + 1$

D) $3x$

> **HINT** *Add the terms in the numerator, and then divide each term by the denominator.*

4. Simplify.

$$(x + 4)(2x - 3) - (4x + 5)$$

A) $-x - 6$

B) $x^2 - 6x + 5$

C) $2x^2 - 9x - 7$

D) $2x^2 + x - 17$

> **HINT** *Use FOIL to multiply, and then subtract.*

ReKap

A polynomial is a mathematical expression that is a sum of terms. The terms can be numbers (constants), variables, or the product of constants and variables. When a constant is multiplied by a variable, the constant is called the coefficient of the variable.

The terms of a polynomial are called like terms if they have the same variable raised to the same power. Constants are also considered like terms. Like terms can be added together to simplify a polynomial.

Remember the following points as you add and subtract polynomials:

- Remember, a variable with no coefficient can be written with a coefficient of 1.

- Rewrite any subtraction in a polynomial as addition of a negative term to help you keep track of which signs go with which numbers.

Remember the following points as you multiply and divide polynomials:

- When you multiply terms with the same variable, add the exponents together.

- Remember, a variable with no exponent can be written with an exponent of 1.

- When you divide terms with the same variable, subtract the exponent of the divisor from the exponent of the dividend. In fraction form, subtract the exponent of the denominator from the exponent of the numerator.

- If the variables have coefficients, multiply or divide the coefficients, and multiply or divide the variables.

? Why would you need to combine like terms to find a sum or difference? Why might you need to combine like terms to find a product or quotient?

_____

_____

_____

Answers

Guided Practice

1. Step 1: $3x^2$ and x^2; $8x$ and $-10x$; -9 and 5

    Step 2: Add the coefficients

    Step 3: $4x^2 - 2x - 4$

    Answer: (C) $4x^2 - 2x - 4$

2. Step 1: multiply each term in the trinomial by the monomial

    Step 2: multiply the coefficients together and multiply the variables together

    Step 3: add the exponents together

    Answer: (D) $10x^3 - 6x^2 + 14x$

3. Step 1: $18x^2 + 12x$

    Step 2: $\dfrac{18x^2}{2x} + \dfrac{12x}{2x}$

    Step 3: divide the coefficients and subtract the exponents in the variables

    Answer: (C) $9x + 6$

Independent Practice

1. **Answer: (A) $-y^2 - 3y + 4$**

    The like terms are $4y^2$ and $-5y^2$, $-6y$ and $3y$, and 12 and -8.

    Rewrite to group like terms: $4y^2 + (-5y^2) + (-6y) + 3y + 12 + (-8)$

    Add coefficients of like terms: $(4 + (-5))y^2 + (-6 + 3)y + (12 + (-8)) = -y^2 - 3y + 4$

2. **Answer: (D) $6x^4 - 3x^3 + 15x^2$**

    Multiply each term in the trinomial by $3x^2$: $(3x^2)(2x^2) + (3x^2)(-x) + (3x^2)(5)$

    Multiply coefficients and variables: $(3 \times 2)(x^2 \times x^2) + (3 \times -1)(x^2 \times x) + (3 \times 5)(x^2)$

    Add exponents to multiply: $6x^{2+2} - 3(x^{2+1}) + 15x^2$

    Simplify: $6x^4 - 3x^3 + 15x^2$

3. **Answer: (C) $3x+1$**

    Start by adding the polynomials in the numerator.

    The like terms are x^2 and $5x^2$, and $6x$ and $-4x$.

    Rewrite the numerator, grouping like terms: $x^2 + 5x^2 + 6x + (-4x) = 6x^2 + 2x$.

    Break apart the numerator to divide: $\dfrac{6x^2}{2x} + \dfrac{2x}{2x}$

    Divide in each part: $3x + 1$.

Answers

4. **Answer: (D) $2x^2 + x - 17$**

    Use FOIL to multiply the first two binomials:

    $(x)(2x) + (x)(-3) + 4(2x) + (4)(-3) = 2x^2 - 3x + 8x - 12$

    Combine like terms: $2x^2 + (-3 + 8)x - 12 = 2x^2 + 5x - 12$

    Subtract $(2x^2 + 5x - 12) - (4x + 5)$

    Distribute the negative sign: $2x^2 + 5x - 12 - 4x - 5$

    Rewrite to group like terms: $2x^2 + 5x - 4x - 12 - 5$

    Combine like terms: $2x^2 + (5 - 4)x + (-12 - 5) = 2x^2 + x - 17$

ReKap

To find a sum or difference, combining like terms allows you to add or subtract the coefficients. When multiplying and dividing, you combine the like terms and then add or subtract the exponents.

3

MATH • LESSON 8

Expressions, Equations, and Inequalities

Suppose a nurse on a hospital staff works eight-hour shifts and that she must work 160 hours per month. How would you determine how many shifts she must work in the month? You can write and solve algebraic equations or inequalities to find unknown quantities in such problem situations.

Common Uses in Health Care

- finding unknown amounts of medicine based on given dosage information

- solving problems related to pay and scheduling

Key Terms/Formulas

- **addition principle** – a principle that allows you add the same amount to both sides of an equation or inequality

- **algebraic equation** – an equation that includes at least one algebraic expression

- **algebraic expression** – an expression that includes at least one variable

- **equation** – a mathematical statement that says that two expressions have equal values

- **inequality** – a mathematical statement that says that one expression is less than, less than or equal to, greater than, or greater than or equal to another expression

- **multiplication principle** – a principle that allows you to multiply by the same amount on both sides of an equation or inequality

- **solution** – the solution(s) of an algebraic equation or inequality is the set of values that make the statement *true*

	Beginning	Accrued	Used	Balance
Annual Leave	0.00	0.00	0.00	0.00
Sick Leave - Future	0.00	0.00 0.00	0.00 32.00	0.00 -32.00
Admin. Leave	0.00	0.00	0.00	0.00
LWOP			0.00	
Comp. Leave	0.00	0.00	0.00	0.00
Seminar			0.00	
Jury Duty			0.00	
Military Leave	0.00	0.00	0.00	0.00
AWOL			0.00	
FFLA	0.00	0.00	0.00	0.00
FMLA	0.00	0.00	0.00	480.00

Equations and Inequalities

Equations are mathematical sentences that use the "=" sign. You can write an equation to give the value of an expression or variable, or to show that expressions or quantities have the same value. Here are a few *true* equations:

$5 = 5$

$2 + 4 = 6$

$3 + 6 = 1 + 8$

Algebraic equations involve variables:

$x = 3$

$2x = 8$

$3x + 6 = 4x$

Inequalities compare the values of numbers or expressions that are not necessarily equal. You would write an inequality with one of the following four symbols:

Symbol	Meaning	Example	Translation
>	Greater than	$6 > 5$	6 is greater than 5
<	Less than	$2x < 6$	$2x$ is less than 6
≥	Greater than or equal to	$2 + 4 \geq x$	$2 + 4$ is greater than or equal to x
≤	Less than or equal to	$2 + x \leq 3x$	$2 + x$ is less than or equal to $3x$

Solving Equations & Inequalities

The solution(s) of an algebraic equation or inequality is the set of values that make the statement true.

For instance, the solution of the equation $2x = 6$ is $x = 3$, since $2x$ has a value of 2×3, or 6 when $x = 3$.

Algebraic inequalities can have many solutions. Take the inequality $x > 4$. Since $5 > 4$ and $6 > 4$, both 5 and 6 are part of the *solution set* of $x > 4$. In fact, any number greater than 4 is part of that solution set.

To find the solution of an algebraic equation or inequality with one variable, you can perform operations in order to get a new equation or inequality that has the variable alone on one side.

Use the addition principle when an equation involves a sum or difference with a variable. For instance, the equation $x + 35 = 77$ shows a sum with the variable x on the left.

In this equation, x is added to 35. To get the variable x alone on one side, you must *undo* that operation with the inverse operation. The inverse of adding 35 is subtracting 35. So, subtracting 35 from the left side of the equation will *cancel out* the + 35. Make sure that whatever you do to one side of the equation, you also do to the other. Subtract 35 from both sides.

$x + 35 = 77$

$x + 35 - 35 = 77 - 35$ Subtract 35 from both sides.

$x = 77 - 35$ Simplify on the left.

$x = 42$ Simplify on the right.

Your goal should always be to reach an equation with a variable on one side and a number on the other.

Other equations and inequalities call for the multiplication principle. When the variable is multiplied or divided by a number, use this principle to *undo* the multiplication or division and get the variable alone on one side.

Take the inequality $25x < 200$. The variable is multiplied by 25. Perform the inverse operation to undo the $25 \times$ on the left. Divide by 25 on both sides to get the variable alone on one side.

$25x < 200$

$\dfrac{25x}{25} < \dfrac{200}{25}$ Divide by 25 on both sides.

$x < \dfrac{200}{25}$ Simplify on the left.

$x < 4$ Simplify on the right.

The solution is $x < 4$.

There is one condition to keep in mind: When you multiply or divide both sides of an inequality by a negative number, you must change the direction of the inequality sign (> becomes <, or vice versa, and ≥ becomes ≤, or vice versa).

For instance, the steps to solving $-\dfrac{x}{3} < 6$ with the multiplication principle are shown below. Notice how the direction of the inequality sign is reversed because you are multiplying by a negative.

$-\dfrac{x}{3} < 6$

$-\dfrac{x}{3}(-3) < 6(-3)$ Multiply both sides by -3.

$-\dfrac{x}{3}(-3) > 6(-3)$ Reverse the direction of the inequality sign.

$1x > 6(-3)$ Simplify on left.

$x > -18$ Simplify on right.

The solution to the inequality is $x > -18$.

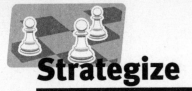

Strategize

Use Reverse Order of Operations to Isolate the Variable

Many equations and inequalities require both the addition and multiplication principles. Consider the equation $3x + 36 = 60$. In this equation, x is multiplied by 3 *and* has 36 added to the result. You must undo each operation by using each of the two principles, one after another, to get x alone and solve the equation.

To decide in which order to undo the operations, use the *reverse* of the order of operations (PEMDAS) that you used to simplify expressions in Lesson 2. Remember the reverse order of operations as SADMEP. It means that you undo subtraction/addition, then division/ multiplication, and then exponents. Lastly, you deal with any operations inside parentheses.

To solve $3x + 36 = 60$, then, apply the addition principle first to undo $+ 36$. Then apply the multiplication principle to undo $3 \times$.

$$3x + 36 = 60$$
$$3x + 36 - 36 = 60 - 36 \quad \text{Subtract 36 from both sides.}$$
$$3x = 60 - 36 \quad \text{Simplify on the left.}$$
$$3x = 24 \quad \text{Simplify on the right.}$$
$$\frac{3x}{3} = \frac{24}{3} \quad \text{Divide by 3 on both sides.}$$
$$x = \frac{24}{3} \quad \text{Simplify on the left.}$$
$$x = 8 \quad \text{Simplify on the right.}$$

Be careful not to apply the principles in the wrong order. The result of using the wrong order could actually appear as an incorrect answer choice on a test!

If you are dealing with an equation or inequality that has variables on both sides, then you will have to use addition or multiplication not just with numbers, but also with x-terms (products of x and a number, like $5x$ or $-7x$, for instance).

To approach the solution to an equation like $5x = 4x + 8$, for instance, you must start by gathering all the x-terms on one side, so that you can then isolate the x. The term $4x$ is added on the right. Subtract $4x$ on both sides to undo this operation.

$$5x = 4x + 8$$
$$5x - 4x = 4x + 8 - 4x \quad \text{Subtract 4x from both sides.}$$
$$x = 4x + 8 - 4x \quad \text{Simplify on the left.}$$
$$x = 8 \quad \text{Simplify on the right.}$$

The solution to this equation is $x = 8$.

Work Backwards

Remember that in a multiple choice question, the answer is one of the four choices already in front of you! If you can figure out which of the four possibilities works, your job is done. You use the strategy *working backwards* by substituting the values given in the answer choices into the equation or inequality.

For instance, imagine you are presented with the following problem.

Solve $6x + 35 = 77$ for x.

   A) 5

   B) 7

   C) 9

   D) 11

Start with C; by beginning with a value near the middle of the answer options, you can figure out whether you should test a smaller or larger answer choice if C is not the correct choice. Substitute 9 for x in the given equation and simplify. If you arrive at a true equation, that must be the right answer. Test $x = 9$:

$$6x + 35 = 77$$
$$6(9) + 35 \overset{?}{=} 77 \qquad \text{Substitute 9 for } x.$$
$$54 + 35 \overset{?}{=} 77 \qquad \text{Multiply.}$$
$$89 \overset{?}{=} 77 \qquad \text{Add.}$$

This last equation is false; 89 is *not* equal to 77! That means C is not the right answer, and you can rule it out.

A smaller value for x would result in a smaller value for $6x + 35$. So, the answer must be A or B. Test choice B, $x = 7$:

$$6x + 35 = 77$$
$$6(7) + 35 \overset{?}{=} 77 \qquad \text{Substitute 7 for } x.$$
$$42 + 35 \overset{?}{=} 77 \qquad \text{Multiply.}$$
$$77 \overset{?}{=} 77 \qquad \text{Add.}$$

This last equation is true; 77 *does* equal 77! We have found the correct answer by working backwards from the answer choices.

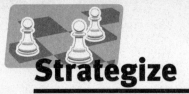

Strategize

Clear Fractions or Decimals

Consider the equation $0.3x + 6 = 0.6$. If it is cumbersome to perform the operations with the decimals, you may opt to use the multiplication principle to *clear* the decimals. In the equation above, two terms have decimals with tenths places. You can multiply both sides by 10 to eliminate the decimals:

$$0.3x + 6 = 0.6$$

$10 \times (0.3x + 6) = 10 \times (0.6)$ Multiply by 10 to clear the decimals.

$\quad 3x + 60 = 6 \qquad\qquad$ Simplify on each side by moving the decimal point.

The solution to $3x + 60 = 6$ is the same as the solution to $0.3x + 6 = 0.6$, so you can solve the equation with the whole numbers instead of the one with the decimals to arrive at the correct answer.

Now consider the inequality $\dfrac{x}{2} - 3 > \dfrac{1}{4}$. You could solve this by working with fractions, but it would be easier to work with whole numbers. Multiply each side by the LCD (least common denominator) of the fractions $\dfrac{x}{2}$ and $\dfrac{1}{4}$. By multiplying both sides by 4, the denominators cancel and the fractions will be cleared.

$$\frac{x}{2} - 3 > \frac{1}{4}$$

$4 \times \left(\dfrac{x}{2} - 3 \right) > 4 \times \left(\dfrac{1}{4} \right)$ Multiply by the LCD, 4, to clear the fractions.

$\quad \dfrac{4x}{2} - 12 > 1 \qquad$ Simplify on each side.

$\quad 2x - 12 > 1$

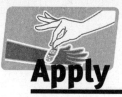

Apply

Let's take a look at an example.

A1. What is the solution of $6x - 31 = 65$?

Step 1: Plan

The variable in this equation is multiplied by 6, and then 31 is subtracted from the result. The order of operations, SADMEP, tells you to undo the subtraction before undoing the multiplication.

Step 2: Add

Perform the inverse of subtracting 31 by adding 31 to both sides. Use the addition principle to do so:

$$6x - 31 = 65$$
$$6x - 31 + 31 = 65 + 31$$
$$6x = 96$$

Step 3: Divide

Perform the inverse of multiplying by 6 by dividing by 6 on both sides. Use the multiplication principle to do so:

$$6x = 96$$
$$\frac{6x}{6} = \frac{96}{6}$$
$$x = 16$$

So, 16 is the solution of $6x - 31 = 65$.

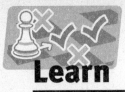

Solving Algebraic Word Problems

Some test questions can be solved by using algebraic equations or inequalities, but you will have to use the wording of the problem to write the appropriate equations or inequalities yourself.

To translate such problems into equations or inequalities that you can then solve, you need to figure out:

- the unknown quantity being asked for

- which operations are performed on the unknown

- whether the correct translation involves an equality symbol, or one of the inequality symbols

Every algebraic word problem involves an unknown quantity that you can represent with a variable in an equation or inequality.

For example, suppose you are told that Jack is five years younger than David, who is 26 years old, and then asked to find Jack's age in years. You could represent this information as a solvable equation. First of all, the *unknown* in this situation is Jack's age. You will need to represent that unknown as a variable (let's say the value of x is his age). Since David is 26 years old, five years older than Jack, you know that David's age in years is five greater than Jack's. So, 26 is $x + 5$:

$$x + 5 = 26$$

Now that you have an equation, you can solve for the unknown on paper.

There are always words and phrases in word problems that tell you which operations are involved. Some common indicators of the four basic operations are given below.

Operation	Common Terms
Addition	more than, total of, altogether, and
Subtraction	fewer than, less than, short of
Multiplication	twice, double, triple, of, times as many, by a factor of
Division	half, per

Word problems also include words or phrases to indicate that you are dealing with a situation in which two quantities are equal. Some of these indicators are shown in the table below.

Sign	Common Terms
=	is, are, is the same as, for a total of

Certain words and phrases are also used to indicate one of the four inequality signs. Some common indicators are shown in the table below.

Sign	Common Terms
>	more than, over
<	fewer than, under, less than
≥	at least, as few as, no less than
≤	at most, no more than

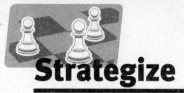

Strategize

Identifying unknowns

In dealing with an algebraic word problem, you should identify the unknown first and pick a variable to represent it. Then, translate the rest of the given information by constructing an equation or inequality around that variable.

Always ask yourself, "What quantity am I trying to find?" That quantity is the variable.

- Suppose that Tricia, who is 30 years old, is at least twice Jane's age. Write an inequality to represent Jane's age.

Ask yourself: What quantity am I trying to find? The question asks for Jane's age. That is your variable, x.

Identify Significant Phrases

You can work at translating word problems by underlining important words and phrases if you are working on a paper and pencil test—words and phrases that represent unknowns, key operations, or comparisons—to use in building up the equation or inequality that represents the situation. When you see phrases familiar from the table, or ones that express similar ideas, mark them, if you are working on a paper and pencil test.

Take this situation, for example:

- The combined weight of a 10-pound suitcase and its contents is over 30 pounds. Write an inequality to represent the weight of the contents of the suitcase.

A few key words here point the way to the correct translation:

- The *combined* weight of a 10-pound suitcase *and* its contents is *over* 30 pounds.

The words *combined* and *and* tell you that two quantities are being added. The word *over* tells you that the sum is greater than 30 pounds. Let your unknown, the weight of the contents, be x. Then $x + 10 > 30$.

Apply

Let's take a look at an example.

A2. A 27-foot long rope is at least 3 feet longer than twice the length of a shorter rope. Write an inequality representing this situation, using the variable x.

Step 1: Identify the unknown

The length of the shorter rope is unknown. So, we'll use the variable x to represent the length of the shorter rope in feet.

Step 2: Translate

Note key words:

A 27-foot long rope is *at least* 3 feet *longer* than *twice* the length of a shorter rope.

The word *twice* tells you that the variable is being multiplied by 2. The phrase *longer than* tells you that 3 feet is being added. So, x is being doubled, which is represented by the term $2x$. The longer rope is at least 3 feet *longer* than that. Represent this by adding 3 to your previous result: $2x + 3$.

Finally, you are told that the length of the longer rope, 27 feet, is *at least* $2x + 3$. So $2x + 3$ is less than or equal to 27.

Step 3: Write

Putting all of that together, you can find that $2x + 3 \leq 27$ represents this situation.

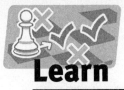
Learn

Absolute Value Equations and Inequalities

We first introduced the idea of absolute value in Lesson 1. Algebraic expressions can involve absolute values, so you might be faced with absolute value equations or inequalities to solve.

Take a basic absolute value equation, $|x| = 8$. This equation is true when $x = 8$ *and* when $x = -8$ because $|8|$ and $|-8|$ is equal to 8. Likewise, most absolute value equations, except a few special cases that you most likely will not see on the test, will have two solutions. The general pattern for translating an absolute value equation into two regular equations is:

- If $|y| = n$, then $y = n$ and $-y = n$. (here, n is a number and y is the variable)

Similarly, absolute value inequalities have two separate sets of solutions. For instance, consider the inequality $|x| > 8$. Any positive number greater than 8 (such as 9, 20, or 1,000, to name a few) is a solution, and any negative number that is less than −8 (such as −9, −20, or −1,000, to name a few) is a solution. Therefore, we would say that the solution of $|x| > 8$ is $x > 8$ or $x < -8$. All absolute value inequalities can be translated into two regular inequalities. The general pattern for translating absolute value inequalities into two regular inequalities is:

- If $|y| > n$, then $y < -n$ or $y > n$. (here, n is a number and y is the variable)
- If $|y| < n$, then $y > -n$ and $y < n$. (here, n is a number and y is the variable)

These patterns also work for inequalities using *or equal to*:

- If $|y| \geq n$, then $y \leq -n$ or $y \geq n$.
- If $|y| \leq n$, then $y \geq -n$ and $y \leq n$.

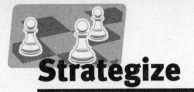

Strategize

Converting Absolute Value Equations

The key to solving equations with absolute value bars is to translate them into equations without absolute value expressions. Each absolute value equation represents two equations. Use the pattern for absolute value equations, given above, to write the two regular equations. Remember that:

- One equation shows the expression inside the absolute value bars, as is.
  - ‰ For instance, the equation $|x + 1| = 2$ represents $x + 1 = 2$. The expression $x + 1$ is the expression inside the absolute value bars in $|x + 1|$.

- The other equation shows the opposite of the expression inside the absolute value bars.
  - ‰ The equation $|x + 1| = 2$ also represents $-(x + 1) = 2$. The expression $-(x + 1)$ is the opposite of the expression inside the absolute value bars in $|x + 1|$.

The solution to each equation is also a solution to the absolute value equation. So, your solution would look like "x = [First solution] and x = [Second solution]".

Take the equation $|x + 4| = 12$. The expression inside the absolute value bars is $x + 4$.

- Solving with the term inside the bars, as is, means solving $x + 4 = 12$. The solution to this equation is $x = 8$. So, $x = 8$ is one solution to $|x + 4| = 12$.

$$x + 4 = 12$$

$x + 4 - 4 = 12 - 4$ Subtract 4 from both sides.

$$x = 8$$

- Solving with the opposite of the term inside the bars means solving $-(x + 4) = 12$. Distribute the negative sign to write: $-x - 4 = 12$. The solution to this equation is $x = -16$. So, $x = -16$ is the other solution to $|x + 4| = 12$.

$$-(x + 4) = 12$$

$-x - 4 = 12$	Distribute the negative sign.
$-x - 4 + 4 = 12 + 4$	Add 4 on both sides.
$-x = 16$	
$x = -16$	Divide both sides by -1.

Converting Absolute Value Inequalities

To solve an absolute value inequality, translate the inequality into two separate inequalities without absolute value expressions. Use the appropriate pattern for the type of absolute value inequality, greater than or less than, to write the two regular inequalities.

Take the inequality $|x + 6| > 15$. The expression inside the absolute value bars is $x + 6$. This is a *greater than* symbol, so use the pattern $y < -n$ or $y > n$, where y is the expression inside the bars, $x + 6$.

- One inequality is $x + 6 > 15$, which has the solution $x > 9$.

   $x + 6 > 15$

   $x + 6 - 6 > 15 - 6$ Subtract 6 from both sides.

   $x > 9$

- The other inequality is $x + 6 < -15$, which has the solution $x < -21$.

   $-(x + 6) > 15$ Write an inequality with the opposite of the expression inside the bars.

   $(x + 6) < -15$ Divide both sides by –1, reversing the inequality sign.

   $x + 6 < -15$ Drop the parentheses.

   $x + 6 - 6 < -15 - 6$ Subtract 6 from both sides.

   $x < -21$

The solution to $|x + 6| > 15$ is $x < -21$ or $x > 9$.

Now take the inequality $|x + 6| \leq 15$. The expression inside the absolute value bars is again $x + 6$. This is a *less than or equal to* symbol, so use the pattern $y > -n$ and $y < n$, where y is the expression inside the bars, $x + 6$.

- One inequality is $-15 \leq x + 6$, which has the solution $-21 \leq x$.

- The other inequality is $x + 6 \leq 15$, which has the solution $x \leq 9$.

The solution to $|x + 6| \leq 15$ is $x \leq -21$ and $x \leq 9$. These inequalities can be combined into the compound inequality: $-21 \leq x \leq 9$.

Apply

Let's take a look at an example.

A3. What are the solutions of $|5x - 10| + 20 > 15$?

Step 1. Plan

This is an absolute value inequality involving an absolute value expression with a variable that is *greater than*. You will use the pattern $y < -n$ or $y > n$. Then, you can solve each resulting inequality.

Step 2. Isolate the Absolute Value Expression on One Side

Make sure you get the absolute value expression by itself on one side before writing the two regular inequalities. Subtract 20 from both sides to get $|5x - 10| > -5$. Here, the y in the pattern $y < -n$ or $y > n$ is stands for the variable expression $5x - 10$.

Step 3. Write and Solve Two Inequalities

Using the pattern for *greater than*, the two inequalities are $5x - 10 < 5$ and $5x - 10 > -5$. The solutions are $x < 3$ and $x > 1$, respectively. This can be written as the compound inequality $1 < x < 3$.

Guided Practice

1. **What is the solution of 8x + 12 > 4?**

   A) $x < -2$

   B) $x < 1$

   C) $x > -1$

   D) $x > 2$

   STEP 1: What principle should you apply first?

   _____

   _____

   STEP 2: What principle should you apply next?

   _____

   _____

   STEP 3: What is the solution?

   _____

   _____

Guided Practice

2. A 3,000 gram block is 300 grams heavier than 12 lighter blocks of the same size. Which equation represents this situation?

   A) $12x - 300 = 3,000$

   B) $12x + 300 = 3,000$

   C) $300x - 12 = 3,000$

   D) $300x + 12 = 3,000$

STEP 1: What is the unknown?

_____

_____

STEP 2: What expression can be used to represent the combined weight of the *12 lighter blocks?*

_____

_____

STEP 3: What operation should you use to represent *300 grams heavier?*

_____

_____

3. What are the solutions of $|3x - 12| = 6$?

   A) –6 and –2

   B) –6 and 2

   C) –2 and 6

   D) 2 and 6

STEP 1: How can you apply a pattern to convert this equation into two equations without absolute value bars?

_____

_____

STEP 2: What is the solution to the first equation?

_____

_____

STEP 3: What is the solution to the second equation?

_____

_____

Independent Practice

1. **What is the solution of $6x + 7 = 2x - 5$?**

   A) -3

   B) -2

   C) 2

   D) 3

   HINT *Get all the x-terms on one side and all the constants on the other.*

2. **The value of 64 is at least 8 more than twice another number.**

   A) $2y - 8 \leq 64$

   B) $2y - 8 \geq 64$

   C) $2y + 8 \leq 64$

   D) $2y + 8 \geq 64$

3. **What are the solutions of $|4x| + 20 < 44$?**

   A) $x < -16$ and $x > 16$

   B) $x < -16$ and $x > 6$

   C) $-6 < x < 16$

   D) $-6 < x < 6$

ReKap

Remember these key points about working with equations and inequalities:

- To solve, use the addition and multiplication principles to perform inverse operations on both sides, in order to get the variable alone on one side.

- Translate situations in word problems to equations and inequalities by keeping track of operations performed on the unknown.

- Solve an absolute value equation or inequality by converting it into two related statements without absolute value brackets.

? What is the solution of $4.5y - 15 = 45 - 3y$?

Answers

Guided Practice

1. Step 1: Subtraction/addition comes first in SADMEP, so apply the addition principle first. Subtract 12 from both sides.

    Step 2: Multiplication/division come next in SADMEP, so apply the multiplication principle next. Divide by 8 on both sides.

    Step 3: $x > -1$

    Answer: (C) $x > -1$

    TIP: You might be tempted to change the direction of the inequality sign. However, you are dividing by a positive number here. You would change the direction of the direction of the sign if you were multiplying by -8 rather than 8.

2. Step 1: The mass of the lighter block is the unknown.

    Step 2: $12x$

    TIP: Since there are 12 lighter blocks, their combined weight is $12x$ grams.

    Step 3: You should use $+ 300$.

    TIP: Since the heavier block weighs 300 grams more than $12x$, the sum of $12x$ and 300 is a total of 3,000 grams. So, $12x + 300 = 3,000$.

    Answer: (B) $12x + 300 = 3,000$

3. Step 1: Use the pattern $y = n$ and $-y = n$. The absolute value equation can be converted into the two equations $3x - 12 = 6$ and $-(3x - 12) = 6$.

    Step 2: To solve $3x - 12 = 6$, add 12 to both sides to get $3x = 18$. Then divide both sides by 3 to get $x = 6$.

    Step 3: Begin solving $-(3x - 12) = 6$ by distributing the negative on the left side, to get $-3x + 12 = 6$. Subtract 12 from both sides to get $-3x = -6$. Then divide both sides by -3 to get $x = 2$.

    Answer: (D) 2 and 6

Independent Practice

1. **Answer (A) -3**

    Get the variable x on just one side by subtracting $2x$ from both sides:

    $$6x + 7 - 2x = 2x - 5 - 2x$$
    $$4x + 7 = -5$$

    Subtract 7 from both sides:

    $$4x + 7 - 7 = -5 - 7$$
    $$4x = -12$$

    Divide both sides by 4:

    $$\frac{4x}{4} = \frac{-12}{4}$$
    $$x = -3$$

2. **Answer: (C) $2y + 8 \leq 64$**

    When y represents another number, 8 more than twice that amount is $2y + 8$. Since 64 is at least $2y + 8$, 64 is greater than or equal to $2y + 8$. So, $2y + 8$ is less than or equal to 64.

3. **Answer: (D) −6 < x < 6**

Start by isolating the absolute value expression.

$|4x| + 20 < 44$

$|4x| < 24$ Subtract 20 from both sides.

Use the pattern for less than, $y > -n$ and $y < n$ to write $4x > -24$ and $4x < 24$. Divide by 4 on both sides of each to get the solutions $-6 < x < 6$.

ReKap

Multiply both sides by 10 to get $45y - 150 = 450 - 30y$

Add 30y to both sides to get $75y - 150 = 450$.

Add 150 to both sides to get $75y = 600$.

Divide both sides by 75 to get $y = 8$.

MATH • LESSON 9

Representations of Data

How much does it hurt? Many medical practices and hospitals use a chart showing faces that represent levels of pain to help patients quantify their pain on a scale from 0 (no pain) to 10 (worst pain imaginable). The patient's pain level can then be plotted on a graph to show how it improves over time, or to identify any patterns, such as increased pain levels at night. In fact, graphs can be used to display a wide variety of medical data.

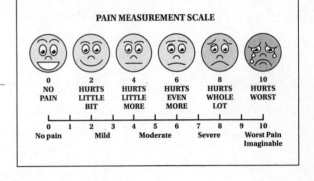

Common Uses in Health Care

- representing results of an experiment or study

- plotting heights or weights on a growth chart

- representing vital signs over time

Key Terms/Formulas

- **bar graph** – a representation of data in which each category is shown as a bar, the height of which indicates the number of data values in the category

- **circle graph (pie graph)** – a representation of data in which each category is shown as a sector of a circle, the size of which indicates the part of the whole that the category represents

- **dependent variable** – the variable whose values are the outputs that result from inputting the independent variable

- **independent variable** – the variable whose values are the inputs

- **frequency** – the number of times a data value occurs in a set

- **histogram** – a representation of data in which the data values are arranged in intervals and each interval is shown as a bar, the height of which indicates the number of data values in the interval

- **interval** – a range of data values

- **line graph** – a representation of data in which each data value is plotted as an ordered pair and the points are joined with lines

- **ordered pair** – a set of coordinates in the order (x, y) that describe the location of a point

- **sector** – a section of a circle graph

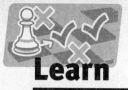
Line Graphs

Line graphs compare the values of an independent variable, the inputs, to the corresponding values of the dependent values, the outputs. Line graphs usually show how data change over time. The independent variable is generally a unit of time, such as hours, days, months, or years.

The data are plotted as ordered pairs (x, y), where x is a value of the independent variable and y is the corresponding value of the dependent variable, and the points are joined by line segments. You can use the line segments to predict or estimate the value of the dependent variable at a particular value of the independent variable.

Some line graphs show more than one data set. For example, the double-line graph below shows the pain levels of two patients with similar conditions, but taking different medications.

- The independent variable, time (in hours), is shown along the horizontal axis. These are the x-values.

- The dependent variable, pain level, is shown along the vertical axis. These are the y-values.

- The graph for Patient 1 shows the ordered pairs (0, 9), (1, 9), (2, 8), (3, 7), (4, 5), (5, 3), and (6, 2).

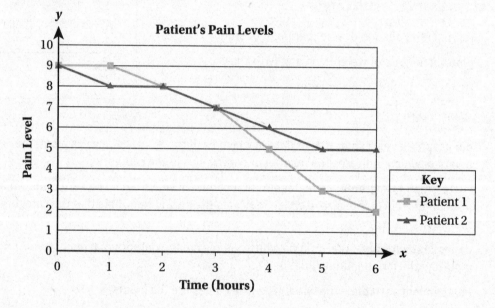

Circle Graphs

Circle graphs, also called *pie graphs*, show how the sizes of categories relate to the whole and to each other. Each piece of the pie, or sector, of the circle represents a category. You can quickly compare the sizes of the categories based on the sizes of the sectors. The sectors can be labeled directly, or given in a key.

The sectors can be labeled with a quantity, a percent, or both. If the graph presents the number in each category, you can find the total and then calculate the percent for each category. If the graph presents the percent in each category and you know the total number of data values represented in the graph, you can use the percent equation to find the number in each category.

The circle graph below shows the number of times each of 260 patients visited the doctor last year.

- The key shows the number of doctor visits represented by each sector.

- Each sector is labeled with the number of data values and the percent that the sector represents. For example, 22 patients visited the doctor 0 times last year, which represents about 8% of the total number of patients.

Number of Doctor Visits Last Year

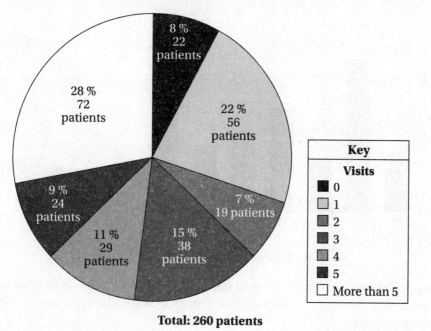

Total: 260 patients

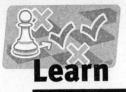
Bar Graphs

Bar graphs, like circle graphs, compare the number of data values in different categories. Each category is represented by a bar, and the height of the bar indicates the number of data values in that category. You can quickly compare the sizes of the categories based on the heights of the bars. The bars in a bar graph generally do not touch each other.

If the categories are listed along the horizontal axis, you can read the vertical axis to find the number of data values that each bar represents. Similarly, if the categories are listed along the vertical axis, you can read the horizontal axis to find the number of data values in a category.

The bar graph below represents the number of times each patient visited the doctor last year. Notice that this graph shows the same data as the circle graph in the previous example.

- The categories are shown along the horizontal axis. In this case, the categories are the numbers of doctor visits.

- The number of patients is shown on the vertical axis. Notice that the vertical axis is labeled at intervals of 10. The lines between the labels are at intervals of 2.

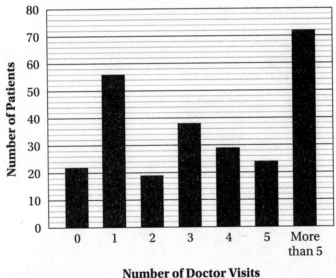

Some bar graphs show more than one data set. For example, a bar graph could show the same categories in different years, or at different hospitals. A key usually indicates which bars represent which data sets.

Histograms

Histograms resemble bar graphs, but show a different type of data. Histograms compare the frequency of data in different intervals, rather than in different categories. For example, a histogram might compare the number of data values in different age ranges, which might be more useful than comparing the number of data values for each age. The intervals are shown along the horizontal axis, and the intervals should all be the same size. Unlike bar graphs, the bars in histograms should touch.

For example, the histogram below shows the ages of patients who visited a pediatrician's office last week.

- The intervals are shown along the horizontal axis. Notice that each interval includes 4 different ages.

- The frequencies, or numbers of patients, are shown on the vertical axis. Notice that the vertical axis is labeled at intervals of 10. The lines between the labels are at intervals of 2.

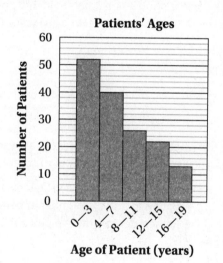

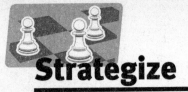

Strategize

Analyze the Graph

Regardless of the type of graph presented in a problem on the test, you will need to analyze it closely.

- Identify the categories shown on a bar graph. Determine which categories are needed to solve the problem.

- Read the scale of the graph to make sure you are reading the graph accurately. If the values on the vertical axis (or on the horizontal axis of a line graph) do not have an interval of 1, take particular care.

- Identify the intervals of a histogram. Determine which intervals are needed to solve the problem.

- Find the total number of data values shown on a circle graph by finding the sum of the data values in each category.

- Read the key of a double-bar or double-line graph to identify which line or set of bars represents which data set. Determine which set (or sets) you will need to solve the problem.

Use the Percent Equation

Recall that the whole, the part, and the percent are related by the following equation:

percent · whole = part

In the case of a circle graph, the whole is the total number of data values and the part is the number of data values in a particular category (or sector of the graph).

For example, suppose that a circle graph shows 200 data values, each of which represents a person. You can use the percent equation to find the number of people in a category whose sector represents 18% of the circle. Remember to write the percent as a decimal by moving the decimal point two places to the left.

$18\% = 0.18$

percent · whole = part

$$0.18 \cdot 200 = x$$

$$36 = x$$

So, there are 36 people in the category.

Predict Before You Peek

All of the information you will need to answer a question can be found in the graph. So, before you look at the answer choices, solve the problem yourself. Be careful, though. The incorrect answer choices are often the results of common errors.

Eliminate

If you are unsure how to solve a problem, or are running short on time, start by eliminating the answer choices that you know are incorrect.

For example, because the relative sizes of the sectors correspond to the relative size of the percents they represent, you can compare the sizes of the sectors to help you eliminate answer choices.

The difference between two categories on a bar graph cannot be greater than the larger category. So, if you are asked to find the difference between two categories, eliminate any answer choices that are greater than the larger category. Similarly, the sum of two categories must be greater than the larger category, so eliminate any answer choices that are less than the larger category.

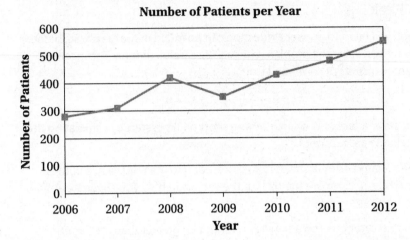

Number of Patients per Year

A1. The graph above shows the number of unique patients seen each year in a family practice. Between which two years was the increase in number of patients the greatest?

Step 1: Analyze the Graph

The graph shows the number of patients per year.

The years are shown along the horizontal axis, with an interval of 1 year.

The number of patients is shown along the vertical axis, with an interval of 100 patients.

Step 2: Identify the Greatest Increase

The greatest increase is the greatest change in the height from one point to another. This occurs between the second and third points, counting from the left. The increase is from about 300 to about 420.

Step 3: Read the Horizontal Axis

The greatest increase occurs between 2007 and 2008.

Favorite Exercise Activities

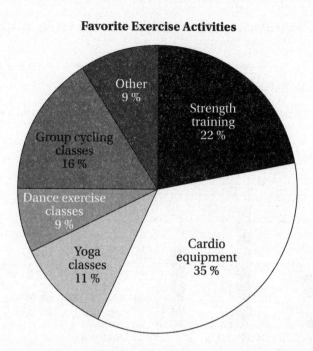

A2. The graph above shows the favorite exercise activities of gym members. If 230 gym members were surveyed, about how many said strength training was their favorite activity?

Step 1: Analyze the Graph

The graph shows the favorite exercise activities of gym members.

There are 6 categories.

The graph shows the percent for each category.

22% of members chose strength training.

Step 2: Find the total amount paid.

percent · whole = part

Step 3: Calculate the Number of Data Values

$0.22 \cdot 230 = x$

$50.6 = x$

About 51 gym members said strength training was their favorite activity.

Guided Practice

Let's work through a few examples together. Look back at the lesson content as often as necessary to help you apply the concepts and strategies you learn.

The next two questions are based on this bar graph.

The graph below shows the results of a survey asking men and women about the highest level of education they had completed.

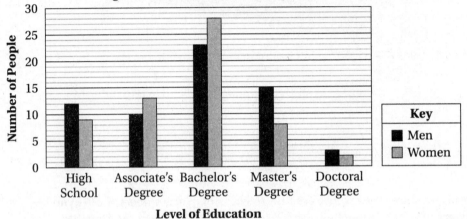

1. **How many more men than women listed high school as their highest level of education completed?**

   A) 3

   B) 9

   C) 12

   D) 21

STEP 1: How many men listed high school as their highest level of education completed?

_____

STEP 2: How many women listed high school as their highest level of education completed?

_____

STEP 3: How many more men than women listed high school as their highest level of education completed?

_____

2. Which statement about the number of master's degrees and associate's degrees is correct?

A) Two more people listed master's degrees than associate's degrees as the highest level of education completed.

B) Two more people listed associate's degrees than master's degrees as the highest level of education completed.

C) Four more people listed master's degrees than associate's degrees as the highest level of education completed.

D) The same number of people listed associate's degrees as master's degrees as the highest level of education completed.

STEP 1: How many men and women listed associate's degree?

_____

STEP 2: How many men and women listed master's degree?

_____

STEP 3: How do the numbers in each category compare?

_____

Guided Practice

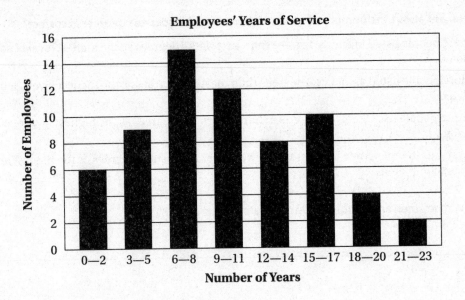

Employees' Years of Service

3. The graph above shows the number of years of service of employees at a local business. How many employees have served for more than 5 years and fewer than 15 years?

A) 35

B) 50

C) 51

D) 54

STEP 1: Which intervals should be included?

_____

STEP 2: What is the number of employees within each interval?

_____

STEP 3: How many employees have served for more than 5 years and fewer than 15 years?

_____

Independent Practice

You are ready to show what you know! Answer the questions below without looking back at the lesson content. Use the Hints to help you.

---

1. The results of a survey asking people the number of days they exercised last week are shown in the table below. In a circle (pie) graph that displays the same data, what part of the circle will represent "1 day"?

Number of Days Last Week	Number of People
0	7
1	5
2	9
3	12
4	8
5	6
6	2
7	1

A) $\dfrac{1}{10}$

B) $\dfrac{1}{8}$

C) $\dfrac{1}{6}$

D) $\dfrac{1}{5}$

HINT Find the *whole*. Then find the part of the whole that will represent *1 day*.

Independent Practice

Use the line graph below to answer the next two questions.

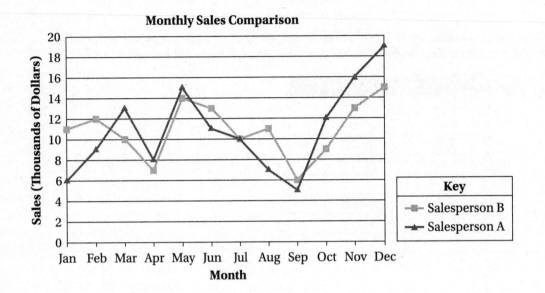

2. In which month was the difference between Salesperson A's and Salesperson B's sales the greatest?

A) August

B) December

C) January

D) November

HINT *Read the graph. For which month are the two points farthest apart?*

3. In which month were Salesperson B's sales twice as much as Salesperson B's September sales?

A) February

B) July

C) October

D) September

HINT *Make sure you are looking at the correct line on the graph.*

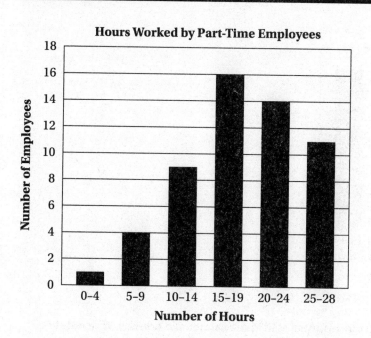

Hours Worked by Part-Time Employees

4. The graph above shows the number of hours worked last week by a group of part-time employees. Which two intervals had the same number of employees?

A) 0–9 hours and 10–14 hours

B) 0–14 hours and 20–24 hours

C) 0–14 hours and 15–19 hours

D) 5–14 hours and 20–28 hours

HINT ⟩ *If an interval includes more than one interval from the graph, find the sum of the frequencies of the included intervals.*

Independent Practice

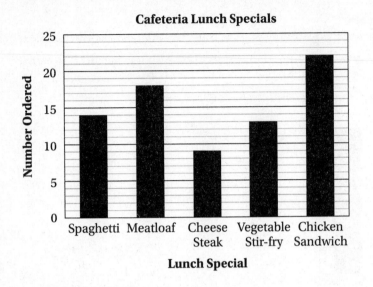

Cafeteria Lunch Specials

5. The bar graph above shows the number of each lunch special sold in the cafeteria in one day. Which statement is true?

A) The meatloaf was the most popular special.

B) Twice as many meatloaf specials as cheese steak specials were ordered.

C) The same number of spaghetti specials and vegetable stir-fry specials were ordered.

D) The number of chicken sandwich specials ordered was the same as the combined number of spaghetti and cheese steak specials.

HINT *Read the height of each bar. Then, compare the numbers as described in the answer choices.*

ReKap

Line Graphs

- Compare the values of an independent variable to the corresponding values of the dependent values (outputs).
- Usually show how data change over time, so the independent variable is generally a unit of time, such as hours, days, months, or years.
- The data are plotted as ordered pairs (x, y), and the points are joined by line segments.
- Some line graphs show more than one data set.

Circle Graphs (Pie Graphs)

- Show how the sizes of categories relate to the whole and to each other.
- Each piece of the pie, or sector, of the circle represents a category.
- The sectors can be labeled directly, or given in a key, or both.
- The sectors can be labeled with a quantity, a percent, or both.
- If the graph presents the number in each category, you can find the total and then calculate the percent for each category. If the graph presents the percent in each category and you know the total number of data values represented in the graph, you can use the percent equation to find the number in each category.

Bar Graphs

- Compare the number of data values in different categories.
- Each category is represented by a bar, and the height of the bar indicates the number of data values in that category.
- The bars generally do not touch each other.

Histograms

- Compare the frequency of data in different intervals, rather than in different categories.
- The intervals are shown along the horizontal axis, and the intervals should all be the same width.
- The bars in histograms should touch.

> **?** **How are bar graphs like circle graphs and histograms? How are bar graphs different from circle graphs and histograms?**
>
> _____
>
> _____
>
> _____

Answers

Guided Practice

1. Step 1: 12

   Step 2: 9

   Step 3: 12 – 9 = 3

   Answer: (A) 3

2. Step 1: 10 men + 13 women = 23 people

   Step 2: 15 men + 8 women = 23 people

   Step 3: The numbers in each category are equal.

   Answer (D): The same number of people listed associate's degrees as master's degrees as the highest level of education completed.

3. Step 1: 6 – 8, 9 – 11, and 12 – 14

   Step 2: 6 – 8: 15; 9 – 11: 12; 12 – 14: 8

   Step 3: 15 + 12 + 8 = 35

   Answer: (A)

Independent Practice

1. **Answer: (A) $\frac{1}{10}$**

   A circle graph shows parts of the whole.

   Ask: Which column contains the data you need to sum up to find the whole? ["Number of People"]

   Find the sum of the number of responses to find the whole: 7 + 5 + 9 + 12 + 8 + 6 + 2 + 1 = 50.

   Read the table to find the number who responded *1 day*: 5

   Write the ratio of *1 day* to the whole: $\frac{5}{50}$

   Write the fraction in simplest terms: $\frac{1}{10}$

2. **Answer: (C) January**

   The greatest distance between points seems to occur in January.

   In January, Salesperson A had sales of $6,000 and Salesperson B had sales of $11,000.

   Subtract: $11,000 – $6000 = $5000.

   Check August: $11,000 – $7,000 = $4,000

   Check November: $16,000 – $13,000 = $3,000

   Check December: $19,000 – $15,000 = $4,000

3. **Answer: (A) February**

   Read the graph to find Salesperson B's September sales: $6,000

   Multiply September sales by 2: 2($6,000) = $12,000

   Read the vertical axis to find $12,000 and look across to find the month in which Salesperson B's sales were $12,000: February

4. **Answer: (B) 0 – 14 hours and 20-24 hours.**

   The interval 0–9 hours includes 0–4 hours and 5–9 hours. Add the frequencies: 1 + 4 = 5.

   The interval 10–14 hours has a frequency of 9, so choice A is incorrect.

   The interval 0–14 hours includes 0–4 hours, 5–9 hours, and 10–14 hours. Add the frequencies: 1 + 4 + 9 = 14.

   The interval 20–24 hours has a frequency of 14, so choice B is correct.

   The interval 15–19 hours has a frequency of 16, so choice C is incorrect.

   The interval 5–14 hours includes 5–9 hours and 10–14 hours. Add the frequencies: 4 + 9 = 13.

   The interval 20–28 hours has a frequency of 11, so choice D is incorrect.

5. **Answer: (B) Twice as many meatloaf specials as cheese steak specials were ordered.**

   The chicken sandwich was the most popular, 22 were sold. Eliminate Choice A. This was more than the combined number of spaghetti (14 sold) and cheese steak specials (9 sold). Eliminate Choice D. More spaghetti specials were ordered than were vegetable stir-fry specials, eliminate Choice C.

ReKap

Bar graphs are like circle graphs because they show data broken down into categories. Bar graphs are like histograms because the height of the bar in a bar graphs shows the number of data values in that category, just as the height of the bar in a histogram shows the number of data values in that interval.

Bar graphs are different from circle graphs because they do not show how the size of each category relates to the whole. They are different from histograms because they show categories of data instead of intervals and the bars do not touch each other.

3

MATH · LESSON 10
Other Topics

Have you ever read a pharmaceutical prescription that seemed to be written in code? Prescriptions can be difficult for a layman to read because doctors often use abbreviations (sometimes for Latin words) and Roman numerals instead of the more familiar, Arabic numerals. In fact, Roman numerals are used in a variety of medical terminologies. In this lesson, you will also learn about estimation strategies and operations with money.

Common Uses in Health Care

- estimation strategies: ordering medical supplies, converting units of measurement

- working with money: office management and budgeting, billing

- Roman numerals: pharmaceutical prescriptions, cancer stages

Key Terms/Formulas

- **Arabic numerals** – the numerals we use in the modern world; also referred to as *standard* numerals

- **digit** – a single number, 0–9; digits make up numbers with multiple decimal places

- **estimation** – finding an approximate answer to a computation

- **place value** – the value of a digit in a number, given by the position of the digit relative to the decimal point

- **Roman numerals** – ancient numeric system that uses Latin letters

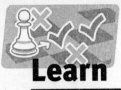

Learn

Estimation Strategies

Some items on the test may not require an exact answer. These types of items tend to use words like *approximately* or *about* in the question stem. If an exact answer is not needed, you can estimate the answer. Estimation is also a useful way to check whether your exact computations are accurate.

To estimate properly, you must have some understanding of place values. The place value of a digit is given by the position of the digit relative to the decimal point. The names of the place values in the number in 987,654.321, for instance, are shown in the chart below.

9	8	7,	6	5	4	.	3	2	1
hundred thousands (100,000s)	ten thousands (10,000s)	thousands (1,000s)	hundreds (100s)	tens (10s)	ones (1s)	decimal point	tenths (0.1s)	hundredths (0.01s)	thousandths (0.001s)

Note that the place values correspond to powers of 10 (10, 100, 1,000, etc.).When talking about place values, use language like:

- The ones digit in 987,654.321 is 4. So, the digit 4 has the value 4×1, or 4.

- The hundredths digit in 987,654.321 is 2. So, the digit 2 has the value 2×0.01, or 0.02.

- The thousands digit in 987,654.321 is 7. So, the digit 7 has the value $7 \times 1,000$, or 7,000.

We will refer to place values when discussing estimation strategies below.

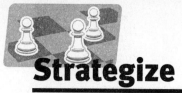

Strategize

Rounding

Instead of working with numbers that have non-zero digits in each place, you can round each number to a particular place before performing computations.

To round a number to a given place, look at the digit in the place just to the right of the given place.

- If that digit is 1, 2, 3, or 4, keep the digit in the given place and change all digits to its right to 0.

- If that digit is 5, 6, 7, 8, or 9, increase the digit in the given place by 1 and change all digits to its right to 0.

For example, consider the number 13,581.

To round to the nearest...	Look at the...	The digit is...	Round the number...
ten	ones digit	1	down to 13,580
hundred	tens digit	8	up to 13,600
thousand	hundreds digit	5	up to 14,000
ten-thousand	thousands digit	3	down to 10,000

Compatible Numbers

To estimate using compatible numbers, choose numbers that are close to the numbers you are given, but are easier to work with. This may require you to round some numbers up and some numbers down, or to round each number to a different place.

For example, to estimate $412 \div 58$, you could choose to divide the compatible numbers 420 and 60, because the numbers divide evenly. Since $420 \div 60 = 7$, you can estimate that $412 \div 58$ is about 7.

Process of Elimination

Process of elimination is a useful strategy for multiple-choice questions, because it helps you eliminate incorrect answer choices to narrow down the options for the correct answer choice.

When you estimate an answer, you get an idea of how large or small the answer should be. Use your estimate to eliminate any answer choices that are much too large or much too small. Then, if more than one answer choice remains, you can perform the exact calculation to identify the correct answer. Before you perform the exact calculation, you greatly increase your odds of answering correctly when you can eliminate any obviously incorrect answers!

Apply

A1. Amanda drove 987 miles over a three-day period. Her total driving time was 18.5 hours. Approximately what was her average speed?

Step 1: Write an Expression

To find the average speed, divide the total distance by the driving time.

$987 \div 18.5$

Step 2: Choose Compatible Numbers

Since you must divide to find the answer, choose numbers that will divide evenly.

987 is close to 1,000

18.5 is close to 20

Step 3: Compute with the Compatible Numbers

$1,000 \div 20 = 50$

Amanda's speed was approximately 50 miles per hour.

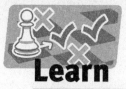

Learn

Working with Money

Working with money uses the same concepts as operations with decimals.

To add or subtract amounts of money, set up the problem vertically and align the dollar amounts on the decimal point. You will almost always have digits in the tenths and hundredths places. Remember to write ".00" after any whole-dollar amount.

- For instance, to add $3.47 to $10.52, set up the problem as shown below:

    ```
      3.47
    +10.52
    ```

- The sum of $3.47 + $10.52 is equal to $13.99.

To multiply an amount of money by a decimal or a whole number, multiply the digits without considering the decimal point. Then, count the total number of digits to the right of the decimal point in the factors. Your product will have the same number of digits to the right of the decimal point.

- For instance, to multiply $5.65 by 3, first disregard the decimal points. Multiply 565 × 3 to get 1695. In the factors 5.65 and 3, there are 2 digits altogether to the right of the decimal points. That means you must place a decimal point in your answer so that there are 2 places to the right of it: $16.95

To divide an amount of money by a whole number, place the decimal point in the quotient directly above the decimal point in the dividend.

- For instance, to divide $14.40 by 3, set up the problem as shown below, so that the decimal points in the dividend (the number under the division bar) and the quotient (your answer) are aligned: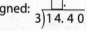

- To find the digit in the box, divide 14 by 3. Then continue on applying the steps you have learned to complete the long division.

If there is a decimal in the divisor, multiply both the divisor and the dividend by the same power of 10 to eliminate the decimal point in the divisor.

- For instance, to divide $14.40 by $3.60, start by looking at the divisor, $3.60. There are two digits to the right of the decimal point, so multiply 3.60 by 100 to get rid of the decimal point: 3.60 × 100 = 360.

- Next, to make sure the decimal point is placed correctly in the answer, multiply the dividend, $14.40 by the same power of 10: 14.40 × 100 = 1440.

- So, $14.40 ÷ $3.60 can be rewritten as 1440 ÷ 360. Then perform long division to find the answer.

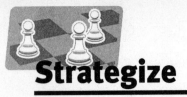

Strategize

Choose the Sign

A word problem involving money may use unfamiliar terms to indicate whether you should add or subtract the amount.

Clues to Add	Clues to Subtract
Credit	Debit
Deposit	Withdrawal

For example, if a monthly report shows total debits of $46,318 and total credits of $62,894, the income was $62,894 − $46,318 = $16,576.

Align Decimal Points

To add or subtract amounts of money, align the decimal points and subtract place by place. Remember to write all of the amounts as decimals to hundredths.

Your groceries cost $17.38, including tax. What change will you receive if you pay with a $20 bill?

Align the decimal points and subtract place by place. Regroup if necessary.

$$
\begin{array}{r}
\$\,{}^{1}\cancel{2}\,{}^{9}\cancel{0}\,{}^{9}\cancel{0}.\cancel{0}\,{}^{1}0 \\
-\ 1\ \ 7\ .\ 3\ 8 \\
\hline
\$\ \ \ \ 2\ .\ 6\ 2
\end{array}
$$

Process of Elimination

You can estimate the answer to a question involving money by rounding or using compatible numbers. Then, eliminate unreasonable answer choices.

If five friends equally split a dinner bill of $92.12, what was each friend's share?

Round the dinner bill to $100 and divide: 100 ÷ 5 = 20.

Eliminate any answer choices that are not near $20.

Apply

A2. Aurora bought three T-shirts for $8.95 each. She paid with two $20 bills. How much change did she receive?

Step 1: Find the total cost of the T-shirts.

Multiply 3×8.95.

```
  8.95
×    3
26.85
```

Step 2: Find the total amount paid.

Multiply: $2 \times \$20 = \$40$

Step 3: Find the change.

Subtract the total cost from the total amount paid.

Write $40 as $40.00 and align the decimal points.

$$\overset{3}{\cancel{4}}\,\overset{9}{\cancel{0}}.\,\overset{9}{\cancel{0}}\,\overset{1}{\cancel{0}}\,.$$

```
 $4 0 . 0 0
-2 6 . 8 5
 $1 3 . 1 5
```

Aurora received $13.15 in change.

A3. For a construction project, Gavin bought 9 gallons of paint for $23.28 per gallon from one supplier and 17 gallons of paint for $18.72. About how much did Gavin pay in total for the paint?

Step 1: Estimate the cost of paint from the first supplier.

9 gallons of paint is about 10 gallons.

$23.28 is about $20.

$10 \times \$20 = \$200$

Step 2: Estimate the cost of paint from the second supplier.

17 gallons of paint is about 15 gallons.

$18.72 is about $20.

$15 \times \$20 = \$300$

Step 3: Estimate the total cost of paint.

$\$200 + \$300 = \$500$

Gavin paid about $500 for paint.

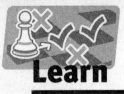
Roman Numerals

The basic symbols used in Roman numerals are shown below.

1	5	10	50	100	500	1,000
I	V	X	L	C	D	M

To write Roman numerals, follow these rules:

- There is no Roman numeral for 0.

- Roman numerals cannot include more than three of the same symbol.

- Each numeral can be modified by adding or subtracting specific other numerals:

    X can be modified by I and V

    L can be modified by X

    C can be modified by X

    D can be modified by C

    M can be modified by C

- To show addition, lower-value numerals are shown to the right of the higher-value numeral. For instance, VI represents 5 + 1, or 6.

- To show subtraction, lower-value numerals are shown to the left of the higher-value numeral. For instance, IV represents 5 – 1, or 4.

- The only numerals that can be placed to the left of a higher numeral in order to indicate subtraction are I, X, C, M, (1, 10, 100, 1,000) or any greater powers of 10.

The table below shows some numbers written in standard numerals and Roman numerals.

Standard Numeral	Roman Numeral	Standard Numeral	Roman Numeral
1	I	9	IX
2	II	10	X
3	III	20	XX
4	IV	30	XXX
5	V	40	XL
6	VI	50	L
7	VII	75	LXXV
8	VIII	125	CXXV

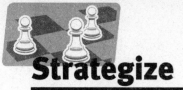
Strategize

Use Expanded Form

To write a standard number using Roman numerals, start by writing the number in expanded form. In expanded form, a number is shown as the sum of the values of its digits.

For example, $3{,}471 = 3{,}000 + 400 + 70 + 1$

Next, use Roman numerals to represent each component of the expanded form.

$3{,}000 = 1{,}000 + 1{,}000 + 1{,}000 = MMM$

$400 = 500 - 100 = CD$

$70 = 50 + 10 + 10 = LXX$

$1 = I$

Finally, combine the Roman numerals.

$3{,}471 = MMMCDLXXI$

Stop at Three

When you write a number using Roman numerals, remember that any Roman numeral is never used more than three times in that number. If you find you need to write the same numeral more than three times, use the next-largest numeral instead, writing a smaller numeral to the left to show subtraction. For instance:

- If you write 4 as IIII, you would have too many Is. So, bump I up to V. Record an I to the left of V to indicate subtraction: $4 = IV$.

- If you write 9 as VIIII, you would have too many Is. So, bump V up to X. Record an I to the left of X to indicate subtraction: $9 = IX$.

- If you write 140 as CXXXX, you would have too many Xs. So, bump X up to L. Record an X to the left of L to indicate subtraction: $140 = CXL$.

Break Apart and Translate

To change from Roman numerals to standard numerals, expand the Roman numeral into its component groupings and translate each numeral or group of numerals. Then, add those values together.

If any single Roman numeral in the number is followed by a numeral that is greater than it, group those numerals into a pair.

- For example:

  $MCDXVI = M + CD + X + V + I$

  $\qquad\quad = 1{,}000 + 400 + 10 + 5 + 1$

  $\qquad\quad = 1{,}416$

Because $C = 100$ and $D = 500$, and yet C is to the left of D, we paired C and D together into CD while breaking the numerals apart.

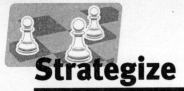

Strategize

If any Roman numeral is repeated 2 or 3 times in a row, group the repeated numerals.

- For example:

MCCCVII = M + CCC + V + II

= 1,000 + 300 + 5 + 2

= 1,307

When breaking the Roman numeral apart, the three Cs are grouped together and the two Is are grouped together.

Apply

A4. Write MMLXXXIV as a standard number.

Step 1: Break Apart the Roman Numeral

Group XXX because X is repeated. Group IV because I < V and yet I is to the left of V in the number.

MMLXXXIV = MM + L + XXX + IV

Step 2: Translate Each Component

MM = 1,000 + 1,000 = 2,000

L = 50

XXX = 10 + 10 + 10 = 30

IV = 5 − 1 = 4

Step 3: Write the Standard Number

2,000 + 50 + 30 + 4 = 2,084

Guided Practice

Let's work through a few examples together. Look back at the lesson content as often as necessary to help you apply the concepts and strategies you learn.

1. A caterer prepares 204 portions of salmon for a banquet. Each portion weighs about 5 ounces, or about 142 grams. About how many grams of salmon did the caterer prepare?

   A) 30,000 g

   B) 10,000 g

   C) 3,000 g

   D) 1,000 g

   STEP 1: What operation do you need to perform?

   _____

   STEP 2: What compatible numbers can you use?

   _____

   STEP 3: What is the product of the compatible numbers?

   _____

Guided Practice

2. An interest-free checking account has a balance of $2,819.45 on March 1. During the month of March, there are three withdrawals for $101.25 each, one withdrawal of $2,569.10, one withdrawal of $1,064.37, and two deposits of $2,335.91 each. What is the account balance on March 31?

A) $1,420.64

B) $2,084.85

C) $3,554.05

D) $11,428.59

STEP 1: What was the total amount withdrawn?

_____

STEP 2: What was the total amount deposited?

_____

STEP 3: What was the ending balance?

_____

3. Which is equal to 3,309?

   A) MMMCDIX

   B) MMMCCCIX

   C) MMMCCCXC

   D) MMMXXXIV

STEP 1: How can you write 3,309 in expanded form?

_____

STEP 2: Will you use addition or subtraction of Roman numerals for each part of the expanded form?

_____

STEP 3: How can you represent 3,309 using Roman numerals?

_____

_____

Independent Practice

You are ready to show what you know! Answer the questions below without looking back at the lesson content. Use the Hints to help you.

---

1. **Population density is the average number of people per square mile in a given area. Last year, the population of a county with area 684 square miles had a population of 342,906. Choose the best estimate of the population per square mile of the county.**

   A) 400 people per square mile

   B) 500 people per square mile

   C) 4,000 people per square mile

   D) 5,000 people per square mile

   > HINT *Divide the population by the area to find the population per square mile. Round each number or choose compatible numbers before dividing.*

2. **Christopher Columbus arrived in the New World in 1492. How is this year written using Roman numerals?**

   A) MCDXLII

   B) MCDXCII

   C) MCCCCXCII

   D) MCDCCXCII

   > HINT *Write the year in expanded form. Remember to stop at three.*

3. **A part-time employee at a retail store earns $10.25 per hour. During one pay period, she works 18 hours. Her deductions during that pay period are $27.68 for federal income tax, $14.76 for state income tax, and $14.11 for payroll taxes. What was her take home pay for the pay period?**

   A) $66.80

   B) $127.95

   C) $184.50

   D) $241.05

   > HINT *A deduction is an amount that is taken away. Use subtraction to represent deductions.*

ReKap

Estimation

- Use estimation when an exact answer is not needed or to check whether your answer is reasonable.

- To estimate, round the numbers or choose compatible numbers that are easy to work with.

- After you estimate, use process of elimination to narrow down the answer choices.

Working with Money

- To solve problems involving money, apply your understanding of operations with decimals.

- Round answers to the nearest cent (hundredth) if needed.

- Words like *deduction*, *debit*, and *withdrawal* should be represented with subtraction.

- Words like *credit* and *deposit* should be represented with addition.

Roman Numerals

- The basic symbols used in Roman numerals are shown below.

1	5	10	50	100	500	1,000
I	V	X	L	C	D	M

- Never use more than three of the same numeral to represent a place value.

- Write standard numbers and Roman numerals in expanded form to change from one system to the other.

? **How can you use estimation to help you solve a problem that involves working with money?**

_____

_____

_____

Answers

Guided Practice

1. Step 1: multiplication

    Step 2: 200 and 150 are compatible numbers to use

    Step 3: $200 \times 150 = 30,000$

    Answer: (A) 30,000 g

2. Step 1: The total amount withdrawn is $3,937.22 (three withdrawals of $101.25 each, and then two additional withdrawals of $2,569.10 and $1,064.37 each)

    Step 2: The total amount deposited is $4,671.82 (two deposits of equal amounts, $2,335.91)

    Step 3: $2,819.45 - $3,937.22 + $4,671.82 = $3,554.05

    Answer: (C) $3,554.05

3. Step 1: $3,309 = 3000 + 300 + 9$

    Step 2: MMM + CCC + IX (addition, addition, subtraction)

    Step 3: MMMCCCIX

    Answer: (B) MMMCCCIX

Independent Practice

1. **Answer: (D) 5,000 people per square mile**

    Choose compatible numbers: 684 is close to 700 and 342,906 is close to 350,000.

    $350,000 \div 700 = 5,000$

    TIP: Be careful when multiplying and dividing the compatible numbers and make sure that you have written the correct number of zeros in the problem and the answer. If you had skimmed the answer choices, you might have chosen B because it begins with a 5.

2. **Answer: (B) MCDXCII**

    Write 1492 in expanded form: $1,000 + 400 + 90 + 2$

    $1,000 = M$

    $400 = CD$

    $90 = XC$

    $2 = II$

    $1492 = MCDXCII$

    Choice A is incorrect because MDCXLII = M + DC + XL + II = $1,000 + 400 + 40 + 2 = 1,442$.

    Choices C and D are incorrect because they use four Cs instead of CD. Remember that no Roman numeral can appear more than 3 times in a row.

3. **Answer: (B) $127.95**

    Find the total wages: $18 \times \$10.25 = \$184.50$

    Find the total deductions: $\$27.68 + \$14.76 + \$14.11 = \$56.55$

    Subtract the deductions from the wages: $\$184.50 - \$56.55 = \$127.95$

ReKap

Estimations can help solve problems that involve working with money as often variables include dollars and cents. Rounding to whole numbers, or even ten-cent intervals can make the addition, subtraction, multiplication, and division easier. Questions on the admissions test are multiple choice, estimating should allow one to eliminate 1 or 2 or 3 answer choices.

UNIT
4 Science

4 SCIENCE · LESSON 1
Scientific Reasoning

Science is at the heart of health care. It is a process that uses experimentation, technology, and mathematics to develop theories that continually evolve as technology advances and discoveries are made. This lesson will reintroduce you to the scientific method and how it is utilized to develop and use techniques in medicine. So let's get scientific!

Common Uses in Health Care

- the development of new treatment protocols
- the creation of new medicines
- the treatment of individual patients

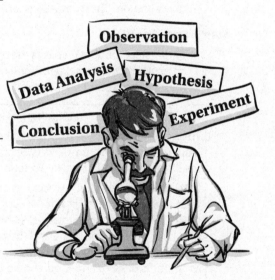

Key Terms/Formulas

- **conclusion** – a statement that analyzes the data

- **control** – the group that does not receive the experimental protocol

- **data** – measurements and observations

- **experiment** – a carefully designed procedure

- **hypothesis** – a testable statement

- **inference** – a conclusion based on the assumption of something being true

- **model** – usually a graph, chart, or diagram

- **observation** – a problem that needs to be solved

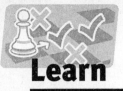

Learn

SCIENCE IS A METHOD

When some people hear the word science, they think of the large body of knowledge that has been discovered by scientists over the centuries. But science is not a body of knowledge contained in some huge collection of books. Science is a method. Specifically, it is a method of investigating things that are observable and measurable. When you encounter a phenomenon that makes you curious, you can use science to learn about it. Below are the five basic steps of the scientific method.

There is no official list of steps that makes up the scientific method. You may encounter slightly different wordings of the scientific method in other texts. The spirit of the method is the same across the board.

Step 1: Observation

In this step, a scientist notices something that sparks his or her curiosity or identifies a problem that needs to be solved.

Step 2: Hypothesis

In this step, the scientist formulates a testable statement, called a *hypothesis*, based on his or her original observation. Another way to think about a hypothesis is that it is a temporary explanation of the observation that will be tested in later steps of the investigation. These later steps will determine if the hypothesis is correct or incorrect.

Step 3: Experiment

In this step, the scientist tests the hypothesis using a carefully designed procedure, called an *experiment*. In an experiment, measurements and observations are collected. These measurements and observations become the *data* that the scientist will later analyze.

Designing an Effective, Ethical Experiment

The gold standard in medical experimentation is the randomized, double-blind, placebo-controlled study. This type of study is considered to be good science, so the results of these studies are taken seriously.

In this type of study, the participants are randomly assigned to one of two groups, the treatment group or the control group. This is called *randomization*. There must be only one difference between the treatment group and the control group: the treatment group receives the medicine and the control group does not. Usually, the control group receives a *placebo*, which is a false treatment such as a sugar pill. All other variables, such as amounts of sleep and food, should be the same for the two groups.

Such studies will often be *double-blind*, meaning that neither the participants nor the researchers know who has received the placebo and who has received the actual treatment. Double-blind design prevents the researchers and participants from believing that the experimental medicine is having an effect when it actually might not be.

A good experiment will have a large *sample size*, or number of participants. The bigger the sample size and the more similar it is to the real human population, the better. This will make the results more reliable. The experimental procedure must also be recorded in great detail so that other scientists can repeat the experiment and confirm the results.

It's not just good design scientists need to worry about; they must also make sure their experiments are ethical. Experimenters use informed consent forms to let human participants know of the potential risks and benefits of participating in the study. Experimenters who use animals are expected to treat them humanely.

Step 4: Data Analysis

In this step, the scientist finds out more about what the data mean and determines if they are reliable. To be reliable, there needs to be a lot of data, not just a few measurements.

Step 5: Conclusion

In this step, the scientist uses the results of his or her data analysis to determine whether the data support his hypothesis. Scientists must often make **inferences** to form conclusions because they cannot always directly observe what they are attempting to study.

Scientific Models

Conclusions help scientists develop models. Scientific **models** usually take the form of diagrams, graphs, or charts. They are constructed from data gained through experimentation and they enable scientists to predict the results of future tests of the same phenomenon. Models are continually changed and refined as new technologies emerge and more data are collected. Because models change, it is important to realize their limitations. The predictions that models imply should not be too broadly applied.

Math and Technology: The Scientist's Most Important Tools

The knowledge we gain through the scientific process is greatly enhanced by the application of math and technology. Without math and technology, scientists would be limited in their ability to advance their theories and refine their models.

Technology is often used by scientists to enhance their senses and improve communication. Before the microscope was invented, biologists could not observe the cells that make up living tissue. Before the telescope was invented, astronomers could not observe the distant celestial objects that allow them to more fully understand the universe. As technology advances with inventions like spectrometers and sophisticated medical imagers, scientists can peer ever deeper into the nature of reality. Also, advances in communication technologies such as the Internet speed up the pace of scientific progress by enabling scientists to instantly share their discoveries with one another.

Math is the language of science. It is used to demonstrate the validity of data, to create models, and to make predictions about the future. Sometimes scientists create whole new branches of mathematics to describe their observations, such as when Isaac Newton invented calculus to complement his study of motion.

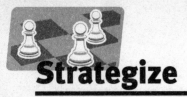

Strategize

Reflect

To help yourself remember the steps of the scientific method, think of the last time you used them. We all use the scientific method—practically on a daily basis—to learn about the world around us.

Think about the first time you encountered a hot stove as a child. You likely made the *observation* (step 1) that the stove looked different because there was a bright flame coming out of it. You *hypothesized* (step 2) that since the stove looked different, it would feel different to the touch. You may have conducted a simple *experiment* (step 3) to test your hypothesis by touching the stove. You *analyzed the data* (step 4) from your experiment by evaluating the sensation of heat, and perhaps pain, that you felt while touching the stove. Finally, you drew the *conclusion* (step 5) that you should not again touch the stove when a bright flame is coming out of it.

Thinking about the incident described above, and other times where you used the scientific method to learn something simple about the world, can demystify the method and help you remember the steps more easily.

Apply

Here are some examples of questions you might see when you take the admissions test.

A1. A scientist is studying the effects of a medication to determine its efficiency in lessening the severity of migraine headaches. How can the scientist be sure that she produces reliable results?

A) She uses a large number of participants in the study.

B) She publishes her findings in a peer-reviewed journal.

C) She forms a hypothesis before beginning the experiment.

D) She records and analyzes her data in a computer-generated chart.

Step 1: Reread and Realize:

What is the question asking you to do?

Realize: The question is asking how the scientist can produce reliable results.

Step 2: Remember:

Remember how to design a reliable experiment.

Step 3: Rule Out:

Eliminate the choices that are not about designing an experiment.

Choice B is about what happens after the experiment is over.

Choice C is about the steps of the scientific method.

Choice D is about recording data.

This means the correct answer is A!

Apply

A2. A biologist is studying how saltwater fish are affected by the temperature of the water. He conducts an experiment in the lab to determine how the temperature of water affects the amount of dissolved oxygen in a saltwater solution. He performs several trials and averages the data. His results are shown in the data table below.

Temperature of Water			
Average Concentration of Dissolved Oxygen in mg/L	32°C	21°C	8°C
	8.6	7.2	5.0

What can the biologist conclude from his results?

A) Saltwater fish thrive in water with higher temperatures.

B) Saltwater fish are unaffected by the temperature of the water.

C) The amount of dissolved oxygen in saltwater is unaffected by temperature.

D) The amount of dissolved oxygen in saltwater increases as temperature increases.

Step 1: Reread and Realize:

What is the question asking you to do?

It is asking you to form a conclusion based on the biologist's results.

Step 2: Remember:

A conclusion analyzes the data of the experiment.

Step 3: Rule Out:

Eliminate the answer choices that do not support the data. Look at each choice and compare it to the information given.

Choices A and B: The data does not mention anything about the effects of water temperature on saltwater fish. You can eliminate these two.

Choice C: You can see that the amount of dissolved oxygen changes with the temperature. Therefore, you can rule out this choice.

That leaves you with Choice D, the correct answer!

Guided Practice

1. A group of researchers is designing a study to test the effect of a specially formulated, vitamin-infused drink on the duration of the common cold in the general population. They gather 200 participants, 165 women and 35 men. They randomly assign 100 participants to the control group and 100 participants to the treatment group. During the trial, the members of the control group will receive a placebo drink and the members of the treatment group will receive the vitamin-infused drink. In what way could the design of this experiment be improved?

   A) More participants should have received the vitamin-infused drink.

   B) More participants should have received the placebo drink.

   C) More men should have been gathered for the experiment.

   D) More women should have been gathered for the experiment.

STEP 1: Reread and Realize

Reread the question. What is the question asking you to do? Write down the details of the question that are related to the answer choices.

_____

_____

_____

STEP 2: Remember

Reread the section about designing a good experiment. Think about what makes up a good experiment. What makes an experiment's results reliable?

_____

_____

_____

STEP 3: Rule-out

Try to eliminate the final incorrect answer choice. Hint: Reread the paragraph about sample size. Which answer choice can you now eliminate and why?

_____

_____

_____

_____

2. Which option describes a researcher using technology to help make observations that cannot normally be detected by the senses?

A) a doctor installing an artificial heart into a heart transplant patient

B) a chemist using a computer to perform fast calculations on her data

C) an astronomer using a radio telescope to detect non-visible radiation from space

D) a zoologist comparing a lizard to pictures in a book to identify its species

STEP 1: Reread and realize

On the lines provided, write the purpose of the technology you must identify to answer the question.

_____

_____

_____

_____

STEP 2: Remember

On the lines below, identify the piece of technology included in each option and describe its purpose.

_____

_____

_____

_____

STEP 3: Rule-out

On the lines below, list the options you can eliminate because the technologies are not being used to extend the senses of a researcher. Which option is left?

_____

_____

_____

_____

Guided Practice

3. The model below shows how a population of the bacterium *Staphylococcus aureus* responds to an increasing concentration of the antibiotic erythromycin.

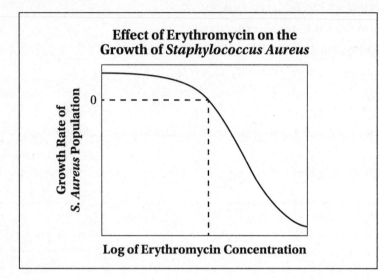

Which prediction is supported by the model?

A) Erythromycin can shrink a population of *Staphylococcus aureus*.

B) Erythromycin can shrink a population of any species of bacteria.

C) Any antibiotic can shrink a population of *Staphylococcus aureus*.

D) Any antibiotic can shrink a population of any species of bacteria.

STEP 1: Reread and Realize

Look at the chart carefully. What is the name of the antibiotic used in the model? What is the name of the bacterium?

_____

_____

_____

STEP 2: Remember

Reread the portion of the lesson text about models. What does the text have to say about applying the predictions made by models too broadly?

_____

_____

_____

STEP 3: Rule-out

Eliminate the answers that go beyond the scope of the information in the model. Which answer choice is left?

_____

_____

_____

_____

Independent Practice

1. A group of researchers wants to improve upon an existing chemotherapy protocol for early-stage breast cancer in women. The researchers gather a group of 1,000 women with early-stage breast cancer and randomly divide them into two groups of equal size. What treatments should each group receive?

   A) The treatment group should receive the experimental protocol and the control group should receive the existing protocol.

   B) The treatment group should receive the existing protocol and the control group should receive the experimental protocol.

   C) Both groups should receive the experimental protocol.

   D) Both groups should receive the existing protocol.

   HINT *The objective of this study is to compare a new protocol to an existing protocol, so the existing protocol must be included in the study as the control treatment.*

2. A researcher is designing an experiment to compare a new conductor material to the most commonly used conductor in transistors. Which procedure would be best to include in his experiment?

   A) Measure the resistance of the new conductor 10 times and compare it to the known resistance of the existing conductor.

   B) Measure the resistance of the new and old conductors 10 times each under the same conditions and compare the two results.

   C) Measure the resistance of the new conductor 50 times and compare it to the known resistance of the existing conductor.

   D) Measure the resistance of the new and old conductors 50 times each under the same conditions and compare the two results.

3. Repeated use of antibiotics causes bacteria to become resistant to them. During the 20th century, the bacterium *Staphylococcus aureus* became highly resistant to penicillin. Which model accurately reflects the development of penicillin resistance in *S. aureus*?

A)

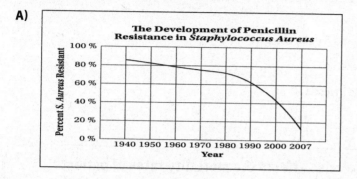

B)

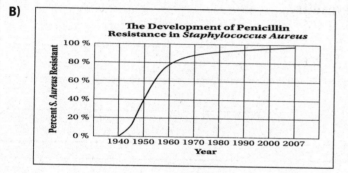

C)

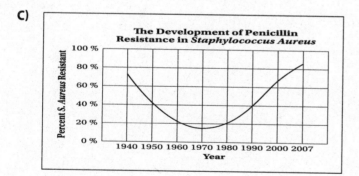

D)

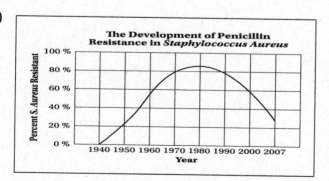

ReKap

In this lesson, you learned that science is a method of investigating things that are measurable and observable. Remember the following:

- The steps of the scientific method are: observation, hypothesis, experiment, analyzing data, and drawing conclusions.

- A good experiment must be reliable, ethical and free of bias.

- Models can change as new evidence is gathered.

- Technology plays an integral part in scientific investigation.

> **?** **A doctor is investigating how exercise affects the mortality rates of patients who have suffered a heart attack. Explain how she can plan and carry out this investigation to produce reliable results.**
>
> _____
>
> _____
>
> _____
>
> _____

Answers

Guided Practice

1. Step 1: Figure out how the design of the experiment could be better.

   Step 2: A good experiment will have a large sample size, or number of participants, reflective of the population. Reliable results can be reproduced.

   Step 3: Choice D can be eliminated, as there are more women than men gathered. More, an equal number of participants received the vitamin-infused drink as did the placebo, eliminate Choice A and B.

   Answer: (C) More men should have been gathered for the experiment.

2. Step 1: The purpose of technology is to help make observations that cannot normally be detected by the senses.

   Step 2: In (A), the technology is the artificial heart for the purpose of replacing a damaged heart; (B) computer, fast calculations, (C) radio telescope, detecting non-visible radiation; (D) book, to identify species.

   Step 3: Eliminate Choices A, B, and D because the technology is not being used to extend the senses of the researcher.

   Answer: (C) an astronomer using a radio telescope to detect non-visible radiation from space

3. Step 1: The antibiotic is erythromycin; the bacterium, *Staphylococcus aureus*.

   Step 2: Predictions from models should not be used broadly.

   Step 3: Eliminate Choices B, C, and D – all go beyond the scope of the information in the model.

   Answer: (A) Erythromycin can shrink a population of *Staphylococcus aureus*.

Independent Practice

1. **Answer: (A) The treatment group should receive the experimental protocol and the control group should receive the existing protocol.**

   In this case, the original protocol takes the place of the placebo, since the point of the study is to improve upon the protocol.

2. **Answer: (D) Measure the resistance of the new and old conductors 50 times each under the same conditions and compare the two results.**

   Every experiment must have a control group, so the existing conductor should be included in this procedure. The larger the sample size or greater number of trials, the better.

3. **Answer: (B)**

   Choice B is the only model to illustrate only an increase in resistance. Answer choice A shows decreasing resistance over time. Choice C shows resistance decreasing before it increases, and Choice D shows resistance that increases but then decreases.

ReKap

To produce reliable results, the investigation should include a large, randomly selected sample that is representative of the population. More, the investigator should record results in great detail so the experiment can be repeated.

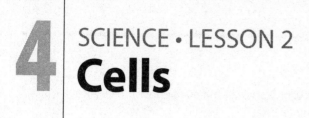

SCIENCE · LESSON 2
Cells

What does a human have in common with seaweed? They might not look similar, but humans and seaweed are both made up of cells. All living organisms are made of cells, from the simple single-celled bacteria to the giant blue whales.

Understanding how cells work and knowing the different types of cells are essential skills in biology and health care. Knowing how cells function will help you to understand how the body works.

Common Uses in Health Care

- interpreting red and white blood cell counts

- using antibiotics to inhibit growth of bacterial cells

- understanding organelle-based diseases such as cystic fibrosis

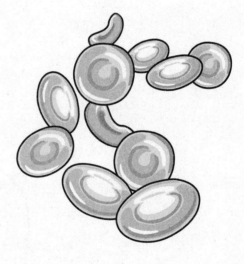

Key Terms/Formulas

- **active transport** – movement of substances against the concentration gradient

- **autotroph** – organism that makes its own food

- **cellular respiration** – process used by cells to release energy from glucose

- **heterotroph** – organism that cannot synthesize its own food

- **organelles –** *small organs* or functional parts of a cell

- **passive transport** – movement of substances with the concentration gradient

- **photosynthesis** – process used by cells to form glucose, using energy from the sun

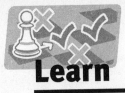

Cell Structure

We can group cells into two basic categories: prokaryotes and eukaryotes. Prokaryotes are bacteria, while eukaryotes are plant and animal cells.

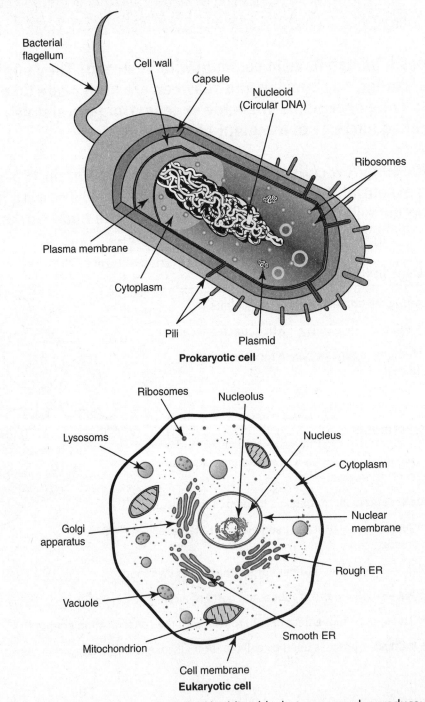

Prokaryotic cell

Eukaryotic cell

Both types of cells use energy and chemical building blocks to grow and reproduce; however, they use different processes and cell structures, called *organelles*, to accomplish these goals.

There are many different organelles to remember. It helps to summarize them by function and cell type:

Function	Prokaryote Organelles	Eukaryote Organelles	Similarities/Differences
Hold and protect cell contents	Cell membrane	Cell membrane	Both are semi-permeable.
	Cell wall	Cell wall (only in plants)	Plant cell walls are made of cellulose; prokaryote cell walls are made of various other polysaccharides and proteins.
Supports cell contents	Cytoplasm	Cytoplasm	Gel-like protein fluid.
DNA storage	Nucleoid	Nucleus	Nucleoid is a cluster of DNA in the cytoplasm; nucleus is bound by membranes.
Protein synthesis	Ribosomes	Ribosomes	Smaller and free-floating in prokaryotes; larger and attached to ER in eukaryotes.
		Golgi apparatus	Refines and finishes proteins made by eukaryotic ribosomes.
		Endoplasmic reticulum (ER)	Moves eukaryotic proteins within the cell or out of the cell.
Locomotion	Flagella	Flagella or cilia	Prokaryotic flagella are single fibers; eukaryotic flagella and cilia are bundles of microtubules.
Assembling ribosome parts		Nucleolus	Prokaryote ribosomes assembled entirely in the cytoplasm; eukaryote ribosomes subunits assembled in the nucleolus and transported out of the nucleus for final assembly.
Producing cellular fuel (ATP)		Mitochondria	Metabolism of food occurs in the cytoplasm and cell membrane of prokaryotes; eukaryotes have a specific membrane-bound organelle for the purpose.
Photosynthesis		Chloroplasts	Chloroplasts are only found in plant cells; photosynthesis occurs in sites on the cell membrane in photosynthetic prokaryotes.
Storage		Vesicles	Prokaryotes store compounds in the cytoplasm; eukaryotic cells use vacuoles, lysosomes, and peroxisomes to store water, enzymes, toxic chemicals, and other compounds.

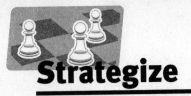

Strategize

Reread, Remember, Rule Out

To succeed on questions about organelles,

Step 1: Always **reread** the question. Figure out what the question is asking you to do.

Step 2: Remember which organelles are in which type of cells.

Step 3: Using the information you remembered, predict the correct organelles and function, and **rule out** the choices that do not match.

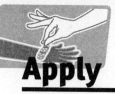

Apply

A1. Many antibiotics work by interfering with protein synthesis in bacteria. Which organelle would these antibiotics most likely affect?

A) Cell membrane

B) Golgi Apparatus

C) Mitochondrion

D) Ribosome

STEP 1: Reread and Realize

What is the question asking? Reread the question and put the two parts together—it is asking which organelle is involved with protein synthesis in bacteria, which are prokaryotes.

STEP 2: Remember

Which organelle is involved in protein synthesis in prokaryotes? The ribosomes.

A2. The antibiotics mentioned in Example 1 do not affect human cells—why?

STEP 1: Reread and Realize

What is the question asking? Reread the question and incorporate your answer to Example 1. Why wouldn't the ribosomes in humans (eukaryotes) be affected by the same things as the ribosomes in prokaryotes?

STEP 2: Remember

How are the ribosomes in eukaryotes different from those in prokaryotes? They are larger, and attached to the ER. Both of these differences suggest that eukaryote and prokaryote ribosomes could react differently to antibiotics.

STEP 3 Rule Out

Based on what you remembered, predict the correct answer. Then, look at each answer choice and see if the organelle matches the function described in the question.

Choice A: The cell membrane allows materials in and out of the cell. It is not involved in protein synthesis.

Choice B: The Golgi apparatus is involved in protein synthesis, but only in eukaryote cells. Bacteria are prokaryotic.

Choice C: Mitochondria supply energy for the cell.

We ruled out choices A, B, and C. Therefore, the correct answer is D, ribosomes, which is what we predicted from Step 2.

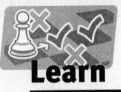

Passive and Active Transport

All cells need to transport materials in and out to live. Eukaryotic cells also need to transport materials in and out of their organelles. This transport can either be passive (no energy needed from the cell) or active (the cell must put energy into the process).

All molecules are in constant, random motion. The motion of liquid and gaseous molecules causes them to spread out evenly in their container. You can see this when you add a drop of dye to a glass of water. The dye molecules spread out until they are evenly distributed throughout the water. The motion of the dye molecules is random, but the net motion of the molecules is from high concentration to low concentration, until the concentration is equal everywhere.

Passive Transport

When there is a net movement of substances from high to low concentration, it is called *passive transport*. It is also often referred to as *diffusion*. *Osmosis* is a special term used to describe diffusion of water through a semi-permeable membrane. There will always be a net movement of water through a semi-permeable member if the concentration of water is different on each side of the membrane.

We don't usually indicate the concentration of water in a solution; instead, we indicate the concentration of solute (the material dissolved in the water). This can be a source of confusion when talking about osmosis, since it is the water that moves and not the solute. Therefore, water will move from where it has a higher concentration (low concentration of solute) to where it has a lower concentration (high concentration of solute). Trace the movement of water in the cells below, and verify that the water is moving from high concentration (low solute concentration) to low concentration (high solute concentration):

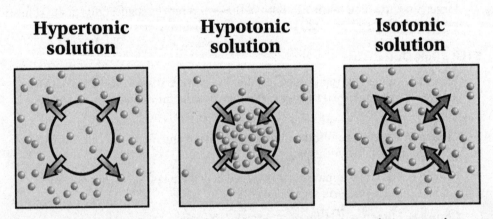

Arrows represent direction that water moves via osmosis.

The environments shown above are described as *hypotonic* (low solute concentration), *hypertonic* (high solute concentration), and *isotonic* (equal solute concentration inside and outside the cell).

Active Transport

Cells often need to move substances from a low concentration to a high concentration. They do this in a process called active transport. For example, the concentration of nutrients outside a cell might be lower than the concentration in the cytoplasm, so the cell must use energy to move nutrients across the membrane, against the direction in which the substances would normally move. Cells accomplish this using transport proteins, which act like pumps, in their membranes. When energy is supplied to the transport protein, it binds to the substance on one side of the membrane and then releases it on the other side of the membrane.

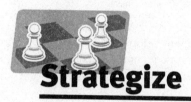

Strategize

Visualize

You can remember the differences between passive and active transport by visualizing the concentration differences:

- Passive moves *downhill* from high to low, and therefore needs no added energy.

- Active moves *uphill* from low to high, and therefore needs added energy.

You can avoid confusion about hypo-, hyper-, and isotonic solutions by visualizing the concentration of water in the solution:

- **Hypotonic:** Solute concentration is lower, therefore water concentration is higher; water will move from the extracellular space to the intracellular space.

- **Hypertonic:** Solute concentration is higher, therefore water concentration is lower; water will move from the intracellular space to the extracellular space.

- **Isotonic:** Solute concentration is the same, therefore water concentration is the same; no net movement of water in or out of the cell.

You can remember hypo-, hyper- and iso- by looking at other words you already know. For example:

- Hypo- (under) is used in *hypodermic needle* which is a needle that goes *under* the skin.

- Hyper- (over) is used in *hyperactive* which describes an *over*active child.

- Iso- (same) is used in *isometric* which describes an exercise in which your body parts stay in the *same* position.

A3. A researcher places a red blood cell into distilled water. She observes that water moves into the cell, and then movement ceases. Which statement best describes this observation?

A) The cell has undergone active transport.

B) The cell has undergone passive transport.

C) The cell has become hypertonic.

D) The cell has become hypotonic.

STEP 1: Reread and Realize

What is the question asking? Reread the question and put the two parts together—it is asking whether the water was moving from a high concentration to a low concentration (passive) or from a low concentration to a high concentration (active).

STEP 2: Visualize and Remember

Distilled water has no solutes -it contains only one water molecule- while a cell has proteins and salts in its cytoplasm. The water was moving from high concentration of water to low concentration of water, or going *downhill*.

Hypotonic solution

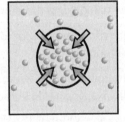

STEP 3: Rule Out

Since the water was moving *downhill*, we can predict that the cell has undergone passive transport (osmosis). Let's rule out the other choices to be sure.

Choice A: In active transport, water will move from a low concentration to a high concentration. This is the opposite of what has happened in the question.

Choice C: The water stopped moving into the cell, so this means that concentration has become equal, or isotonic.

Choice D: The water stopped moving, so this means that concentration is equal, or isotonic inside and outside of the cell.

Therefore, the correct answer is B, passive transport!

Apply

A4. A scientist places a red blood cell into distilled water and observes water moving into the cell. In this case, the distilled water is _____ to the red blood cell.

A) Active

B) Hypotonic

C) Hypertonic

D) Passive

STEP 1: Reread and Realize

Which choice fits best into the given statement? You need to figure out if the concentration of solute is higher in distilled water or in the red blood cell.

STEP 2: Visualize and Remember

When the concentration of water is higher, the concentration of solute is lower. Since water is moving into the cell, that means that the concentration of solute is higher inside the cell.

STEP 3 Rule Out

Based on what you remembered in Step 2, the distilled water would be hypotonic to the red blood cell because its concentration of solute is lower.

Let's rule out the other choices to be sure.

Choice A: *Active* is a type of transport. It doesn't describe the relationship of the distilled water to the cell.

Choice C: In a hypertonic environment, the concentration of solute would be higher in the distilled water. This would mean the water would move out of the cell and into the distilled water. This is the opposite of what is happening.

Choice D: *Passive* is a type of transport. Like *Active*, it doesn't describe a relationship between the distilled water and the red blood cell.

Therefore, the correct answer is Choice B, *hypotonic*.

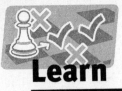

Learn

Cellular Respiration and Photosynthesis

All cells need energy, in the form of *ATP* (adenosine triphosphate) to live. The basic way they access ATP is by processing glucose; plants (autotrophs) make their own glucose, but animals and non-photosynthetic bacteria (heterotrophs) must consume plants (or other animals) to obtain that glucose. Autotrophs use photosynthesis to make the glucose; both autotrophs and heterotrophs use cellular respiration to release the ATP. Photosynthesis and cellular respiration are mirror images of each other—photosynthesis backwards looks like cellular respiration and vice versa. In prokaryotes, both processes are done in the cell membrane or cytoplasm, but in eukaryotes, each process is done by a specific organelle. Look at the following table for a comparison:

	Photosynthesis	Cellular Respiration
Organelle	Chloroplasts	Mitochondria
Main chemical	Chlorophyll	Citric acid derivatives
Reactants	CO_2, H_2O, photons (sun energy)	$C_6H_{12}O_6$ (Glucose), O_2
Products	$C_6H_{12}O_6$ (Glucose), O_2	CO_2, H_2O, ATP (energy for cells)

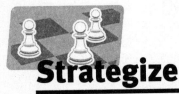

Strategize

Reread and Realize, Remember, Rule Out

When you are answering questions about cellular respiration and photosynthesis, use these steps to successfully find the correct answer.

- **Reread** the question and find details that help you to **realize** what the question is asking you to do.

- Next, **remember** the facts about cellular respiration and photosynthesis that are related to the question. This will allow you to predict the correct answer.

- Finally, use the facts you remembered to help you **rule out** the incorrect answer choices.

Apply

A5. Why can plants live for days without sunlight, but animals can't live without oxygen for more than a few minutes?

A) Plants can make and store glucose, but animal cells cannot store energy.

B) Plants have mitochondria to provide energy, but animal cells do not contain mitochondria.

C) Plants use carbon dioxide to produce oxygen, and animal cells use oxygen to produce carbon dioxide.

D) Plants produce water as a product of photosynthesis, and animal cells produce water as a product of cellular respiration.

STEP 1: Reread and Realize

What is the question asking? Reread the question and put the two parts together—it is asking for the difference between how a plant uses sunlight and how an animal uses oxygen.

STEP 2: Visualize and Remember

Why do plants need sunlight? To produce glucose. Why do animals need oxygen? To turn glucose into energy for their cells. Plants can store glucose, but animals can't store energy, so a plant can last much longer without making glucose than an animal can without energy.

STEP 3 Rule Out

You figured out from Step 2 that A is probably the correct answer, but let's look at all the other choices to be sure.

Choice B: Plants have mitochondria which are the *powerhouse* of the cell, but animal cells also have mitochondria.

Choice C: This statement is true, but it is unrelated to why animal cells cannot survive without oxygen for more than a few minutes. Don't be tricked because the choice uses the word *oxygen*.

Choice D: Water is not a product of photosynthesis; glucose and oxygen are the products. Water is a product of cellular respiration, but this is unrelated to the question.

Therefore, Choice A is correct.

Guided Practice

Let's work through a few examples together. Look back at the lesson content as often as necessary to help you apply the concepts and strategies you learned.

1. Which of the following describes a structure found in a human cell but not in a bacterial cell?

   A) chloroplasts

   B) DNA

   C) mitochondria

   D) ribosomes

   STEP 1: Reread and realize

   What is the question asking you to do? Reread the item and find the important details.

   _____

   _____

   STEP 2: Remember

   Which structures are found in prokaryotes?

   _____

   _____

   _____

   _____

   STEP 3: Rule out

   Using your answer from Step 2, go through each answer choice. Which ones can you eliminate?

   _____

   _____

   _____

   _____

2. **Which of the following requires the input of energy?**

A) A cell shrivels up when placed in a very concentrated salt water solution.

B) When hot water is added to cold water, the temperature of the water gradually becomes a uniform temperature throughout.

C) An intestinal cell has a higher concentration of glucose than the fluid passing through the intestine, and more glucose continues to move into the cell.

D) When a semi-permeable membrane is used to separate two samples of distilled water, the same amount of water passes across the membrane in each direction.

STEP 1: Reread and realize

What is the question asking you to do?

_____

_____

STEP 2: Remember

In which direction (high to low or low to high) is the net movement of substances in active transport?

_____

_____

_____

_____

STEP 3: Rule out

Which choices can you eliminate? Determine which ones describe a concentration difference as a result. The choices that do not can be eliminated.

_____

_____

_____

_____

Guided Practice

3. The presence of which substance would indicate a eukaryotic cell is an autotroph?

   A) ATP

   B) chlorophyll

   C) glucose

   D) oxygen

STEP 1: Reread and realize

What is the question asking you to do? Reread the question and find the details that tell you.

_____

_____

STEP 2: Remember

Which substances are required for photosynthesis?

_____

_____

STEP 3: Rule out

Determine which answer choices can be eliminated. Are there substances that are used by both plants and animals?

_____

_____

_____

_____

Independent Practice

1. A researcher immerses a skin cell in a solution, and the cell swells up and then bursts. This suggests that the solution was _____ to the cell.

   A) hypotonic

   B) hypertonic

   C) isotonic

   D) keytonic

   HINT *Remember that the solution is described by the concentration of its solute, but water moves according to the concentration of water.*

2. A scientist is looking at a cell under a microscope. She observes these organelles: cell wall, ribosomes, and mitochondria. Which type of cell is the researcher most likely viewing?

   A) bacteria

   B) plant

   C) animal

   D) human

   HINT *Remember which structures are shared by all cell types and which are not.*

3. Which of the following best describes how plant cells access ATP?

   A) They use energy from sunlight and carbon dioxide to form glucose.

   B) They use passive transport to draw it in from a hypotonic solution.

   C) They consume other organisms that contain the ATP molecule.

   D) They combine carbon dioxide and water to produce citric acids.

   HINT *What do plants do that animal cells do not?*

ReKap

In this lesson you reviewed the structure of cells, how materials are transported into and out of cells, and the processes of cellular respiration and photosynthesis. Remember:

- There are two types of cells, prokaryotic and eukaryotic.

- Cell organelles are *little organs* that perform functions vital to the cell.

- Active transport requires energy and passive transport does not.

- Solutions can be hypotonic, hypertonic, or isotonic to a cell.

- Cellular respiration and photosynthesis are processes that help cells to acquire energy in the form ATP.

? **How will having knowledge about cells help you to better understand a patient's diagnosis?**

_____

_____

_____

_____

Answers

Guided Practice

1. Step 1: The question is asking you to identify what is in a human cell and not in a bacterial cell.

   Step 2: Prokaryotes contain DNA and ribosomes (of those listed above).

   Step 3: Eliminate Choices B and D (see above). Eliminate Choice A, as chloroplasts are found only in plant cells.

   Answer: (C) mitochondria

2. Step 1: The question is asking you to figure out which choice needs energy added.

   Step 2: The net movement of substances in active transport is from low to high concentration.

   Step 3: Eliminate Choice A (reflective of osmosis, diffusion of water through a semi-permeable membrane, a form of passive transportation – water moves from an area of higher concentration [cell] to lower concentration [surrounding solution]) and Choices B and D (neither describes a concentration difference as the result).

   Answer: (C) An intestinal cell has a higher concentration of glucose than the fluid passing through the intestine, and more glucose continues to move into the cell.

3. Step 1: The question is asking for you to state which choice shows that a eukaryotic (plant and animal) cell is an autotroph (plant).

   Step 2: Carbon dioxide, light energy, and water are required for photosynthesis.

   Step 3: Eliminate Choices A (all cells use ATP), C and D (glucose and oxygen are components of both photosynthesis and cellular respiration).

   Answer: (B) chlorophyll

Independent Practice

1. **Answer: (A) hypotonic**

   The cells swelled, so water moved from the solution into the cell. The water concentration in the solution was higher, so the solute concentration in the solution was lower. Hypo = under.

2. **Answer: (B) plant**

   Determine first if it is prokaryotic or eukaryotic and then continue to narrow, if needed. Cell wall: prokaryotes and some eukaryotes (plants). Ribosomes: prokaryotes and eukaryotes. Mitochondria: eukaryotes. Plants are eukaryotes and then have cell walls.

3. **Answer: (A) They use energy from sunlight and carbon dioxide to form glucose.**

   ATP is accessed by the processing of glucose. To process glucose, the cell must first obtain it. Plant cells make glucose through the process of photosynthesis. Sunlight and carbon dioxide are the reactants in photosynthesis, and glucose is a product.

ReKap

Knowledge about cells and transport can help to understand flow of solutes and fluid.

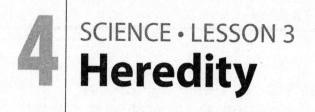

SCIENCE • LESSON 3
Heredity

Genetics and heredity have a powerful influence on patient responses to treatment. It is important that health care professionals have a thorough understanding of the nature of DNA and the patterns of heredity so that they can understand and explain the variation that so often confounds health care practices. This lesson will reacquaint you with these concepts.

Common Uses in Health Care

- testing for and treating genetic diseases

- predicting the spread of genetic diseases through families

- developing new treatments for genetic diseases and other diseases

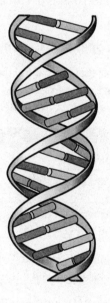

Key Terms/Formulas

- **allele** – one of two or more variations of a single gene

- **amino acid** – the building block of a protein

- **chromosomes** – large strands of DNA in the nucleus that each contain several genes

- **deoxyribonucleic acid (DNA)** – the primary genetic material inside human cells

- **gene** – a short segment of DNA that codes for a single protein, or trait

- **genotype** – the gene combination present in a cell for a given trait

- **heterozygous** – having two different alleles for a trait

- **homozygous** – having two of the same alleles for a trait

- **meiosis** – reproductive cell production process

- **mitosis** – cell replication process

- **phenotype** – the visible characteristic determined by genotype

- **Punnett square** – a graphical tool used to calculate the probabilities of inheritance

The Basics of DNA

DNA determines our characteristics and influences our health. DNA, which stands for *deoxyribonucleic acid*, is just one of the family of molecules, called *nucleic acids*, that contain our genetic information. The other primary nucleic acid is RNA, or *ribonucleic acid*, and it has a variety of roles that are different from DNA.

DNA exists in the nucleus of our cells in very long strands called *chromosomes*. Our various genes are spread along the lengths of chromosomes. Genes are short segments of DNA that code for *proteins*, which are what ultimately give us our traits. A strand of DNA takes on a characteristic shape, called a double helix, which you can see in the image on the first page of this lesson.

All nucleic acids are long chains of smaller molecules called nucleotides that are bonded together. Each *nucleotide* is itself composed of three smaller parts: a pentose sugar, a phosphate group, and a nitrogenous base. DNA and RNA molecules differ in two key ways: first, the sugar portion of an RNA nucleotide contains an extra oxygen atom that DNA nucleotides do not have; second, strands of RNA contain the base uracil instead of the thymine that is present in DNA strands.

Nitrogenous Bases and the DNA Code

Recall that the central rungs of the DNA double helix are each a bonded pair of nitrogenous bases, sometimes called *letters* because the sequence of these bases makes the DNA code. You may remember that there are several nitrogenous bases with differing properties.

The Two Types of Nitrogenous Bases		
Type of base	Purine	Pyrimidines
Names of specific bases	guanine (G), adenine (A)	cytosine (C), thymine (T, DNA only), Uracil (U, RNA only)
Number of rings in structure of the base	2	1

Purines only bond to pyrimidines and vice versa. Specifically, the letter A always bonds with T (or U in RNA), and the letter G always bonds with C.

From DNA to Protein

Proteins are created from the information in the DNA code through the processes of *transcription* and *translation*. The table below shows a comparison of the two processes.

Distinguishing between Transcription and Translation		
Name of process	Transcription	Translation
Order of occurrence during protein production	first	second
Purpose	to copy information from DNA to mRNA (m is for messenger)	to build a protein from the information in mRNA
Where in the cell it occurs	nucleus	rough endoplasmic reticulum, carried out by ribosomes

Each group of three DNA letters is called a *codon*, and each codon codes for an amino acid. *Amino acids* are the building blocks of proteins. They are linked together as translation takes place. There are twenty primary amino acids and sixty-four codons. Most amino acids have more than one codon associated with them.

Up Close

The Role of DNA in Evolution by Natural Selection

Recall that evolution is the changing of a population of organisms over time. This change originates in the DNA of these organisms; it must originate in the DNA since genes produce an organism's traits. Mutations can give rise to new versions of genes, called *alleles*, that then give rise to variations on traits.

How do DNA Mutations Occur?

Mutations occur because of errors made during DNA replication or because of mutagens such as chemicals and UV light. Mutations can occur in all types of cells, but only the ones that occur in germ cells, such as sperm and egg cells, will be passed on to future generations. The enzyme that replicates DNA, called DNA polymerase, inserts an incorrect nucleotide approximately 0.1% of the time. Most mutations are not beneficial (cancer, for instance, is usually the result of random mutations), so human cells have ways to reduce mutation rates. DNA polymerase checks its work as it adds new nucleotides to a DNA strand and this reduces the mutation rate to between one in a billion and one in a trillion nucleotides. Other mechanisms, such as mismatch repair and excision repair, exist to further reduce the mutation rate.

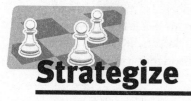

Strategize

Tips and Tricks

Remembering the details about the structure and properties of nucleic acids can be tricky. Below are a few devices to help you out.

D is for double-stranded: In our cells, DNA is double-stranded (picture the double helix) and RNA is usually single-stranded (picture just one side of the double helix). Just remember that the D in DNA stands for double-stranded.

Deoxy means without oxygen: The fact that the sugar in DNA nucleotides lacks an oxygen atom that is present in RNA nucleotides is right there in the name of DNA. The sugar is called ribose, hence *deoxyribo*nucleic acid, which can be translated as "nucleic acid missing an oxygen in its ribose."

Two syllables, two rings: Have trouble remembering that purines have a two-ring structure and pyrimidines have a one-ring structure? Try associating the number of syllables in the word purine with the number of rings a purine has: two.

The word AT is a pair: The only English word that is spelled by the pairing of nitrogenous bases, or letters, is AT, because A pairs with T. This means that G must pair with C.

A1. Which option shows the DNA sequence that would pair with the one below to form a double helix?

5'-AGTCCATG-3'

A) 3'-ACTGGATC-5'

B) 3'-TGACCTAG-5'

C) 3'-TCAGGTAC-5'

D) 3'-CTGAACGT-5'

You need to find the complementary sequences. The correct answer is Choice C. A's bond with T's and G's bond with C's.

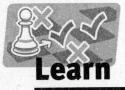

Learn

Heredity

Cell Reproduction

Eukaryote cells grow and divide by a complex process, called *mitosis*. Most of our body's cells are produced through the process of mitosis. *Gametes*, or sex cells (eggs and sperm), are produced by a process called *meiosis*. The phases of meiosis are similar to the phases of mitosis, except that each phase occurs twice: once during Meiosis I and once during Meiosis II. During Meiosis I, *homologous chromosomes*, which are chromosomes from different parents, are pulled apart. During Meiosis II, *sister chromatids*, which are replicated and therefore identical chromosome pairs, are pulled apart.

During meiosis the original cell divides twice and the four resulting cells each contain a single copy of each human chromosome, a condition referred to as *haploid*. A normal body cell contains two of each chromosome, one from each parent, a condition referred to as *diploid*. When a haploid sperm fertilizes a haploid egg, the result is a single diploid cell that contains a unique combination of chromosomes from the two people who produced the gametes. This combining of chromosomes is the basis for heredity.

The Cell Cycle		
Stage	Substage	Description
Interphase	G1	Gene expression and cell growth occur.
	S-phase	DNA is replicated.
	G2	Protein synthesis and further growth occur.
Mitosis	Prophase	Nuclear membrane disappears, centrioles migrate to opposite ends of cell and spindle fibers form.
	Metaphase	Chromosomes align in center of the cell.
	Anaphase	Replicated chromosomes begin to move toward opposite poles of the cell.
	Telophase	Identical chromosome sets are at opposite ends of the cell and new nuclear membranes form around them.
	Cytokinesis	Plasma membrane splits into two separate cells, each containing one of the new nuclei.

Traits Are Passed to Offspring

Every human has two copies of every gene—one copy from each parent. Sometimes the two copies are the same allele and the person is said to be *homozygous* for that trait. Sometimes the two copies are different alleles and the person is said to be *heterozygous* for that trait. Dominant alleles are typically symbolized with capital letters and recessive alleles are symbolized with lowercase letters. Consider the example of hair texture where curly hair is dominant. We'll use the letter C to symbolize the trait. The following table shows the possible *genotypes*, or allele combinations, along with their corresponding *phenotypes*, or visible traits.

Hair Texture Genotypes and their Phenotypes		
Genotype	**Description**	**Phenotype**
CC	homozygous dominant	curly hair
Cc	heterozygous	curly hair
cc	homozygous recessive	straight hair

You can use a tool called a *Punnett square* to calculate the probabilities of two people with known genotypes having children with various genotypes and phenotypes.

Consider two parents who are both heterozygous for cystic fibrosis, a recessive genetic disease. Both parents are healthy, but each of them has a 50% chance of passing the recessive allele to their offspring. A Punnett square can be used to work this problem.

To solve a problem like this, write the genotype of each parent (we'll use the letter *f* to symbolize the gene involved in cystic fibrosis). Both parents are heterozygous, so the mother has the

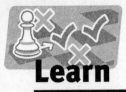

genotype *Ff* and the father has the genotype *Ff*. The figure below shows how to set up and complete the Punnett square for this problem.

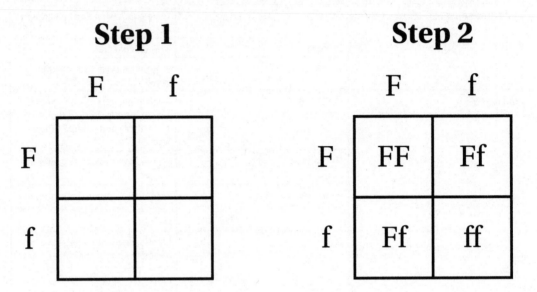

The completed Punnett square shows the four possible allele combinations that these parents can give to their offspring. Each combination has an equal chance of occurring. We are only interested in the homozygous recessive combination, since it will result in a child with cystic fibrosis. The Punnett square shows that 1 in 4 children will have that combination, so the probability is 0.25.

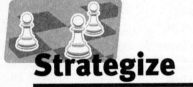

Strategize

Remember:

I'll Peel More Apples Tomorrow

This phrase will help you to remember the order of the phases of mitosis and meiosis

- **I**nterphase = Chromosome doubling

- **P**rophase = Ready to move

- **M**etaphase = Lining up

- **A**naphase = Pulling apart

- **T**elophase/Cytokinesis = Separate cells form.

In meiosis, the cycle is done twice.

Use Squares!

When you asked to determine the probability of offspring receiving a certain trait, use a Punnett square to figure it out.

Apply

A2. A researcher is observing liver cells under a microscope. He notices that the chromosomes have separated and are moving towards opposite sides of the cell.

What phase of mitosis is he most likely observing?

A) anaphase

B) metaphase

C) prophase

D) telophase

This question is asking you to determine the phase of mitosis that the researcher is looking at. Reread the part of the question that describes his observation.

STEP 1: Remember

In mitosis, body cells reproduce. In each part of mitosis, something distinct happens.

STEP 2: Rule Out

Eliminate the answer choices that do not fit with the researcher's observations.

Choice B: In metaphase, the chromosomes are lined up in the center of the cell.

Choice C: In prophase, the nuclear membrane disintegrates.

Choice D: In telophase, the cell has completed the division process.

This means the answer is **A: Anaphase**.

A3. Curly hair is dominant over straight hair. What is the probability that a straight-haired mother and a curly-haired father with a heterozygous genotype will have a curly-haired child? Use the letter *C* to symbolize the gene.

A) 0

B) 25%

C) 50%

D) 75%

STEP 1: Reread and Realize

Reread the problem to determine the parents' genotypes. The mother is straight-haired, which is the recessive phenotype. Therefore, she must have the homozygous recessive genotype, or *cc*. The father is heterozygous, so his genotype is *Cc*.

STEP 2: Use Squares!

Use a Punnett square to solve the problem.

Two of the four genotype combinations in the square are homozygous recessive, which will lead to children with straight hair. The other two are heterozygous, which will lead to children with curly hair. Since two out of four offspring will have curly hair, the chance is 50%, or a probability of 0.5. The correct answer is Choice C.

Guided Practice

Let's work through a few examples together. Look back at the lesson content as often as necessary to help you apply the concepts and strategies you learned.

1. A student is examining the cells of a plant root through a microscope. She notices a cell without a nucleus that has chromosomes lined up neatly down the middle.

   Which phase of the cell cycle is she likely witnessing?

   A) anaphase

   B) prophase

   C) metaphase

   D) telophase

   STEP 1: Reread the question

   What is the question asking you to do? Reread the item and find the important details.

   _____

   _____

   _____

   _____

   STEP 2: Remember

   What happens during each phase of mitosis?

   _____

   _____

   _____

   _____

   STEP 3: Rule Out

   Which choices can you eliminate and why?

   _____

   _____

2. Dimples are a dominant trait. The letter *D* symbolizes the allele for dimples.

Which option shows the heterozygous genotype and its matching phenotype?

A) genotype: Dd; phenotype: dimples

B) genotype: Dd; phenotype: no dimples

C) genotype: DD; phenotype: dimples

D) genotype: DD; phenotype: no dimples

STEP 1: Reread the question

What is this question asking you to do?

_____

_____

_____

_____

STEP 2: Remember

What does heterozygous mean? What are the definitions of genotype and phenotype?

_____

_____

_____

_____

STEP 3: Rule Out

Eliminate the incorrect answers. Why are these options incorrect?

_____

_____

_____

_____

Guided Practice

3. Tulip color is a trait governed by incomplete dominance. Homozygous dominant tulips are red. Homozygous recessive tulips are white. Heterozygous tulips are pink.

What is the probability that a red tulip will be produced by breeding a pink tulip with a white tulip?

A) 0

B) 25%

C) 50%

D) 75%

STEP 1: Reread the question

On the lines below, write the details you can pick out of the question. Specifically, write the genotype that the breeder wants to produce and the genotypes the question proposes that she breed together. Use the letter *R* to represent the gene for tulip color.

_____

_____

_____

STEP 2: Use Squares!

Use the Punnett square below to predict the results of breeding a pink tulip with a white tulip.

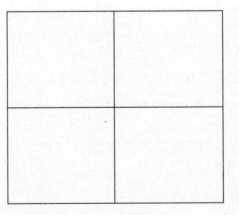

STEP 3: Rule Out

Eliminate the incorrect answers using the Punnett square.

Independent Practice

1. Which RNA codons would match the DNA sequence below?

   5'-TACCCATTT-3'

   A) AUC, CCU, AAA

   B) AUG, GGU, AAA

   C) UUC, CCA, UUU

   D) UUG, GGA, UUU

   > **HINT** *Remember that the word AT is pair. But this only applies to DNA because in RNA uracil (U) takes the place of thymine (T). So As pair with Us, and Gs still pair with Cs.*

2. Burmese pythons have reticulated skin coloration. This coloration helps them blend in with their environment. On rare occasions, a mutation causes a Burmese python to be born white. The white color does not spread through the population and it remains a very rare occurrence to see a white python in the wild.

   What is the most likely explanation for this?

   A) Collectors of rare animals remove all of the white pythons from the wild because they are valuable.

   B) Natural selection does not favor the white coloration because predator and prey animals can spot the pythons more easily.

   C) The mutation that causes the white coloration also affects a python's ability to constrict and suffocate its prey.

   D) A second random mutation reverses the original mutation, thus removing the white coloration from the population.

   > **HINT** *Would the white color be beneficial for a python when it is hunting?*

3. Jonathan has brown eyes and Cindy has blue eyes. Brown eyes are dominant and blue eyes are recessive.

   What is the probability that they will have a child with blue eyes if Jonathan has the homozygous genotype?

   A) 0%

   B) 25%

   C) 50%

   D) 75%

   > **HINT** *Use the letter B to represent the eye color gene.*

ReKap

In this lesson, you reviewed the structure and importance of DNA and RNA. You also saw how cell division is completed and its importance in heredity. You learned strategies for remembering the parts of the cell cycle and how to determine the probabilities of traits being passed to offspring. Make sure to remember:

- DNA determines our characteristics.

- DNA is made up of nitrogenous bases, which pair with each other.

- Mutations cause changes in characteristics and can be beneficial or harmful.

- Mitosis and meiosis are processes in which cells divide. Meiosis allows combinations of cells from parents to combine into a new individual with unique traits.

- Punnett squares can be used to determine the probability of traits in offspring.

? How will knowing the roles DNA and heredity help you to understand the diagnosis of a patient?

_____

_____

_____

_____

Answers

Guided Practice

1. Step 1: The question is asking you to determine a stage of the cell cycle.

   Step 2: Remember the mnemonic: *I'll Peel More Apples Tomorrow*: prophase: nuclear membrane disappears; metaphase: chromosomes in center of cell; anaphase: chromosomes begin to split; telophase: chromosome sets at opposite ends of cell with new nuclear membranes formed around them; cytokinesis: membrane split into new cells

   Step 3: Eliminate Choices A, B, and D. Choice A is incorrect because during anaphase the chromosomes are beginning to separate and are no longer lined up in the middle of the cell. Choice B is incorrect because the chromosomes have not yet lined up during prophase. Choice D is incorrect because during telophase the two sets of chromosomes are at opposite ends of the cell and nuclear membranes are starting to reform.

   Answer: (C) metaphase

2. Step 1: The question is asking you to figure out the phenotype that would show with a particular genotype.

   Step 2: heterozygous: different alleles; genotype: the combination of alleles; phenotype: the physical trait

   Step 3: Eliminate Choices C and D (homozygous genotypes) and B (the heterozygous genotype will be Dd and that since D is dominant, this is the trait that will show, so Dd shows dimples). This means the correct answer is Choice A.

   Answer: (A) genotype: Dd; phenotype: dimples

3. Step 1: The breeder wants to produce a red tulip (homozygous dominant, *RR*); pink tulip: *Rr*; white tulip: *rr*

   Step 2:

   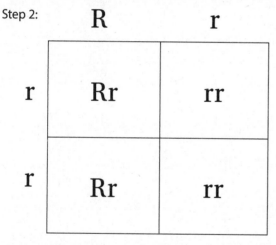

   Step 3: There is a 50% chance of the pink flower contributing the R allele to the offspring, but a 0% chance of the white flower contributing the R allele to the offspring. Eliminate Choices B, C, and D

   Answer: (A) 0%

Answers

Independent Practice

1. **Answer: (B) AUG, GGU, AAA**

2. **Answer: (B) Natural selection does not favor the white coloration because predator and prey animals can spot the pythons more easily.**

   If the white coloration was favored by natural selection, most pythons would be white and they wouldn't be rare.

3. **Answer: (A) 0%**

   Jonathan: BB; Cindy: bb. A child need only receive one copy of the dominant allele to show the dominant phenotype. Therefore, a heterozygous individual will have brown eyes.

ReKap

Knowing the roles of DNA and RNA help to understand the heredity component of disease.

4

SCIENCE · LESSON 4
Human Body Systems

Understanding how the human body systems work and how they are related are essential skills in biology and health care. For example, a patient with high blood pressure might have a condition affecting his circulatory system, but it can also be due to problems with his endocrine, digestive, excretory, or nervous systems.

Common Uses in Health Care

- recognizing symptoms of damage to one or more body systems
- understanding how damage to one system could affect another system
- understanding the importance of vital organs to human health

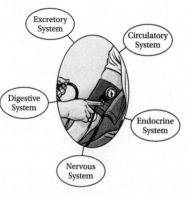

Key Terms/Formulas

The main body systems are:

- **circulatory –** system of organs and tissue that distribute substances throughout the body
- **digestive –** system of connected organs and tissue that breaks down food and expels solid waste
- **endocrine –** system of tissue that releases chemicals that control functions
- **excretory –** system of organs and tissue that collects and expels chemical waste
- **integumentary –** system of skin, hair, and nails to contain and protect the other systems
- **lymphatic –** system of tissues that distributes white blood cells and excess fluid throughout the system
- **muscular –** system of muscles and connective tissue for moving the body
- **nervous –** system of tissue that senses and controls the body
- **reproductive –** system of organs and tissue for producing offspring
- **respiratory –** system of organs and tissue that supplies oxygen and removes carbon dioxide from the body
- **skeletal –** system of bones and connective tissue for supporting the body

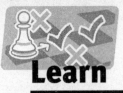

Hierarchy of Structure

Moving from most simple to most complex, we can describe humans as:

- **atoms** – mostly carbon, hydrogen, oxygen, and nitrogen

- **molecules** – atoms bonded together in certain ratios and arrangements, such as a glucose molecule

- **cells** – molecules combined in complex structures to make cell walls, DNA, organelles, etc.

- **tissues** – sets of similar cells with a certain purpose, such as skin cells

- **organs** – sets of tissues that work together for complex functions, such as the liver, filtering out and breaking down toxins in the blood

- **body systems (or organ systems)** – set of organs that accomplish several complex functions, such as the digestive system (breaking down food and absorbing water and nutrients)

- **human (or organism)** – the living being that is the result of all of the body systems working together

Reproduction

Let's look at how the function of reproduction fits into the hierarchy. Humans have a set of organs (such as the ovaries or testes) that make up their reproductive system. These organs are made of tissue, and they are also connected by tissues (*epithelial*, *connective*, *muscle*, and *nervous*). The tissues are made of protein, carbohydrate, and fat molecules, which are made of atoms.

The reproductive system is the one system that humans can survive without. Male and female reproductive systems have the same purpose: to prepare and transport eggs or sperm. The end goal is for an egg and a sperm to meet and combine their genetic material (each one half of the parent's genetic material) to start the growth of a new human. It helps to compare the parts of the male and female systems to remember similarities and differences:

Male		Female	
Organ or Tissue	**Purpose**	**Organ or Tissue**	**Purpose**
Testes	Production of sperm	Ovaries	Production of eggs
Prostate	Production of semen		
		Fallopian tube	Transports fertilized egg
		Uterus	Protects and nourishes growing baby
Penis/Urethra	Passage for sperm to exit the male system	Vagina	Passage for sperm to enter the female system; also passage for baby to exit system

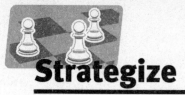

Strategize

Reread, Remember, Rule Out

To succeed on questions about hierarchy of structure in body systems:

Step 1: Always **reread** the question. Figure out what the question is asking you to do.

Step 2: **Remember** the order of the levels.

Step 3: Using the information you remembered, predict the correct level, and **rule out** the choices that do not match.

Apply

A1. A patient has a yeast infection—a fungal overgrowth that causes irritation in the surface layers of her vagina, characterized by redness and itching. Which best describes the level in the hierarchy of structure that is being affected?

- **A)** Body system
- **B)** Molecules
- **C)** Organ
- **D)** Tissues

STEP 1: Reread and Realize

What is the question asking? Reread the question—it is asking about the "surface layers of her vagina" which you would probably describe as "membranes" or "skin."

STEP 2: Remember

The affected membranes or skin are part of the vagina, which is part of the reproductive system.

STEP 3: Rule Out

Based on what you remember, rule out any choice that does not fit—since the question is asking about a part of an organ, the answer cannot be "organ" or anything above organ on the hierarchy, so you can rule out choices A and C. Membranes and skin are tissues, so choice D is the best answer. Choice B is too specific for the question, as the question did not indicate whether molecules were being changed. Choice D is the correct answer.

Learn

Physical Support Systems

The integumentary, skeletal, and muscular systems provide support for the body.

Integumentary System: The integumentary system contains and protects all of the body systems. It is composed of the skin, hair, nails, and mucus membranes, and it has three main functions:

- **Protection:** It provides a barrier both against physical injury and against infections by viruses or bacteria.

- **Containment:** It holds all the tissues and fluids in the body and keeps them from drying out (or being waterlogged).

- **Temperature regulation:** It allows body heat to be released or retained as needed.

Skeletal System: Bones provide the framework for supporting and protecting the body's organs and tissues. The skeletal system also contains *cartilage*, which is used to support flexible areas such as ears or cushion areas where bones meet, and *ligaments*, which connect bones and joints together.

Muscular System: Muscles support the body and allow the body to move around. Muscles are connected to each other and to bones by *tendons*. Some muscles move bones (such as arm and leg muscles) and some move organs (such as tongue muscles or eye muscles).

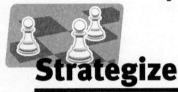

Strategize

Reread, Remember, Rule Out

To succeed on questions about the body systems that provide physical support:

Step 1: Always **reread** the question. Determine what the question is asking you to do.

Step 2: **Remember** the three physical support systems, their function, and how they interact.

Step 3: Using the information you remembered, predict the system, organ in the system, or function, and **rule out** the choices that do not match or are not the best match.

Apply

A2. Botulism is a dangerous condition caused by the presence of a certain strain of bacteria in the body. A severely affected patient cannot walk, swallow, or breathe. Which system is most affected by botulism?

A) Integumentary

B) Muscular

C) Skeletal

D) Reproductive

STEP 1: Reread and Realize

What is the question asking? Reread the question—it is asking which system would affect the movement of the entire body, including the parts involved with swallowing and breathing.

STEP 2: Remember

All three systems work together to move the body; a failure in which system would have the most effect on those types of movement?

STEP 3: Rule Out

Based on what you remember, rule out any choice that does not fit or is not the best match—all three systems could prevent walking (skin that won't stretch, bones that are broken, or muscles that won't contract) but bones and skin are less involved in swallowing and breathing than are muscles, so choices A and C are not as good a match as choice B, and can be ruled out. D can be eliminated because the reproductive system is unrelated to movement.

Tissue Types and Their Descriptions

Tissue type	Description
Epithelial tissue	Epithelium serves two functions. It can provide covering (such as skin tissue) or produce secretions (such as glandular tissue). Epithelial tissue commonly exists in sheets and does not have its own blood supply. Subsequently, epithelium is dependent on diffusion from the nearby capillaries for food and oxygen. Epithelial tissue can regenerate easily if well nourished. Epithelial tissues are classified according to two criteria : number of cell layers and cell shape. Simple and stratified epithelial tissues vary in relation to the number of cell layers. Simple epithelium contains one layer of cells. It is found in body structures where absorption, secretion, and filtration occur. Stratified epithelium has more than one layer of cells and serves as protection . The shape of epithelial cells includes squamous, cuboidal, and columnar.
Connective tissue	Connective tissue is found throughout the body; it serves to connect different structures of the body. Connective tissue commonly has its own blood supply; however, there are some types of connective tissue, such as ligaments, that do not. The various types of connective tissue include bone, cartilage, adipose (fat), and blood vessel.
Muscle tissue	Muscle tissue is dedicated to producing movement. There are three types of muscle tissue: skeletal, cardiac, and smooth. Skeletal muscle supports voluntary movement since it is connected to bones in the skeletal system. Voluntary movements are consciously controlled by the brain. Smooth muscle is under involuntary control, which means it cannot be consciously controlled. It is found in the walls of hollow organs, such as intestines, blood vessels, bladder, and uterus. Like smooth muscle, cardiac muscle movement is involuntary. Cardiac muscle is found only in the heart.
Nervous tissue	Nervous tissue provides the structure for the brain, spinal cord, and nerves. Nerves are made up of specialized cells called neurons that send electrical impulses throughout the body. Support cells, such as myelin, help protect nervous tissue.

Nutrition/Waste Removal Systems

All body systems need nutrients and water to keep their cells alive, and they need to get rid of the waste produced by those cells

- **Digestive System**: The digestive system makes the nutrients and water available for use; each part of the digestive system has a specific purpose:

  - **Mouth:** Entry point for food—teeth break the food into smaller parts and saliva from salivary glands lubricates and holds it together during swallowing. *Enzymes* in the saliva begin to break carbohydrates, such as starches, down into glucose.

  - **Esophagus:** Once the food is swallowed, it is moved through the digestive tract by *peristalsis*—rhythmic contractions in the muscles. The food is moved down the esophagus by peristalsis, not gravity—people can swallow without gravity because of peristalsis.

  - **Stomach:** Peristalsis churns the food, breaking it down into smaller parts, and the stomach lining releases protein enzymes and hydrochloric acid, which start to break down proteins. The stomach protects its own tissues from the enzymes and acid with mucus. Glucose and amino acids can be absorbed by the stomach, as well as water.

  - **Small intestine:** The pancreas secretes bicarbonate to neutralize the acid, and enzymes that will finish breaking down carbohydrates and proteins, as well as fats. The fats first must be mixed with bile from the gallbladder, to keep the fat and the enzymes from separating (like oil and water do). Carbohydrates are broken down into *monosaccharides*, such as glucose; proteins are broken down into *amino acids*; fats are broken down into *lipids*. The nutrients are then absorbed by the small intestine. Since the nutrients can only be absorbed by the surface cells of the small intestine, the more cells that are available, the better. By having small folds or projections, called *villi* and *microvilli*, in the surface, the small intestine can make more cells available to absorb nutrients. Additional water is also absorbed by the small intestine.

  - **Large intestine:** Whatever is left of the food as it exits the small intestine then moves through the large intestine (*colon*) where water is removed. The feces, which contain indigestible food (such as fiber) and unabsorbed nutrients, exit through the anus. More water is absorbed in the large intestine—the dryness of the feces is a result of the time spent in the large intestine.

- **Excretory System:** When cells break down proteins and nucleic acids, the waste produced contains nitrogen. These nitrogen-containing wastes are converted to *urea* before being excreted from the body.

  - **Kidneys:** Urea is filtered out of the blood by the kidneys and concentrated in the urine, along with other waste materials. The kidneys also control the amount of certain elements, such as sodium and potassium, in the blood, and therefore are important in controlling blood pressure.

  - **Bladder:** Holds urine (water, urea, and other wastes) for disposal. Urine reaches the bladder through ureters and leaves through the urethra.

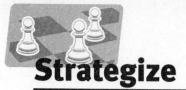

Strategize

Reread, Remember, Rule Out

To succeed on questions about the body systems that provide nutrition and waste removal:

Step 1: Always **reread** the question. Determine what the question is asking you to do.

Step 2: **Remember** the parts of the digestive and excretory systems, their functions (and the order in which they perform those functions), and how they interact.

Step 3: Using the information you remembered, predict the system, organ in the system, or function, and **rule out** the choices that do not match or are not the best match.

Apply

A3. When their blood glucose levels drop, diabetics often need to chew on tablets to bring up the blood glucose quickly. Which of these best explains how the glucose gets into the blood?

A) Glucose is absorbed in the stomach and small intestine, where it diffuses into the blood.

B) Glucose is absorbed in the mouth, where it is dissolved by saliva, and passes into the blood.

C) Glucose is broken down in the small intestine, and enters the blood by the excretory system.

D) Glucose is broken down in the stomach, where it then flows to the heart and is mixed into the blood.

STEP 1: Reread and Realize

What is the question asking? Reread the question—it is asking the pathway(s) by which glucose gets from the digestive system to the circulatory system.

STEP 2: Remember

Follow glucose through the digestive system. Starches and carbohydrates are broken down into glucose, beginning in the mouth, but glucose does not need to be broken down further. The breakdown of starches and carbohydrates continues in the stomach and small intestine, and glucose is absorbed in both places. Glucose diffuses through the cells in the lining of the stomach and small intestine into the blood, where it is circulated to the rest of the body.

STEP 3: Rule Out

Based on what you remember, rule out any choice that does not fit—since glucose does not need to be broken down, you can rule out choices C and D. Choose the answer among the remaining choices that best fits what you remember—choice A fits the best, as glucose absorption starts in the stomach.

Apply

A4. A doctor injects a radioactive dye into a patient and then takes x-ray images in order to study a particular body system in the patient. Which is the best explanation of the system being studied?

A) Excretory system, because the kidneys filter out substances from the blood, therefore the dye will be concentrated there, making the kidneys more visible.

B) Digestive system, because the small intestine will absorb the dye from the blood, making the tissues in the small intestine more visible.

C) Excretory system, because the dye will break down in the digestive system but not in the excretory system, therefore the excretory system will be more visible.

D) Digestive system, because blood passes through the digestive system in order to pick up nutrients, therefore the blood vessels around the digestive system will be move visible.

STEP 1: Reread and Realize

What is the question asking? Reread the question—it is asking in which system would more of the dye end up, so that it is more visible on the x-ray image.

STEP 2: Remember

The digestive system breaks food down so that nutrients and water can enter the blood; the excretory system filters substances that aren't nutrients out of the blood so that they can be expelled from the body. Is the dye a nutrient?

STEP 3: Rule Out

Based on what you remember, rule out any choice that does not fit or is not the best match—choice B can be excluded because the blood absorbs substances from the small intestine, not the other way around. Choice C can be excluded, because the dye might enter the excretory system from the blood, but not the digestive system, so that is not a good explanation. In choosing between choices A and D, notice that choice D does not provide a way in which one system would be more visible than any other part of the body that has blood. Choice A has a correct explanation of how the excretory system works and also explains how part of the excretory system would become more visible.

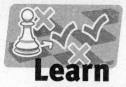

Learn

Material Movement

Respiratory System: All body systems need oxygen to release ATP from glucose to provide energy that keep their cells alive, and they need to get rid of the carbon dioxide produced. Humans move air in and out of the lungs to both take in oxygen and release carbon dioxide:

- **Air passages:** Air comes in through the nose or mouth, travels down the *trachea*, which splits into two tubes (*bronchi*). These lead to the lungs and split into smaller tubes (*bronchioles*) and then air sacs (*alveoli*). The air then exits the same way, but in reverse.

- **Lungs:** The surface area of the lungs is much greater on the inside than on the outside, since the alveoli divide the lungs into smaller and smaller compartments, each adding its own bit of surface. Oxygen diffuses from the inhaled air through the surface cells, while carbon dioxide diffuses out, to be released when the air is exhaled.

Circulatory System: All of the cells in each body system need oxygen and nutrients delivered, and carbon dioxide, excess nutrients, and waste taken away. These materials are carried in the blood, which is moved by the heart pumping. Oxygen and carbon dioxide are transported by red blood cells between the lungs and the rest of the body. Waste is transported to the liver and kidneys for processing. Excess nutrients are stored (excess glucose is converted to *glycogen* and fat, for example).

- **Arteries:** Blood is pumped away from the heart through arteries, which branch out into smaller and smaller blood vessels (*arterioles*).

- **Capillaries:** Passive and active transport of oxygen, nutrients, carbon dioxide, and wastes occur in capillaries, which are the smallest blood vessels.

- **Veins:** Blood moves from the capillaries, merging into larger blood vessels (*venules*) and then into veins, which transport the blood back toward the heart.

- **Heart:** Blood is pumped in two circuits through four chambers. Oxygen-rich blood comes from the lungs to the left side of the heart, entering through one chamber (*left atrium*) and exiting through another chamber (*left ventricle*) to the major artery (*aorta*) which carries it to rest of the body. Oxygen-poor blood comes back from the body to the right side of the heart, entering through one chamber (*right atrium*) and exiting through another chamber (*right ventricle*). One-way valves prevent blood from flowing backward into each atrium (*mitral* on the left and *tricuspid* on the right) and from flowing backward into each ventricle (*aortic* on the left and *pulmonary* on the right).

Keep the many parts of the circulatory system straight with memory aids:

- <u>A</u>rteries move blood <u>a</u>way from the heart.

- Blood moves through the chambers in alphabetical order: <u>a</u>trium to <u>v</u>entricle.

- Blood moves from the <u>l</u>ungs to the <u>l</u>eft side of the heart.

- Blood moves from the <u>r</u>est of the body to the <u>r</u>ight side of the heart.

- Ventricle valves indicate where the blood is heading: pulmonary valve = lungs, aortic valve = aorta.

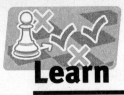

Learn

Lymphatic System: Lymph fluid, containing white blood cells, circulates between tissues and lymph nodes in vessels, much like those in the circulatory system. The lymphatic system, however, does not have a central pump. The lymphatic system also moves excess fluid (mostly water) from the tissues back into the circulatory system; when this movement slows or stops, the tissues swell, producing *edema*.

- **White blood cells:** Various types of white blood cells recognize and attack viruses, bacteria, parasites, and other foreign bodies, as well as dead cells from the body.

- **Lymph nodes:** Collection of lymph tissue that filters fluid to prevent infection from entering the circulatory system. These swell when fighting an infection; *tonsils*, which are two large lymph nodes in our throats, can become very swollen and sore, causing the typical sore throat associated with a cold.

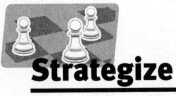

Strategize

Reread, Remember, Rule Out

To succeed on questions about the body systems that move materials:

Step 1: Always **reread** the question. Determine what the question is asking you to do.

Step 2: **Remember** the parts of the circulatory, respiratory, and lymphatic systems, what they move (and the order in which materials move through them), and how they interact.

Step 3: Using the information you remembered, predict the system, organ in the system, or material, and **rule out** the choices that do not match or are not the best match.

Apply

A5. During exercise, muscle cells increase the amount of ATP they break down to produce energy. Which systems must speed up immediately for the muscle cells to be able to break down more ATP?

- **A)** Circulatory and lymphatic systems
- **B)** Respiratory and lymphatic systems
- **C)** Respiratory and circulatory systems
- **D)** Circulatory, respiratory, and lymphatic systems

STEP 1: Reread and Realize

What is the question asking? Notice the word *immediately* in the question—it is suggesting that, while all of the systems might need to speed up over a period of time to support the muscle cells, certain systems must speed up at the same time as the muscle cells speed up their breakdown of ATP.

STEP 2: Remember

Breaking down ATP is the goal of cellular respiration—the reactants are glucose and oxygen, and the products are carbon dioxide and water. The cells will need to receive more glucose and oxygen, and get rid of carbon dioxide.

STEP 3: Rule Out

Based on what you remembered, rule out any choices that don't fit. The lymphatic system does not move glucose, oxygen, or carbon dioxide, so it is not immediately needed (although it will be needed to provide fluid balance over time), so choices A, B, and D can be eliminated. The respiratory and circulatory systems provide oxygen and glucose to cells, and remove carbon dioxide, so choice C is the best answer.

A6. Which has a greatest concentration of oxygen?

A) the muscle cells in the fingers

B) the blood passing through the alveoli

C) the air touching the surface of the alveoli

D) the blood moving the through the capillaries of the fingers

STEP 1: Reread and Realize

What is the question asking? Reread the question—it is asking you to compare the concentration of oxygen in each part and choose the one that would be greatest.

STEP 2: Remember

Oxygen moves into the lung tissues, blood, and cells by diffusion, which means it moves from higher concentration to lower concentration. The highest concentration will be at the the beginning of the respiratory/circulatory cycle.

STEP 3: Rule Out

Based on what you remember, order the choices and rule out any choice that is in the end of the respiratory/circulatory cycle. If you order the choices in terms of the direction of the oxygen flow, you will have C, B, D, A. The concentration of oxygen must be highest in the air touching the surface of the alveoli in order for oxygen to diffuse into the tissues and then the blood. As the blood moves away from the lungs, through the body, it will have a lower and lower concentration of oxygen, therefore choice C is the correct answer.

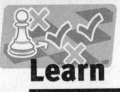

Control and Communication

Finally, all of the body systems need to communicate effectively. This is accomplished through electrical signals produced by the nervous system and chemical signals produced by the endocrine system.

Nervous System: The central nervous system (CNS) consists of the nerves in the brain (*cranial*) and the *spinal cord*. These nerves coordinate and process signals to and from the peripheral nervous system (PNS) which consists of the nerves that extend beyond the CNS. The nerves in the PNS control and communicate with both involuntary (*autonomic*) functions, such as respiration, digestion, reproduction, circulation, and voluntary (*sensory-somatic*) functions, such as movement and touch. The nervous system responds both to electrical signals received (*senses*—touch, taste, smell, hearing, vision) and chemical signals from the endocrine system.

Endocrine System: Glands in the endocrine system secrete chemical signals, or *hormones*, to regulate growth and metabolism. Some common hormones include: *insulin* (digestive system) and *estrogen* and *testosterone* (reproductive system). Glands secrete hormones in response to hormones secreted by other glands, or in response to signals from the nervous system.

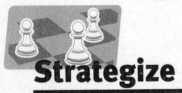

Strategize

Reread, Remember, Rule Out

To succeed on questions about the body systems that provide control and communication:

Step 1: Always **reread** the question. Determine what the question is asking you to do.

Step 2: **Remember** the nervous and endocrine systems, their function, and how they interact.

Step 3: Using the information you remembered, predict the system, organ in the system, or function, and **rule out** the choices that do not match or are not the best match.

Apply

A7. Which of these is an example of the nervous and endocrine systems interacting?

A) A person touches a finger to a hot stove and pulls her hand back without thinking.

B) The thought of a cold day causes signals to be sent to the skin, causing goose bumps to form.

C) The production of one chemical to stimulate storage of glucose also stimulates the production of another chemical that suppresses appetite.

D) A baby nursing causes signals to be sent to the mother's brain, which causes certain chemicals to be made that increase the production of milk.

STEP 1: Reread and Realize

What is the question asking? Reread the question—it is asking for an example of the nervous and endocrine systems working together.

STEP 2: Remember

The nervous system works by receiving sensory signals and sending out instructions by electrical signals in the nerves, while the endocrine system works by sensing and sending chemical signals.

STEP 3: Rule Out

Based on what you remember, rule out any choice that does not fit or is not the best match—you will be looking for an example that contains both sensory or nerve signal instructions plus chemical signals. Choice A involves sensory signals and nerve signal instructions, but no chemical signals. Choice B involves only nerve signal instructions. Choice C involves only chemical signals. Choice D involves both sensory and chemical signals, so it is the best example.

Guided Practice

1. As a result of chronic inflammation and infection, some or all of a person's large intestine might need to be removed. Which of the following materials would be ineffectively absorbed?

   A) amino acids

   B) glucose

   C) lipids

   D) water

STEP 1: Reread and realize

What is the question asking you to do? Reread the item and find the important details.

_____

_____

STEP 2: Remember

In which parts of the digestive system are each of the choices absorbed (there may be more than one for each)?

_____

_____

_____

_____

STEP 3: Rule out

Using your answer from Step 2, go through each answer choice. Which ones can you eliminate?

_____

_____

_____

_____

2. Where does blood go immediately after it exits the left ventricle?

A) lungs

B) left atrium

C) right ventricle

D) rest of the body

STEP 1: Reread and realize

What is the question asking you to do?

_____

_____

STEP 2: Remember

Pick a starting point, such as the lungs, and list the parts of the heart or body that the blood travels through in its circuits.

_____

_____

_____

STEP 3: Rule out

Which choices can you eliminate? Only one choice should appear in your list immediately after the left ventricle.

_____

_____

_____

Guided Practice

3. A patient has swollen and sore lymph nodes in one armpit. Which of the following does this symptom most likely indicate?

   A) The patient has poor circulation in that arm.

   B) The patient has an infection in or near that arm.

   C) The patient has low blood sugar.

   D) The patient has nerve damage.

STEP 1: Reread and realize

What is the question asking you to do? Reread the question and find the details that tell you.

_____

_____

STEP 2: Remember

What system do lymph nodes belong to, and what are the functions of that system?

_____

_____

STEP 3: Rule out

Determine which answer choices can be eliminated. If more than one choice fits in with the function of the system, determine which choice is more closely associated with the functions of the lymph nodes.

_____

_____

_____

_____

Independent Practice

1. A loud noise startles a person and his heart beats faster for several seconds. Which of the following describes the part of the nervous system most involved with the change in the startled person's heart rate?

   A) Autonomic

   B) Central

   C) Peripheral

   D) Sensory-somatic

   HINT   *Remember that your nervous system is a set of systems, some of which may have a subset of systems.*

2. A blood test indicates that a patient has a buildup of nitrogen-containing wastes. Which organ is most likely malfunctioning?

   A) Brain

   B) Kidney

   C) Lung

   D) Stomach

   HINT   *Remember that a buildup of waste indicates it is not being removed from the blood.*

3. A chest wound that punctures a lung is very dangerous—one reason, of course, is that only one lung will be providing oxygen. Which of the following best describes another reason that a chest wound is dangerous?

   A) The respiratory system is in a direct circuit with the heart.

   B) The lungs help filter out infections from the rest of the body.

   C) The digestive system will function more slowly if a lung is damaged.

   D) The central nervous system shuts down if the amount of oxygen is reduced.

   HINT   *Which system contains the lungs? With which system does that system work most closely?*

ReKap

In this lesson you reviewed the body systems, their parts and their functions. All of the systems interact, but we can group them by main function:

- Reproductive.

- Physical Support (Integumentary, Skeletal, Muscular).

- Nutrition/Waste Removal (Digestive, Excretory).

- Material Movement (Respiratory, Circulatory, Lymphatic).

- Control and Communication (Nervous, Endocrine).

? **How will having knowledge about body systems help you to better understand a patient's diagnosis?**

_____

_____

_____

_____

Answers

Guided Practice

1. Step 1: The question is asking you to figure out how absorption of materials would be affected if the large intestine was removed.

    Step 2: A - amino acids: stomach and small intestine; B - glucose: stomach and small intestine; C - lipids: small intestine; D - water: large intestine

    Step 3: Eliminate Choices A, B, and C. Choice A is incorrect because amino acids can be absorbed in the stomach, but are mostly absorbed in the small intestine. Choice B is incorrect because glucose can be absorbed both in the stomach and small intestine. Choice C is incorrect because lipids are absorbed in the small intestine only.

    Answer: (D) water

2. Step 1: The question is asking you to remember the path of blood through the heart.

    Step 2: right atrium → right ventricle → lungs → left atrium → left ventricle → rest of the body

    Step 3: Eliminate Choices A, B, and C. Choice A is incorrect, because the blood passes through the right ventricle before heading to the lungs. Choice B is incorrect because the blood passes through the left atrium before the left ventricle, not the other way around. Choice C is incorrect because the blood passes through the right atrium (not the left) before passing through the right ventricle.

    Answer: (D) rest of the body

3. Step 1: The question is asking you to figure out what swollen lymph nodes in an armpit mean.

    Step 2: Lymph nodes belong to the immune system, protecting against and fighting infection.

    Step 3: Eliminate Choices A, C, and D. Choices C and D can be eliminated because they do not directly involve the lymphatic system. Point out that choice A could produce swelling, but it would be generalized, and that the purpose of lymph nodes is to filter out and fight infections.

    Answer: (B) The patient has an infection in or near the arm.

Independent Practice

1. **Answer: (A) Automatic**

    Choice C is incorrect. The PNS contains two systems, and the heart rate is involuntary. Choice B is incorrect because the central nervous system does not control heartbeat. Choice D is incorrect because sensory-somatic nerves control voluntary actions. Choice A is correct because the autonomic system controls automatic functions, such as heartbeat.

2. **Answer: (B) Kidney**

    Nitrogenous waste is processed by the excretory system. Choice A is incorrect because the brain is part of the nervous system. Choice C is incorrect because the lungs are part of the respiratory system. Choice D is incorrect because the stomach is part of the digestive system.

Answers

3. **Answer: (A) The respiratory system is in a direct circuit with the heart.**

   Choice B is incorrect because the lungs are not part of the lymphatic system, which filters out infections. Choice C is incorrect because the digestive system will continue to receive oxygen as long as the other lung is functioning. Choice D is incorrect because shutting down the CNS would produce death—this would not be a response to an injury, although it could be a final result.

ReKap

Knowledge about body systems can help one to understand a patient's diagnosis; one may be able to recognize symptoms of damage to one or more body systems, understand how damage to one system may affect another, and define the importance of given organs to the body's overall function.

4

SCIENCE • LESSON 5
Biological Classification

Biologists estimate that Earth contains just under nine million species of living things, and that number doesn't even include the countless more species of bacteria out there! With so many organisms to keep track of, scientists needed a way to classify them. This lesson is a refresher on how they do it.

Common Uses in Health Care

- diagnosing and treating bacterial, fungal, and protozoan infections

- determining whether cells are healthy or diseased

- discovering how closely related two species are

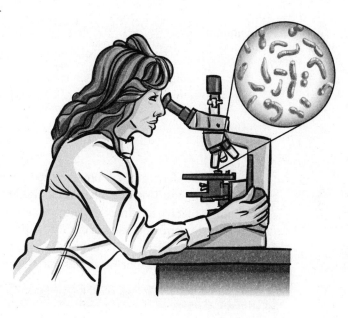

Key Terms/Formulas

- **binomial nomenclature** – the use of an organism's genus and species as its scientific name

- **taxonomic hierarchy** – domain, kingdom, phylum, class, order, family, genus, species

- **taxonomy** – the system biologists use to classify organisms

Biologists have developed a classification system, or **taxonomy**, to categorize the millions of living things that exist on Earth. In the early days of classification, organisms were considered either plants or animals and were classified based on their visible physical characteristics. By the 1970s, scientists recognized five major categories, or *kingdoms*, of living things and had begun to use similarities in DNA sequences to refine the categories. Because of the recent discovery that there are two very different types of bacteria, scientists recognize three major *domains* of organisms, further subdivided into six kingdoms total. The figure below shows how the domains are subdivided into kingdoms.

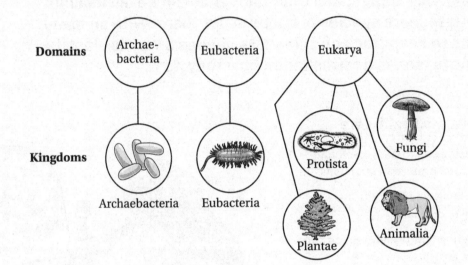

Domains and kingdoms are very broad categories, each containing millions of specific types of living things. To create scientific names for these organisms, scientists had to devise subcategories that are much narrower than domains and kingdoms. They came up with six more categories, each narrower than the last. The eight total categories together are known as the **taxonomic hierarchy**. The table below shows this hierarchy in order from largest to smallest, as well as the names of the specific groups that the gray wolf belongs to as an example.

Taxonomic Level	Gray Wolf Classification
Domain	*Eukarya*
Kingdom	*Animalia*
Phylum	*Chordata*
Class	*Mammalia*
Order	*Carnivora*
Family	*Canidae*
Genus	*Canis*
Species	*Lupus*

Biologists use a combination of an organism's genus and species names as its official scientific name. This naming system is called **binomial nomenclature**. The scientific name of the gray wolf, for example, is *Canis lupus*. A human being is called *Homo sapiens* and a common type of intestinal bacteria is called *Escherichia coli*.

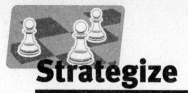

Strategize

Use a Mnemonic

It helps to make a mnemonic to remember the taxonomic levels. The table below shows one mnemonic that is commonly used for this purpose. Try using the empty column on the right to create your own mnemonic.

Taxonomic Level	Mnemonic	Your Mnemonic
Domain	Dear	
Kingdom	King	
Phylum	Phillip	
Class	Come	
Order	Over	
Family	For	
Genus	Good	
Species	Soup	

Identify

Although it is best to consult reputable resources to learn the classifications of organisms, you can often make educated guesses as to which organisms may be closely related. All mammals, for instance, belong to the same class: *Mammalia*. All animals with central nerve cords, like our spinal cord, belong to the same phylum: *Chordata*. Often the name of a group hints at a key characteristic of all of its members.

> **Questions to Ask Yourself**
>
> Which characteristics of organisms would be good for creating different groups?
>
> What mnemonic should I use to remember the taxonomic levels?
>
> When writing a scientific name, did I capitalize the Genus name but not the Species name?

Apply

Here are some examples of problems that deal with biological classification.

A1. **Which list shows four taxonomic levels in order from largest to smallest?**

   A) Family, Order, Class, Phylum

   B) Order, Family, Phylum, Class

   C) Class, Phylum, Family, Order

   D) Phylum, Class, Order, Family

STEP 1: Reread and Realize

What is the question asking you to do?

Realize: The question is asking you to place taxonomic groups in order from largest to smallest.

STEP 2: Remember

Remember the common mnemonic for the taxonomic levels: Dear King Phillip Come Over For Good Soup. If it helps, call to mind the mnemonic you created.

STEP 3: Rule Out

Eliminate the choices that do not match the mnemonic.

Choice A would read "For Over Come Phillip" if the mnemonic were applied.

Choice B would read "Over For Phillip Come" if the mnemonic were applied.

Choice C would read "Come Phillip For Over" if the mnemonic were applied.

The correct answer must be D.

A2. **All of the animals listed below belong to order *Carnivora*, which is an order that contains meat-eating mammals. Which list contains animals that most likely belong to the same family within order *Carnivora*?**

   A) fox, lion, cheetah, grizzly bear

   B) polar bear, black bear, raccoon, tiger

   C) wolf, coyote, fox, dog

   D) jaguar, skunk, spectacled bear, badger

STEP 1: Reread and Realize

What is the question asking you to do?

Realize: The question is asking you identify the animals that most likely belong to the same family within order *Carnivora*.

STEP 2: Remember

Remember that taxonomic groups are often based on common characteristics. Which list contains animals with the greatest number of similarities to one another?

STEP 3: Rule Out

Eliminate the choices that contain animals that are very different from one another.

Choice A contains two cats, a relative of the dog, and a bear, which are all pretty different from one another.

Choice B contains two bears, a cat, and a raccoon, which are all pretty different from one another.

Choice D contains a cat, a bear, a skunk, and a badger, which are all pretty different from one another.

That leaves C as the correct answer, which becomes more apparent when you realize that the animals in this list are all close relatives of the wolf.

WATCH OUT!

Mixing up the middle: The middle four taxonomic levels—phylum, class, order, and family—are the most commonly mixed up because they are the least commonly talked about in everyday life.

Assuming that all organisms with the same characteristic belong to the same group: For instance, sharks eat meat but do not belong to class *Mammalia*, so they do not belong to order *Carnivora*.

Guided Practice

1. Below is the full taxonomic classification of the Nile crocodile.

   Eukarya, Animalia, Chordata, Reptilia, Crocodylia, Crocodylidae, Crocodylus niloticus

   What would be the Nile crocodile's scientific name in the binomial nomenclature system?

   A) *Crocodylus niloticus*
   B) *Chordata reptilia*
   C) *Eukarya animalia*
   D) *Niloticus crocodylia*

STEP 1: Reread

Reread the question. What is the naming system the question is asking about called? How many levels of the taxonomic hierarchy does this system use to generate a scientific name? Which levels are they?

_____

_____

_____

_____

STEP 2: Identify

Write the words given in each answer choice and identify the taxonomic levels they represent.

_____

_____

_____

_____

STEP 3: Eliminate

Write the answer choices that you can eliminate because they contain taxonomic levels other than the genus and species names.

_____

_____

_____

_____

2. **Which of these is the broadest category of organism?**

    A) Class

    B) Family

    C) Genus

    D) Phylum

STEP 1: Reread

Rephrase the question in your own words. What level of the taxonomic hierarchy is the question asking you to identify?

_____

_____

_____

_____

STEP 2: Remember

Write the mnemonic you use to remember the order of taxonomic levels.

_____

_____

_____

_____

STEP 3: Identify

Write the four words from your mnemonic that match the four answer choices. The one that occurs first in the mnemonic represents the broadest category.

_____

_____

_____

_____

Guided Practice

3. The orange peel mushroom is a type of fungus. Which option could be the full taxonomic classification of the orange peel mushroom?

A) *Eukarya, Animalia, Chordata, Mammalia, Carnivora, Ursidae, Ursus arctos*

B) *Eukarya, Fungi, Ascomycota, Pezizomycetes, Pezizales, Pyrenemataceae, Aleuria aurantia*

C) *Eubacteria, Bacteria, Proteobacteria, Gamma Proteobacteria, Enterobacteriales, Enterobacteriaceae, Escherichia coli*

D) *Eukarya, Plantae, Anthophyta, Magnoliopsida, Fagales, Fagaceae, Quercus robur*

STEP 1: Identify Important Information

Write what you know about mushrooms. What type of organism is a mushroom according to the information in the question?

_____

_____

_____

_____

STEP 2: Look for Clues

Scan each option for any words that seem familiar. Write them here.

_____

_____

_____

_____

STEP 3: Identify the Answer

Which of the words you wrote in Step 2 applies to mushrooms? Think about the type of organism a mushroom is.

_____

_____

_____

_____

Independent Practice

1. In the scientific naming system known as binomial nomenclature, which two taxonomic levels are used to identify a specific organism?

    A) domain and kingdom

    B) genus and species

    C) order and family

    D) phylum and class

    HINT *Organisms' scientific names come from the narrowest, or smallest, categories from their complete taxonomic classification.*

2. Which category most likely represents the largest subgroup of class Mammalia?

    A) Genus *Amphechinus*

    B) Family *Erinaceidae*

    C) Order *Insectivora*

    D) Subclass *Eutheria*

    HINT *Think about which of the answer choices contains the broadest category.*

3. Which option could be the full taxonomic classification of a sugar maple tree, which is a type of plant?

    A) *Eukaryata, Protista, Tubulinea, Loboda, Tubulinea, Amoebidae, Amoeba proteus*

    B) *Eukarya, Animalia, Chordata, Mammalia, Rodentia, Muridae, Appodemus, agrarius*

    C) *Eukarya, Plantae, Magnoliophyta, Magnoliopsida, Sapindales, Aceraceae, Acer saccharum*

    D) *Bacteria, Eubacteria, Firmicutes, Baccilli, Bacillales, Staphylococcaceae, Staphylococcus aureus*

    HINT *Can you find some familiar words in the answer choices?*

ReKap

In this lesson, you learned that biologists use a special system to classify organisms. Remember the following:

- Biological classification continues to evolve as scientists discover and learn more about living things.

- Organisms are classified into a hierarchy of taxonomic groups. They are, from largest to smallest: domain, kingdom, phylum, class, order, family, genus, species.

- There are three domains and six kingdoms of organisms.

- Scientists refer to specific organisms by combining their genus and species names; this system is called binomial nomenclature.

? How will understanding taxonomy help you explain to patients why infectious diseases, such as those caused by viruses and fungi, can require treatments other than antibiotics?

_____

_____

_____

_____

Answers

Guided Practice

1. Step 1: The naming system is binomial nomenclature. It uses two levels: genus and species.

   Step 2: A - genus and species; B - phylum and class; C – domain and kingdom; D – species and order

   Step 3: Eliminate Choices B, C, and D

   Answer: (A) *Crocodylus niloticus*

2. Step 1: Identify the level that includes the most organisms.

   Step 2: "Dear King Phillip come over for good soup"

   Step 3: A – come; B – for; C – good; D – Phillip

   Answer: (D) Phylum

3. Step 1: Mushrooms are a type of fungi.

   Step 2: *Animalia, Mammalia, Carnivora, Fungi, Bacteria, Plantae* (answers may vary)

   Step 3: The mushroom is a Fungi.

   Answer: (B) *Eukarya, Fungi, Ascomycota, Pezizomycetes, Pezizales, Pyrenemataceae, Aleuria aurantia*

Independent Practice

1. **Answer: (B) genus and species**

   It wouldn't do much good to refer to an organism by its domain, kingdom, phylum, class, family, or order since so many other organisms will also be grouped in those categories. Therefore we must use the smallest categories: genus and species.

2. **Answer: (D) Subclass** *Eutheria*

   A subclass is a category that can be inserted between class and order, so a subclass is a broader category than an order. Since families and genuses are narrower categories than orders, it follows that the largest subgroup is subclass *Eutheria*.

3. **Answer: (C)** *Eukarya, Plantae, Magnoliophyta, Magnoliopsida, Sapindales, Aceraceae, Acer saccharum*

   Each full taxonomic classification contains some words that should be familiar. Answer A contains the words *Protista* and *Amoeba*, both of which hint at the kingdom of single-celled organisms. Answer B contains the words *Animalia* and *Rodentia*, hinting at an animal that is a rodent; this is in fact the classification of a common field mouse. Answer D contains the word *Bacteria,* which makes it pretty clear that this organism is a bacterium. Answer C, which is correct, contains the word *Plantae* and *Saccharum,* which means "sweet" and refers to the "sugar" portion of the sugar maple's common name.

ReKap

Viruses and fungi may require treatments other than antibiotics; antibiotics affect bacteria, which are a different species.

4 SCIENCE · LESSON 6
Atomic Structure

Small changes in atoms and molecules can make a big difference in the human body. For example, we constantly breathe in air containing *carbon dioxide*, but even small amounts of *carbon monoxide* added to the air we breathe can cause nerve damage and even death.

Common Uses in Health Care

- metabolism and dietary studies
- pharmacy
- toxins and poisons

$NaCl$ $C_6H_{12}O_6$

Fe^{3+}

$NaHCO_3$

Ca^{2+}

O_2 CO_2

Key Terms/Formulas

- **atom** – the smallest unit of an element that still retains the properties of that element

- **atomic number** – number of protons in an atom; all atoms of any one element have the same atomic number

- **average atomic mass** – average of the mass numbers of all the atoms in an element; often close to the mass number of the most abundant isotope

- **bond** – an attraction between elements caused either by sharing or by transferring electrons

- **electron** – negatively charged atomic particle located in shells around the nucleus

- **ion** – an atom that has gained or lost electrons, giving it a negative or positive charge

- **isotope** – a specific atom of an element with a certain number of neutrons; changing the number of neutrons will form a different isotope

- **mass number** – total number of protons and neutrons in an atom

- **molecule** – a group of atoms bonded together in a specific ratio

- **neutron** – neutral atomic particle found in the nucleus

- **proton** – positively charged atomic particle found in the nucleus

- **valence electrons** – outermost electrons in an atom

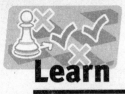

Structure and Properties of Atoms

An **atom** is the smallest particle of an element that still retains the properties of that element. The properties of the element depend on how many *protons*, *electrons*, and *neutrons* there are in that element's atoms. The properties of these particles are summarized in the table:

Particle	Mass	Charge	Location
Proton	about 1 amu	+1	nucleus
Electron	about 1/1840 amu	−1	outside the nucleus
Neutron	about 1 amu	0	nucleus

Note: An amu (atomic mass unit) is a very small measurement of mass; 1 red blood cell has a mass of about 2.7 trillion amus.

All atoms of an element will have the same number of protons, but they can have a different number of neutrons. For example, all gold atoms have 79 protons. Most gold atoms have 118 neutrons, but some can have 116 neutrons, and a few might have 117, 119, or 120 neutrons. The gold atoms that have 118 neutrons will each have a mass of about 197 amu. If the number of neutrons changes, the mass of the atom will change.

When we can specify the number of neutrons in a particular atom, we can also identify which isotope that atom is. Each combination of 79 protons and different numbers of neutron will be a different isotope. We identify the isotope by its *mass number* (number of protons plus number of neutrons); the isotope of gold that has 118 neutrons is gold-197, meaning it has a mass number of 197.

All neutral atoms of an element will have the same number of electrons as protons. For example, all neutral gold atoms will have 79 electrons (equal to the number of protons, so the + and − charges cancel out). If the number of electrons changes, the atom is no longer neutral; it will have a positive or negative charge and will be called an ion. Gold atoms can lose electrons during a reaction, becoming positive ions. Gold ions usually have 78 or 76 electrons, but other numbers are possible. A gold ion with 78 electrons will have a charge of +1, because it has 79 positive charges from the protons and 78 negative charges from the electrons.

Protons and neutrons occupy the *nucleus* in the center of the atom, while the electrons occupy the space outside the nucleus. The distance between the electrons and the nucleus is very large, compared to the size of the nucleus. The electrons move about the nucleus very quickly, and their location can never be precisely determined. However, they tend to occupy certain layers of space around the nucleus; these layers are commonly referred to as *energy levels*.

Each energy level can hold a certain maximum number of electrons; the farther the energy level is from the nucleus, the more electrons it can hold. Each level is designated with a number; level 1 is the one closest to the nucleus. Within each energy level, there are areas in which electrons are most likely to be found; these areas are called *orbitals*, and they are designated by letters. Each orbital can hold a certain maximum number of electrons; *s* orbitals can hold up to 2 electrons, *p* up to 6, *d* up to 10, *f* up to 14.

Each orbital in the diagram must be filled before electrons move into the next orbital (you are not expected to know the exceptions).

It helps to think of the energy levels like floors in a building, and the orbitals like rooms within those floors. Atoms with a few electrons will have only the first few levels occupied, while atoms with many electrons will have more levels occupied, higher up. The order in which the electrons occupy the orbitals follows a pattern (follow the arrow):

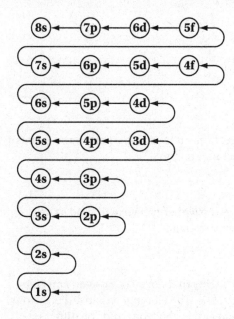

Rather than draw a diagram or table to show how many electrons are in each energy level, we can write the *electron configuration*, using coefficients for the energy levels, letters for the orbitals, and superscripts for the number of electrons in any one orbital. For example, an atom with 17 electrons will have the configuration: $1s^2 2s^2 2p^6 3s^2 3p^5$. Note that you can add up the superscripts to get the total number of electrons. An atom with 19 electrons will have the configuration: $1s^2 2s^2 2p^6 3s^2 3p^6 4s^1$.

The number of electrons in the *s* and *p* orbitals of the outermost energy level of an atom helps us predict the properties of that element. When we group elements by properties, we find that most fall into two groups: metallic and non-metallic.

If the atom has a total of 1, 2, or 3 *s* and *p* electrons in its outer energy level, it is likely to lose them during a reaction, and will become a positive ion (also called a *cation*). These atoms belong to metallic elements; they conduct heat and electricity well, and they are usually shiny and malleable. Most metals are solids at room temperature. Sodium, silver, zinc, and aluminum are examples of metals.

If the atom has a total of 5, 6, or 7 *s* and *p* electrons in its outer energy level, it is likely to try to gain more electrons during a reaction, in order to have a total of 8 combined *s* and *p* electrons, and become a negative ion (also called an *anion*). These atoms belong to non-metallic elements; they do not conduct heat or electricity well, and they are usually dull, brittle solids, or are liquids or gases at room temperature. Nitrogen, sulfur, and bromine are examples of non-metals.

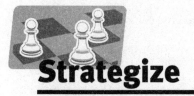

Strategize

Reread, Remember, Rule Out

To succeed on questions about atomic structure and properties:

Step 1: Always **reread** the question. Figure out what the question is asking you to do.

Step 2: **Remember** the relationship between protons, electrons, and neutrons, and how each affects an element's properties.

Step 3: Using the information you remembered, **rule out** the choices that do not match.

Apply

A1. An element has the configuration $1s^2 2s^2 2p^6 3s^2$. Is it a metal or a non-metal and what charge will its ion have?

A) metal, –2

B) metal, +2

C) non-metal, –2

D) non-metal, +2

STEP 1: Reread and Realize

What is the question asking? Reread the question—it is asking whether the element is likely to gain or lose electrons when it becomes an ion.

STEP 2: Remember

Elements with 1, 2, or 3 electrons in their outermost energy level will tend to lose those electrons; elements that lose electrons are metals.

STEP 3: Rule Out

Based on what you remember, rule out any choice that does not fit—you can rule out choices C and D because they are non-metals. The element will lose 2 electrons, so there will be more positive protons than negative electrons and the difference between the number of protons and electrons will be 2, so the charge will be +2. The correct answer is choice B.

A2. Which electron configuration belongs to an element that is a non-conducting gas?

A) $1s^2 2s^2 2p^6 3s^2$

B) $1s^2 2s^2 2p^6 3s^2 3p^1$

C) $1s^2 2s^2 2p^6 3s^2 3p^5$

D) $1s^2 2s^2 2p^6 3s^2 3p^6 4s^1$

STEP 1: Reread and Realize

What is the question asking? Reread the question—it is asking you to identify the electron configuration of a non-metal.

STEP 2: Remember

Non-metals have 5, 6, or 7 electrons in their outermost energy level, while metals have 1, 2, or 3 electrons in their outermost energy level.

STEP 3: Rule Out

Based on what you remember, rule out any choice that does not fit—you can rule out choices A, B, and D because they have 2, 3, and 1 electrons in their outermost energy level. The correct answer is choice C.

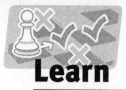

Learn

The Periodic Table and Periodic Trends

We use the periodic table to organize the elements by number of protons and by their electron configuration. This causes them to also form groups with similar properties:

Periodic Table of the Elements

Atomic Number —— 6
Symbol —— C
Atomic Mass —— 12.01

* Numbers in parentheses are the *mass numbers* of the most stable isotope of the element.

1	2	3	4	5	6	7	8	9	10	11	12	13	14	15	16	17	18
1 H 1.008																	2 He 4.003
3 Li 6.941	4 Be 9.012											5 B 10.81	6 C 12.01	7 N 14.01	8 O 16.00	9 F 19.00	10 Ne 20.18
11 Na 22.99	12 Mg 24.31											13 Al 26.98	14 Si 28.09	15 P 30.97	16 S 32.07	17 Cl 35.45	18 Ar 39.95
19 K 39.10	20 Ca 40.08	21 Sc 44.96	22 Ti 47.88	23 V 50.94	24 Cr 52.00	25 Mn 54.94	26 Fe 55.85	27 Co 58.93	28 Ni 58.69	29 Cu 63.55	30 Zn 65.39	31 Ga 69.72	32 Ge 72.61	33 As 74.92	34 Se 78.96	35 Br 79.90	36 Kr 83.80
37 Rb 85.47	38 Sr 87.62	39 Y 88.91	40 Zr 91.22	41 Nb 92.91	42 Mo 95.94	43 Tc (98)	44 Ru 101.1	45 Rh 102.9	46 Pd 106.4	47 Ag 107.9	48 Cd 112.4	49 In 114.8	50 Sn 118.7	51 Sb 121.8	52 Te 127.6	53 I 126.9	54 Xe 131.3
55 Cs 132.9	56 Ba 137.3	57–70	71 Lu 175.0	72 Hf 178.5	73 Ta 181.0	74 W 183.8	75 Re 186.2	76 Os 190.2	77 Ir 192.2	78 Pt 195.1	79 Au 197.0	80 Hg 200.6	81 Tl 204.4	82 Pb 207.2	83 Bi 209.0	84 Po (209)	85 At (210)	86 Rn (222)
87 Fr (223)	88 Ra 226.0	89–102	103 Lr (260)	104 Rf (261)	105 Db (262)	106 Sg (263)	107 Bh (262)	108 Hs (265)	109 Mt (268)	110 Uun (269)	111 Uuu (272)	112 Uub (277)	113 Uut	114 Uuq (289)	115 Uup	116 Uuh	117 Uus	118 Uuo

57 La 138.9	58 Ce 140.1	59 Or 140.9	60 Nd 144.2	61 Pm (145)	62 Sm 150.4	63 Eu 152.0	64 Gd 157.3	65 Tb 158.9	66 Dy 162.5	67 Ho 164.9	68 Er 167.3	69 Tm 168.9	70 Yb 173.0
89 Ac 227.0	90 Th 232.0	91 Pa 231.0	92 U 238.0	93 Np 237.0	94 Pu (244)	95 Am (243)	96 Cm (247)	97 Bk (247)	98 Cf (251)	99 Es (252)	100 Fm (257)	101 Md (258)	102 No (259)

The numbers at the top of each column indicate the *group* (also called a *family*) while the numbers to the left of each row (also called a *period*) indicate the energy level. The elements in a group will have similar endings to their electron configurations. For example, in group 16, oxygen (O) has an electron configuration of: $1s^22s^22p^4$ and sulfur (S) has an electron configuration of $1s^22s^22p^63s^23p^4$. The electrons in the outermost energy level are called valence electrons; therefore, the elements within a group will all have the same number of valence electrons.

Metals: Notice that the metals occupy the left side of the periodic table. Remember that one of the properties of metals is that they have 1, 2, or 3 electrons in their outer energy level (meaning that their configurations end in s^1, s^2, or s^2p^1) and they will lose those electrons when they form ions. Therefore, we can predict that all of the elements in group 1 will form +1 ions, and all of the elements in group 2 will form +2 ions. Groups 3 through 12 are not as simple, as they can also lose or rearrange some of their *d* electrons so that ions of atoms in these groups can have charges from +1 to +6, depending on the conditions the ion is formed in. Metals from these groups are called transition metals.

The ability of transition metals such as iron (Fe), manganese (Mn), and copper (Cu) to form ions with different charges is very important to many vital functions in humans. Hemoglobin, and the enzymes involved in respiration and cell reproduction, all depend on the ability of these ions to change their charge in different environments. Unfortunately, the ability of lead (Pb) to

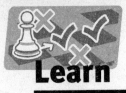

change its charge also makes it able to interfere with those processes—many transition metals are also poisonous.

There are exceptions to every rule. Notice that tin, lead, bismuth, and polonium (Sn, Pb, Bi, and Po) are grouped with the metals, even though they are in groups 14, 15, and 16. However, they behave much like the metals in groups 3 through 12.

Non-metals: Notice that the non-metals occupy the right side of the periodic table. Remember that one of the properties of metals is that they have more than 5, 6, or 7 electrons in their outer energy level (meaning that their configurations end in s^2p^3, s^2p^4, or s^2p^5) and they gain those electrons when they form ions. Therefore, we can predict that all of the elements in group 15 will form –3 ions, all of the elements in group 16 will form –2 ions, and all of the elements in group 17 will form –1 ions.

Notice that carbon (C) is an exception to the rule—it has 4 electrons in its outer energy level, but is included with the non-metals. The properties of carbon (dull, brittle, and non-conductive) are more similar to non-metals than to the other groups. As we will see later, carbon is the main building block in almost every molecule in our bodies; this is mostly because of carbon's electron configuration.

Metalloids: The staircase-shaped group between metals and non-metals contains elements that have both metallic and non-metallic properties. For example, silicon (Si) is shiny and conducts electricity, but it is brittle.

Noble Gases: The farthest group on the right is sometimes included with non-metals, as all of the elements in group 18 are nonconductive gases. However, since they also tend not to form ions or react at all, they are often in a group by themselves.

Since the periodic table arranges elements by number of protons and then by electron configuration, we see trends develop as we move across and down the table.

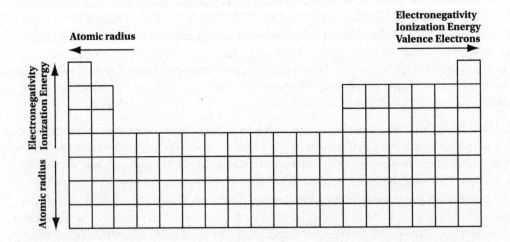

Atomic Radius: The distance from the center of the nucleus to the outer energy level increases as we add energy levels, so radius increases as we move down a group. However, as we increase the number of protons and electrons, we also increase the attraction. So, within an energy level, as the number of protons and electrons increase, the closer the outer energy level is pulled in toward the nucleus, reducing the radius, so radius decreases as we move toward the right in a row.

Electronegativity: Electronegativity is a measure of how much an atom will attract electrons during a reaction. The greater the distance between the nucleus of an atom and an external electron, the less the atom will attract that electron. Therefore, electronegativity will follow the inverse trend of radius: it will decrease as we move down a group and increase as we move toward the right in a row.

Ionization Energy: This is a measure of how much energy is required to remove one electron from an atom. It obviously will increase as electronegativity increases, so ionization energy decreases as we move down a column and increases as we move toward the right in a row.

Valence Electrons: The number of electrons in the outer energy level stays the same as we move up or down in a group, but increases as we move toward the right in a row. The number of valence electrons for the elements (except for the transition metals) is the same as the ones place in the group number. In other words, group 1 elements have 1 valence electron, group 15 elements have 5 valence electrons, and so on.

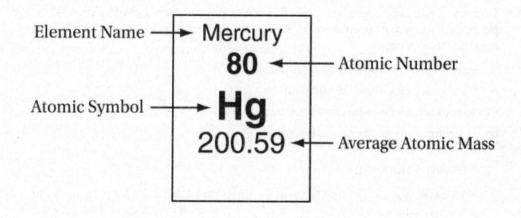

The periodic table usually contains the atom symbols of all the elements and can also contain additional information:

Atomic number: This indicates the number of protons and so is specific to the element. Only carbon has 6 protons, so only carbon has the atomic number of 6.

Atomic symbol: This is a one- or two-letter symbol, and it can be based on the modern name of the element. Many symbols, such as Na for sodium, are based on older names or the sources of the elements. Na comes from natron, which ultimately comes from an ancient Egyptian word for a sodium carbonate mineral. K for potassium comes from kalium, which comes from the Arabic word for wood ashes, which contained potassium hydroxide. Both chemicals were very important in the ancient world and continue to be so today. Knowing where the name comes from can help to remember symbols that don't match the modern name.

Average atomic mass: This is an average of the masses (in amu) of all the atoms of an element found in nature. It is usually close to the mass number of the most common isotope. For example, the most common isotope of nitrogen (N) has a mass number of 14, and the average atomic mass of all the nitrogen atoms is 14.007.

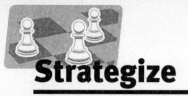

Strategize

Reread, Remember, Rule Out

To succeed on questions about the periodic table and trends:

Step 1: Always **reread** the question. Figure out what the question is asking you to do.

Step 2: **Remember** how the periodic table orders elements by atomic number and electron configuration, and how the trends related to these change across a row or down a group.

Step 3: Using the information you remembered **rule out** the choices that do not match.

Apply

A3. Fluorine-18 is a radioactive isotope of fluorine that is commonly used to detect cancer in the body. It has a mass number of 18. How many protons, electrons, and neutrons does the neutral atom have?

A) 9 protons, 9 electrons, and 9 neutrons

B) 9 protons, 9 electrons, and 10 neutrons

C) 10 protons, 10 electrons, and 9 neutrons

D) 10 protons, 10 electrons, and 8 neutrons

STEP 1: Reread and Realize

What is the question asking? Reread the question—it is asking for the number of protons, electrons, and neutrons for a fluorine atom if the charge is 0 and the mass number is 18.

STEP 2: Remember

The atomic number is the same as the number of protons (and electrons for a neutral atom) and the mass number is the number of protons plus neutrons.

STEP 3: Rule Out

Based on what you remember, rule out any choice that does not fit—since the atomic number of Fluorine is 9, you can rule out choices C and D, because they describe an atomic number of 10. Since the mass number (18) = protons (9) + neutrons, the atom must have 9 neutrons, so you can rule out choice B. (Notice that all the choices had the same number of protons and electrons, so you could not rule out any choices based on charge.) The correct answer is choice A.

Apply

A4. Of the elements that have 7 valence electrons, which has the highest ionization energy?

A) Astatine

B) Fluorine

C) Manganese

D) Nitrogen

STEP 1: Reread and Realize

What is the question asking? Reread the question—it is asking you to identify which of the four elements has 7 valence electrons; of those, it is then asking you to choose the element with the higher ionization energy.

STEP 2: Remember

The ones place of the group number indicates the number of valence electrons in the group for groups 1–2 and groups 13–18 (valence numbers for groups 3–12 do not follow this pattern). Also, ionization energy increases as you go up in a group.

STEP 3: Rule Out

Based on what you remember, rule out any choice that does not fit—since the question is asking for 7 valence electrons, you can rule out choices C and D as they are not in group 17 (group 7 does not necessarily have 7 valence electrons, and an atomic number of 7 does not indicate 7 valence electrons). Since Astatine is at the bottom of group 17, you can rule out choice A. Choice B is the correct answer because fluorine has 7 valence electrons and is at the top of its group.

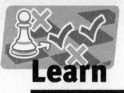

Molecules and Their Properties

Molecules are formed when atoms bond—these bonds are formed when atoms either transfer or share valence electrons. The goal of atoms participating in bonding is to get 8 electrons in their highest energy level (with the exception of elements with atomic numbers less than 6; their goal is to have 2 electrons in their highest energy level, and hydrogen can also have 0 electrons as a goal).

They achieve this by giving away electrons to get down to the next lowest energy level, gaining electrons to get up to the next highest energy level, or sharing electrons with another atom, so that each gets up to the next energy level. We can best see how this works with electron diagrams, although you can also use drawings of valence electrons around atom symbols (called Lewis dot structures) to demonstrate the transfer or sharing of electrons.

Ionic Bonds—electrons are transferred. When a metal and a non-metal atom react, the metal will give up one or more electrons, depending on its configuration, and the non-metal will accept them. For example, when a sodium atom bonds with a chlorine atom, the sodium atom gives up one electron, becoming a positive ion (called a cation) and the chlorine atom accepts it, becoming a negative ion (called an anion). The electron configurations change—notice that each ion has a configuration that has 8 electrons in its highest energy level:

Atom	Electron Configuration	Ion	Electron Configuration
Na	$1s^2 2s^2 2p^6 3s^1$	Na^{+1}	$1s^2 2s^2 2p^6$
Cl	$1s^2 2s^2 2p^6 3s^2 3p^5$	Cl^{-1}	$1s^2 2s^2 2p^6 3s^2 3p^6$

Ionic compounds tend to be very hard and brittle; they have a high melting point and conduct electricity when melted or dissolved in water.

When an atom can donate exactly the number of electrons needed by another atom, they combine in a one-to-one ratio. Since sodium donates one electron, and chlorine accepts one electron, we write the formula NaCl to indicate there is one sodium for each chlorine.

However, if the numbers donated/accepted do not match up, the ratios of the atoms must adjust. Calcium ($1s^2 2s^2 2p^6 3s^2 3p^6 4s^2$) will donate 2 electrons, so when it combines with chlorine, it must combine with 2 chlorines, and the formula will be $CaCl_2$.

Covalent Bonds—electrons are shared. Atoms with higher electronegativity are less likely to donate electrons, so when two non-metals react, they are likely to share the electrons instead. For example, carbon ($1s^2 2s^2 2p^2$) will share electrons with 4 chlorine atoms ($1s^2 2s^2 2p^6 3s^2 3p^5$) to form CCl_4 (carbon tetrachloride, a cancer-causing chemical that used to be used for dry cleaning clothes until it was found to be hazardous). By sharing one electron with each chlorine, and having each chlorine share one in return, carbon seems to have an electron configuration of $1s^2 2s^2 2p^6$ and each chlorine seems to have an electron configuration of $1s^2 2s^2 2p^6 3s^2 3p^6$. Since no electrons are transferred, however, each atom is still neutral.

Seven elements only exist in pure form as covalently bonded diatomic molecules: H_2, N_2, O_2, F_2, Cl_2, Br_2, I_2. All share electrons through single bonds except for nitrogen (triple bond) and oxygen (double bond).

Covalent compounds tend to have low melting points and many are liquids or gases at room temperature. Covalent compounds do not conduct electricity.

Multiple Covalent Bonds—the carbon forms 4 single bonds, one with each chlorine. In each bond, 2 electrons are shared. Atoms can also share 4 and 6 electrons, forming double and triple bonds (2 electrons shared in each bond). Since both the formula and the name of each covalent compound indicate the proportion of the atoms, we can determine how many electrons are shared from the number of valence electrons available.

Hydrocarbons—the ways that carbon can combine with hydrogen are so numerous that a naming system was developed to indicate the number of carbons, hydrogens, and bonds. The names use the same root to indicate the number of carbons, but different endings to indicate if double or triple bonds are present.

The root names from 5 to 10 carbons follow roots used in geometry: pent–, hex–, hept–, oct–, non–, dec–. The root names from 1 to 4 come from older names for compounds and so must be memorized: meth–, eth–, prop–, but–. Names of compounds with all single bonds end in –ane, so a 3-carbon hydrocarbon with no double or triple bonds is propane. Names of compounds with one double bond end in –ene, so a 2-carbon hydrocarbon with one double bond and no triple bonds is ethene. Names of compounds with one triple bond end in –yne, so a 4-carbon hydrocarbon with 1 triple bond and no double bonds is butyne. Names of compounds with combinations of double and triple bonds also follow a pattern.

Alkanes have two hydrogens for every carbon in their formula, plus 2 hydrogens. So propane has the formula C_3H_8. Alkenes have two hydrogens for every carbon, so propene has the formula C_3H_6. Alkynes have two hydrogens for every carbon, minus 2 hydrogens, so propyne has the formula C_3H_4.

Many hydrocarbons retain names from times before this naming system was developed. Ethyne is more commonly known as acetylene, so a welder is more likely to report that he burned himself with an acetylene torch than with an ethyne torch. At some point, chemical names simply must be looked up in a reliable reference for identification.

Hydrogen—hydrogen can either donate an electron or share one (in some circumstances, it can even accept an electron). In most cases, however, hydrogen acts as a non-metal and bonds covalently with other non-metals. In water, for example, 2 hydrogen atoms will share electrons with an oxygen atom to form H_2O, and in methane, 4 hydrogen atoms will share electrons with a carbon atom to form CH_4.

Unshared Electrons—not all of the valence electrons get shared in covalent bonds. For example, oxygen has 6 valence electrons, but only shares 2 of them in a water molecule, one with each hydrogen. The other 4 electrons pair up with each other, so a water molecule has 2 unshared pairs of electrons on the oxygen. This causes water molecules to have a positive side (where the hydrogens are) and a negative side (where the unshared pairs of electrons are). This polar characteristic of the water molecules gives water properties that make it essential to life: it is attracted to itself (cohesion) and is attracted to many surfaces (adhesion) and it can dissolve and transport many ionic and covalent substances.

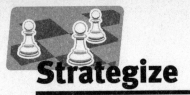

Strategize

Reread, Remember, Rule Out

To succeed on questions about the structure and properties of molecules:

Step 1: Always **reread** the question. Figure out what the question is asking you to do.

Step 2: **Remember** the ways that valence electrons are involved in bonding, and how they affect the properties.

Step 3: Using the information you remembered and **rule out** the choices that do not match or are not the best match.

Apply

A5. Which pair of elements would form a covalent compound?

- **A)** Copper and tin
- **B)** Zinc and chlorine
- **C)** Nitrogen and oxygen
- **D)** Magnesium and sulfur

STEP 1: Reread and Realize

What is the question asking? Reread the question—it is asking you to identify which elements could form covalent bonds with each other.

STEP 2: Remember

Covalent bonds form between two non-metals.

STEP 3: Rule Out

Based on what you remember, rule out any choice that does not fit—since both copper and tin are metals, you can rule out choice A. Zinc and magnesium are metals, so you can rule out choices B and D. Nitrogen and oxygen are both non-metals, so choice C is correct.

Apply

A6. Nitrogen gas molecules contain a triple bond. How many unshared pairs of electrons are in a nitrogen molecule?

A) 2

B) 4

C) 6

D) 8

STEP 1: Reread and Realize

What is the question asking? Reread the question—it is asking how many valence electrons remain after a triple bond is formed between two nitrogen atoms.

STEP 2: Remember

Nitrogen has 5 valence electrons, so there are a total of 10 valence electrons available in the molecule. A triple bond uses 6 valence electrons, so there will be 4 valence electrons left over.

STEP 3: Rule Out

Based on what you remember, rule out any choice that does not fit—there are 4 valence electrons left over, so you can rule out choices C and D, since the molecule won't have more than 4. The question asked for *unshared pairs*, so you would divide by 2; the correct answer is choice A.

Guided Practice

Let's work through a few examples together. Look back at the lesson content as often as necessary to help you apply the concepts and strategies you learned.

1. An atom of an element that is critical to forming certain amino acids has the electron configuration $1s^2 2s^2 2p^6 3s^2 3p^4$ in its neutral state and has a mass number of 34. What is the element name and how many neutrons does it have?

    A) sulfur, with 16 neutrons

    B) sulfur, with 18 neutrons

    C) selenium, with 16 neutrons

    D) selenium, with 18 neutrons

    STEP 1: Reread and realize

    What is the question asking you to do? Reread the item and find the important details.

    _____

    _____

    STEP 2: Remember

    What does the electron configuration tell you? What does the mass number tell you?

    _____

    _____

    _____

    _____

    STEP 3: Rule out

    Using your answer from Step 2, go through each answer choice. Which ones can you eliminate? You can eliminate any choice that does not have the correct number of protons or the correct number of neutrons.

    _____

    _____

    _____

    _____

2. Some ionic compounds can inhibit bacterial growth. Which combination of elements would produce an ionic compound?

A) Silver and chlorine

B) Sulfur and bromine

C) Nitrogen and iodine

D) Phosphorous and oxygen

STEP 1: Reread and realize

What is the question asking you to do? Reread the item and find the important details.

_____

_____

STEP 2: Remember

Which groups on the periodic table combine to form ionic compounds rather than covalent compounds?

_____

_____

_____

_____

STEP 3: Rule out

Which choices can you eliminate? Eliminate any combination that does not match the groups of elements that form ionic compounds with each other.

_____

_____

_____

_____

Guided Practice

3. An atom has 4 valence electrons, and has the lowest electronegativity in its group; it is an atom of which element?

A) Beryllium

B) Carbon

C) Lead

D) Krypton

STEP 1: Reread and realize

What is the question asking you to do? Reread the question and find the details that tell you.

_____

_____

STEP 2: Remember

How does the number of valence electrons indicate a group? What is the trend for electronegativity within a group?

_____

_____

_____

_____

STEP 3: Rule out

Determine which answer choices can be eliminated. Which elements are not in the correct group? Which of the remaining elements do not have the lowest electronegativity in the group?

_____

_____

_____

_____

4. Which of the following hydrocarbons has a triple bond?

A) C_3H_8

B) C_3H_6

C) C_6H_{12}

D C_6H_{10}

STEP 1: Reread and realize

What is the question asking you to do? Reread the question and find the details that tell you.

_____

_____

STEP 2: Remember

What is the ratio between carbons and hydrogens for an alkyne (it can help to remember the ratio for an alkane)?

_____

_____

STEP 3: Rule out

Determine which answer choices can be eliminated. Which formulas do not fit the ratio of carbons to hydrogens for an alkyne?

_____

_____

Independent Practice

1. An ion that is essential to nerve signal transmissions has a +1 charge and 18 electrons—it is an ion of which element?

A) Argon

B) Calcium

C) Chlorine

D) Potassium

HINT ▷ *Remember that the charge equals the protons minus the electrons.*

2. Two elements react and 2 electrons are transferred from an atom of one element to 2 atoms from the other element. Which compound was formed?

A) CO_2

B) $CaCl_2$

C) H_2O

D) Li_2O

HINT ▷ *Remember that electrons being transferred rather than shared indicates a certain type of bond.*

3. Based on periodic trends, which element (excluding hydrogen and the noble gases) has the smallest atomic radius?

A) Astatine

B) Fluorine

C) Francium

D) Lithium

HINT ▷ *Remember that the trend for atomic radius follows both rows and columns.*

4. What is the correct name for a hydrocarbon with the formula C_4H_8?

A) Butane

B) Butene

C) Octane

D) Octene

HINT ▷ *Remember which part of the name is based on the number of carbons and which part indicates the type of bond present.*

ReKap

In this lesson you reviewed:

- the structure of atoms, and how structure affects an atom's properties

- how to use the periodic table to predict an atom's structure and properties

- how number, type, and configuration of atoms in a molecule affects the molecule's properties

- the structure and properties of some common substances

> **?** **How will having knowledge about reading the periodic table and determining the structure and properties of atoms and molecules help you to better understand a patient's diagnosis or treatment?**
>
> _____
>
> _____
>
> _____
>
> _____

Answers

Guided Practice

1. Step 1: Name the element and how many neutrons it has.

    Step 2: Electron configuration indicates the number of electrons (add the subscripts) and mass number indicates the number of protons plus neutrons.

    Step 3: Eliminate Choices A, C, and D. Choices C and D are incorrect because the atom has 16 protons and selenium has 32 protons. Since the mass number is 34 and there are 16 protons, the number of neutrons must be 18.

   Answer: (B) sulfur, with 18 neutrons

2. Step 1: Determine which elements make an ionic compound.

    Step 2: Metal and nonmental compounds combine to form ionic compounds.

    Step 3: Eliminate Choices B, C, and D. Sulfur, bromine, nitrogen, iodine, phosphorous, and oxygen are all non-metals and so can't combine to form ionic compounds—Choice B, C, and D can be eliminated. Silver is a metal, and chlorine is a non-metal, so the correct answer is choice A.

   Answer: (A) Silver and chlorine

3. Step 1: Figure out which element has 4 valence electrons and the lowest electronegativity in its group.

    Step 2: The number of valence electrons indicates the group number. Electronegativity goes down as you move down a group.

    Step 3: Eliminate Choices A, B, and D. Four valence electrons indicate the element is in group 14, so choices A and D can be eliminated (A has an atomic number of 4 but is in group 1; D is in row 4 but not group 4). Choice B, Carbon, is at the top of the group instead of the bottom suggesting it has higher electronegativity than Lead

   Answer: (C) Lead

4. Step 1: Determine which choice has a triple bond.

    Step 2: The ratio between carbon and hydrogen for an alkyne is twice the number of carbons, minus two.

    Step 3: Eliminate Choices A, B, C. For an alkane, the number of hydrogens is twice the number of carbons, plus two. Alkenes have 2 fewer hydrogens than alkanes and alkynes have 2 fewer than alkenes, so the number for hydrogens should be twice the number of carbons, minus 2. Choice A is an alkane; Choices B and C are alkenes.

   Answer: (D) C_6H_{10}

Independent Practice

1. **Answer: (D) Potassium**

   An ion with +1 charge and 18 electrons comes from a neutral atom with 19 electrons (19 − 18 = 1). Choice A is incorrect because argon has 18 electrons when neutral (and does not form ions). Choice B is incorrect because calcium has 20 electrons when neutral (and forms a +2 ion). Choice C is incorrect because chlorine has 17 electrons (and forms a −1 ion).

2. **Answer: (B) CaCl$_2$**

Electrons being transferred indicate an ionic bond so the reaction must be between a metal and a non-metal. Choices A and C are incorrect because they contain only non-metals. Two electrons are transferred from one atom, indicating that the metal has 2 valence electrons. Choice D is incorrect because lithium has only 1 valence electron.

3. **Answer: (B) Fluorine**

Atomic radius decreases as you move toward the right in a row and up in a group. Choices A and C are incorrect because astatine and francium are at the bottom of their groups. Choice D is incorrect because, although lithium is at the top of its group, it is farthest to the left in a row.

4. **Answer: (B) Butene**

The root but indicates the molecule has 4 carbons. Choices C and D are incorrect because they have 8 carbons. The suffix –*ene* indicates that there is a double bond in the molecule, so there will be twice as many hydrogens as carbons without adding or subtracting any hydrogens (or, 2 fewer hydrogens than the alkane, due to the double bond). Choice A is incorrect because it has twice as many hydrogens plus 2.

ReKap

Acid-base chemistry is relevant in health. Understanding the relationship between acids and bases, pH, and buffers is relevant to a patient's level of homeostasis. Knowledge of ionic and covalent bonds and chemistry calculations can lead to a better understanding of metabolic acidosis and oxygen perfusion.

4 SCIENCE · LESSON 7
Chemical Reactions

Chemical reactions are all around us. They occur in nature and in laboratories. Millions of chemical reactions occur inside your body every second. Newly discovered reactions can provide us with the new materials for useful products and breakthrough medications. But what exactly is a chemical reaction? Read on to find out.

Common Uses in Health Care

- understanding the composition of medications
- predicting dangerous drug interactions
- detecting poisons and other contaminating chemicals

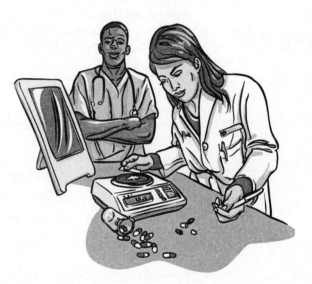

Key Terms/Formulas

- **acid** – a solution that contains more free hydrogen ions than water (pH < 7)
- **base** – a solution that contains fewer free hydrogen ions than water (pH > 7)
- **chemical reaction** – the creation of new substances through the rearrangement of atoms and molecules
- **metabolism** – the sum of all chemical reactions inside a living thing
- **oxidation** – the donation of electrons to another atom or molecule
- **pH** – the measure of how acidic or basic a solution is; ranges from 0 to 14
- **products** – matter that is produced during a chemical reaction
- **reactants** – matter that is consumed during a chemical reaction
- **reduction** – the acceptance of electrons by an atom or molecule
- **salt** – a substance produced by the reaction of an acid with a base

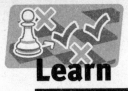

All matter is composed of atoms and molecules. The atoms that make up a sample of matter determine its properties. Matter can undergo physical changes and chemical changes. In a physical change, the observable properties of matter can change, but the arrangement of the atoms that make up the matter does not. One example of a physical change is water freezing.

In a chemical change, the atoms that make up the matter are rearranged and new substances are created. When this happens, we call it a chemical reaction.

Up Close

What is Metabolism?

Living things are jam-packed full of chemicals that react with one another. These reactions serve many purposes: some break down substances and some build new ones; some generate energy and some use energy. The sum of all chemical reactions that occur inside a living thing is called *metabolism*.

All chemical reactions have *reactants*, or substances that are consumed during the reaction, and *products*, which are substances that are created during the reaction. An example of a chemical reaction is the combining of hydrogen gas and oxygen gas to create water. We can symbolize this chemical reaction as follows:

$$H_2 + O_2 \rightarrow H_2O$$
(reactants)   (product)

Atoms are neither created nor destroyed in a chemical reaction, only rearranged. Therefore, the two sides of the chemical reaction must be *balanced*, which means that both sides must have the same types and numbers of atoms. The reaction shown above is not balanced since the left side has two oxygen atoms and the right side has only one. You can balance a chemical reaction by adding coefficients, or numbers, in front of the reactants and products until both sides are equal.

To start balancing the reaction above, first insert the number 2 in front of the product, water.

$$H_2 + O_2 \rightarrow \underline{2}H_2O$$

By doing this, we are saying that the product of this reaction is two water molecules instead of just one. Since each water molecule has a single oxygen atom, we now have the same number of oxygen atoms on both sides: two.

But, now we have a new problem. Since each water molecule has two hydrogen atoms, we have four hydrogen atoms on the right side and only two on the left; hydrogen is now imbalanced. The solution? Simply insert the number 2 before the hydrogen gas molecule on the left side. Since each hydrogen gas molecule has two hydrogen atoms, we will have a total of four atoms.

$$\underline{2}H_2 + O_2 \rightarrow 2H_2O$$

We now have a balanced chemical equation that tells us that two hydrogen gas molecules will react with one oxygen gas molecule to form two molecules of water. We know it's balanced because there are the same numbers of hydrogen and oxygen atoms on both sides of the arrow.

Counting Atoms

To be able to balance an equation, you need to know how to count the atoms in a chemical formula. The chemical formula for a molecule called tricalcium phosphate is shown below.

$$Ca_3(PO_4)_2$$

First determine the types of atoms this molecule contains. Each capital letter indicates an individual type of element, so there are three in this molecule: Ca, P, and O. You can consult the Periodic Table to find that Ca stands for calcium, P stands for phosphorus, and O stands for oxygen.

But how many of each atom are there? The subscripts reveal the amounts. The subscript 3 is attached to the calcium atom, meaning that this molecule contains three calcium atoms (Note: if there is no subscript, that means there is only one of that type of atom). The parentheses around the PO_4 portion of the formula indicates that PO_4 represents a group of atoms (one phosphorus atom and four oxygen atoms) that is repeated in the molecule. How many times is it repeated? The subscript attached to it tells you. In this case, the subscript 2 is attached to the PO_4 group, meaning that this group occurs twice in the molecule. So there are a total of two phosphorus atoms and eight oxygen atoms in this molecule. Let's see what we have come up with:

$$Ca_3(PO_4)_2 = 3 \text{ calcium atoms, 2 phosphorus atoms, 8 oxygen atoms}$$

What if you see a coefficient, or number, added to the beginning of the molecule? That means that there are two of the molecules involved in the reaction. To figure out the number of atoms these molecules contribute, simply multiply the numbers of atoms in a single molecule by the coefficient. Look at this example:

$$2Ca_3(PO_4)_2 = 6 \text{ calcium atoms, 4 phosphorus atoms, 16 oxygen atoms}$$

And that's all there is to counting atoms!

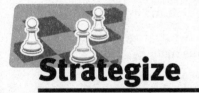

Strategize

Quick Steps for Counting Atoms

1. **Identify** the types of atoms by their symbols.

2. **Write** the number 1 as a subscript after any symbol that does not have a visible subscript. This is a reminder that the absence of a subscript implies that there is only one of that type of atom.

3. If there are parentheses, **multiply** each subscript inside the parentheses by the subscript outside of them. Write the new subscripts in place of the old ones and remove the parentheses.

4. If there is a coefficient before the molecule, **multiply** each subscript by the coefficient. Write the new subscripts in place of the old ones and remove the coefficient.

5. **Read** the subscripts; they now tell you the correct number of each atom in the molecule.

Apply

A1. The reaction between sodium and water is shown below.

$$Na + H_2O \rightarrow NaOH + H_2$$

Which option shows the balanced form of this reaction?

A) $Na + H_2O \rightarrow NaOH + \underline{2}H_2$

B) $\underline{2}Na + H_2O \rightarrow \underline{2}NaOH + H_2$

C) $\underline{2}Na + \underline{2}H_2O \rightarrow \underline{2}NaOH + H_2$

D) $\underline{2}Na + \underline{2}H_2O \rightarrow \underline{2}NaOH + 2H_2$

STEP 1: Reread and Realize

What is the question asking you to do?

Realize: You are being asked to find the balanced form of the equation given in the question.

STEP 2: Count the Atoms

Remember to figure out the types and numbers of atoms on each side of the equation. For example, the left side of the given equation contains one sodium atom, two hydrogen atoms, and one oxygen atom. The right side contains one sodium atom, three hydrogen atoms, and one oxygen atom. The hydrogen atoms are imbalanced. Don't forget to use the Quick Steps for Counting Atoms strategy if you have trouble with this step.

STEP 3: Rule Out

Eliminate the choices that contain imbalances.

Choice A has an imbalance of hydrogen atoms: two on the left and five on the right.

Choice B has imbalances of hydrogen and oxygen atoms: two hydrogens on the left and four on the right; one oxygen on the left and two on the right.

Choice D has an imbalance of hydrogen atoms: four hydrogens on the left and six on the right.

This means the correct answer is C!

 WATCH OUT

Don't forget to balance all the atoms! When beginning to balance a chemical equation, you usually identify a single atom that has unequal amounts. Then you add a coefficient to one side to balance that atom. In many cases, that coefficient serves to *unbalance* another atom. Keep an eye out for this, because balancing equations often takes multiple steps and some trial and error.

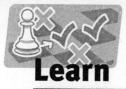

Learn

Types of Chemical Reactions

One common type of chemical reaction is called an oxidation-reduction reaction (commonly called a *redox* reaction). In such a reaction, one reactant undergoes *oxidation*, or the loss of electrons, and the other undergoes *reduction*, or the gaining of electrons. The oxidized reactant becomes a positively charged ion and the reduced reactant becomes negatively charged. In many cases, the two oppositely charged ions then form a compound held together by an ionic bond. Shown below are the oxidation and reduction that happen when copper wire is placed in a solution of silver ions.

Copper atoms lose two electrons, and so are oxidized: $Cu \rightarrow Cu^{2+} + 2$ electrons

Silver ions gain an electron, and so are reduced: $2Ag^+ + 2$ electrons $\rightarrow 2Ag$

Here is the overall reaction: $2Ag^+ + Cu \rightarrow 2Ag + Cu^{2+}$

Redox reactions are involved in many important processes, such as photosynthesis, cellular respiration, and combustion. Batteries also work because of redox reactions; the flow of electrons between the two terminals of a battery occurs because one terminal contains a substance that is oxidized and the other terminal contains a substance that is reduced. When one substance is fully oxidized and the other is fully reduced, the battery will no longer work.

Another important type of reaction is the acid-base reaction. An *acid* is a solution that contains more free hydrogen ions than water. A *base* is a solution that contains fewer free hydrogen ions than water. Acidity is measured using the *pH scale*, which ranges from 0 to 14, with 7 being neutral (water has a pH of 7). Acids have a pH less than 7, and bases have a pH greater than 7.

A neutralization reaction occurs when acids and bases react to form water and a salt. A *salt* is a compound that forms when the negative ion from an acid bonds ionically to the positive ion from a base. A common neutralization reaction is shown below.

$$HNO_3 + KOH \rightarrow KNO_3 + H_2O$$
(acid) (base) (salt) (water)

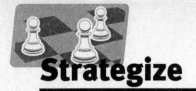

Strategize

Seek Clues

Wondering whether you are dealing with an oxidation-reduction reaction or an acid-base reaction? You can look for specific clues to help you figure it out.

Oxidation-reduction clues:

- Two of the reactants in the equation have clearly switched their ionic charges, like in the example of copper and silver above.

- Half-reactions are shown that have electrons as reactants or products.

Acid-base clues:

- Water is a product. This means that you may be looking at a neutralization reaction.

- A hydrogen ion (H^+), hydroxide ion (OH^-), or both are on the reactant or product side of the equation. These ions are the unmistakable calling cards of strong acids and bases.

A2. In the oxidation-reduction reaction shown below, magnesium atoms are oxidized and oxygen atoms are reduced.

$$2Mg + O_2 \rightarrow 2MgO$$

Which option shows the oxidation half-reaction that is part of the full reaction?

A) $2Mg \rightarrow 2Mg^{2+} + 4$ electrons.

B) $2Mg + 2$ electrons $\rightarrow 2Mg$

C) $2O \rightarrow 2O^{2+} + 4$ electrons

D) $2O + 4$ electrons $\rightarrow 2O^{2-}$

STEP 1: Reread and Realize

What is the question asking you to do?

Realize: You are being asked to identify the half-reaction that shows the oxidation that takes place in the full reaction. **Reread** the question and you'll find the information that magnesium (Mg) is being oxidized.

STEP 2: Seek Clues

Remember that when an atom is oxidized, it loses electrons and gains a more positive charge. Look at the answer choices and try to identify the one that shows magnesium losing electrons and gaining a positive charge.

STEP 3: Rule Out

Eliminate the choices that do not involve magnesium losing electrons.

Choice B shows magnesium gaining electrons and a negative charge, so this cannot be oxidation.

Choice C shows oxygen losing electrons; the supplied information states that magnesium is oxidized, so this cannot be correct.

Choice D shows oxygen gaining electrons and a negative charge; this is the reduction half-reaction, which is not what you are being asked to identify.

This means the correct answer is A!

Apply

A3. **What are the products of a neutralization reaction?**

A) an acid and a base

B) an electron and a proton

C) a positive ion and a negative ion

D) a salt and water

STEP 1: Reread and Realize

What is the question asking you to do?

Realize: The question is asking you what the end results of a neutralization reaction are.

STEP 2: Remember

Remember that a neutralization reaction is a type of acid-base reaction where an acid reacts with a base to create a solution with a pH of 7, which is neutral. Water has a pH of 7.

STEP 3: Rule Out

Eliminate the choices that do not involve water.

Choice A lists the reactants of a neutralization reaction, not the products.

Choice B lists two subatomic particles; although protons are directly involved in acid-base reactions, these are not the products of a neutralization reaction.

Choice C lists two types of ions. Ions are involved in acid-base reactions, but they are not the products of neutralization reactions.

This means the correct answer is D!

 WATCH OUT

Confusing the receiver with the donor: In oxidation-reduction reactions, it's easy to mix up the reactant that is receiving electrons with the reactant that is losing electrons. A handy way to remember the difference is to keep in mind that oxygen *always* receives electrons, and so it oxidizes other reactants by stripping electrons from them. This is why the words oxygen and oxidize have the same root.

Forgetting the salt: It's relatively easy to remember the roles of acids, bases, and water in neutralization reactions. Don't forget about the salt that forms from the leftover ions once the H^+ from the acid and the OH^- from the base have formed water.

Guided Practice

1. Which option shows the names and amounts of atoms contained in the compound shown below?

$Al_2(SO_4)_3$

A) 2 antimony atoms, 1 silver atom, 4 osmium atoms

B) 2 antimony atoms, 3 silver atoms, 12 osmium atoms

C) 2 aluminum atoms, 1 sulfur atom, 4 oxygen atoms

D) 2 aluminum atoms, 3 sulfur atoms, 12 oxygen atoms

STEP 1: Identify

Use the Periodic Table to identify the names of the elements indicated by the symbols in the compound. Remember that a capital letter followed by a lower-case letter is considered a single symbol. Write the names of the elements on the lines below.

_____

_____

_____

_____

STEP 2: Multiply

Multiply the subscripts inside the parentheses by the subscript outside the parentheses. Remember that a subscript of 1 is implied where no subscript is shown, such as after the letter *S* inside the parentheses. Write the results of your multiplication on the lines below.

_____

_____

_____

_____

STEP 3: Count

Read the subscripts to learn how many of each type of atom are in the compound. For the atoms inside the parentheses, use the subscripts that resulted from the multiplication in Step 2.

_____

_____

_____

_____

Guided Practice

2. Which sequence of numbers can you use to balance the chemical equation shown below?

$$\_Hg + \_Br_2 \rightarrow \_Hg_2Br_2$$

A) 1, 1, 1

B) 2, 2, 2

C) 2, 1, 1

D) 1, 1, 2

STEP 1: Count the Atoms

Assume that all coefficients start as 1. Determine the amounts and types of atoms on both sides of the equation. Use the Periodic Table to learn the names of the elements represented by the letters, and the subscripts to determine the amounts of atoms. Write your answer on the lines below.

_____

_____

_____

_____

STEP 2: Locate an Imbalance

Is there a difference between the number of mercury atoms on the two sides of the equations? What about the number of bromine atoms?

_____

_____

_____

STEP 3: Correct the Imbalance

Add a number before a reactant or product to correct the imbalance. For instance, if there are fewer mercury atoms on one side, add a higher number before the mercury symbol on that side. Be sure to check if any other imbalances are caused by adding the number. Write the balanced equation on the lines below.

_____

_____

_____

_____

3. **Which statement describes a substance being reduced?**

   A) Hydrochloric acid and sodium hydroxide combine to form water and a salt.

   B) A chlorine atom gains an electron from a sodium atom and becomes negatively charged.

   C) Methane combusts when it combines with oxygen gas and energy is released.

   D) A zinc atom loses electrons to hydrogen atoms and gains a positive charge.

STEP 1: Reread

Reread the question to identify what you are being asked. Are acids and bases mentioned in the question? What about oxidation or reduction? Write what you are being asked on the lines below.

_____

_____

_____

_____

STEP 2: Define

Consult the text of the lesson and define the process of reduction.

_____

_____

_____

_____

STEP 3: Eliminate

Eliminate answers that do not describe a substance gaining electrons and a negative charge. Which answers can you eliminate? Which one is left?

_____

_____

_____

_____

Independent Practice

1. Which sequence of numbers could be used to balance the equation shown below?

$$\_Li + \_O_2 \rightarrow \_Li_2O$$

   A) 2, 1, 1
   B) 1, 2, 2
   C) 4, 1, 2
   D) 2, 1, 4

   HINT *Start by adding a coefficient to the right side to balance oxygen atoms. Then observe how the balance of lithium atoms has changed and correct it by adding a coefficient on the left side of the equation.*

2. Look at the chemical equation shown below.

$$4Al + 3O_2 \rightarrow 4Al^{3+} + 6O^{2-} \rightarrow 2Al_2O_3$$

   Which statement about aluminum is true?

   A) Aluminum is oxidized in this reaction.
   B) Aluminum is reduced in this reaction.
   C) Aluminum acts as an acid in this reaction.
   D) Aluminum acts as a base in this reaction.

   HINT *How does the charge on the aluminum atoms change and what does this tell you about whether they are gaining or losing electrons?*

3. A neutralization reaction is shown below.

$$2HClO_4 + RbOH \rightarrow RbClO_4 + H_2O$$

   Which compound is a salt?

   A) $HClO_4$
   B) $RbOH$
   C) $RbClO_4$
   D) H_2O

   HINT *Remember that a salt is a product in a neutralization reaction.*

ReKap

In this lesson, you learned how to read chemical formulas, balance chemical reactions, and identify oxidation-reduction and acid-base reactions. Remember the following:

- Chemical formulas show the amounts and types of atoms in a compound.

- Chemical equations must have the same amounts and types of atoms on both sides.

- Oxidation and reduction occur at the same time; for one substance to be reduced, another must be oxidized.

- A pH of 7 is neutral; acids have a pH below 7 and bases have a pH above 7.

- Neutralization reactions occur when an acid and a base react to produce a water and a salt.

? **How will the information in this lesson help you explain to patients why they cannot take certain combinations of drugs at the same time?**

_____

_____

_____

_____

Answers

Guided Practice

1. Step 1: Al = aluminum; S = sulfur; O = oxygen

    Step 2: S: 1 x 3 = 3; O: 4 x 3 = 12

    Step 3: 2 aluminum; 3 sulfur; 12 oxygen

    Answer: (D) 2 aluminum atoms, 3 sulfur atoms, 12 oxygen atoms

2. Step 1: Left side: 2 bromine, 1 mercury; Right side: 2 bromine, 2 mercury

    Step 2: Bromine are balanced; mercury are not

    Step 3: $2Hg + Br_2 + Hg_2Br_2$

    Answer: (C) 2, 1, 1

3. Step 1: Identify an example of a reduction

    Step 2: A reduction is when an atom or molecule gains at least one electron and the charge becomes more negative.

    Step 3: Eliminate Choices A, C, and D. Eliminate Choice A because it describes a neutralization reaction, Choice C because it describes combustion (which is an example of oxidation), and Choice D because it describes oxidation.

    Answer: (B) A chlorine atom gains an electron from a sodium atom and becomes negatively charged.

Independent Practice

1. **Answer: (C) 4, 1, 2**

    Adding the coefficient 2 to the compound on the right side of the equation balances the oxygen atoms (2 on each side); adding the coefficient 4 to the lithium on the left side of the equation balances the lithium atoms (4 on each side).

2. **Answer: (A) Aluminum is oxidized in this reaction.**

    When the charges on atoms change, they are being oxidized or reduced. Since the charge on the aluminum atoms has become more positive, the atoms must have lost electrons and have thus been oxidized.

3. **Answer: (C) $RbClO_4$**

    The products of a neutralization reaction are water and a salt. The products are shown on the right side of the arrow. The two compounds on the right side of the arrow are $RbClO_4$ and H_2O. Since H_2O is clearly water, which means $RbClO_4$ must be the salt.

ReKap

Certain combinations of drugs may react with one another. Understanding redox and acid-base reactions may help to predict and prevent such reactions.

States of Matter

The changing states of matter can have a huge impact on the human body. Ice crystals that form inside cells can damage them. Water that evaporates from human skin can cool an overheated body. Liquid chemicals that give off gaseous fumes can make people sick. How can you recognize the states of matter and predict when a change in state might have consequences for a patient? Read on to find out!

Common Uses in Health Care

- dissolving and precipitating substances during chemical reactions

- using the heat of vaporization to cool overheated patients

- preserving the solid structures of donor organs

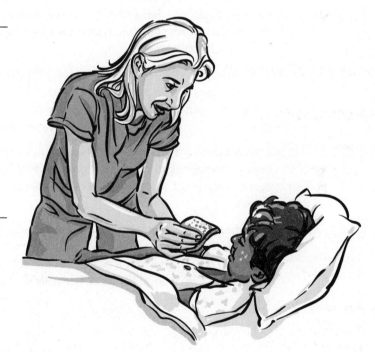

Key Terms/Formulas

- **crystal** – a type of solid with highly ordered atoms or molecules

- **gas** – a state of matter with a variable shape and volume

- **heat** – a type of energy that is transferred during changes in temperature

- **latent heat** – the amount of heat energy a substance must release or absorb to transition between the liquid and gas states

- **liquid** – the state of matter that has a fixed volume but a variable shape

- **phase transition** – the changing of a substance from one state of matter to another

- **solid** – the state of matter that has a fixed volume and shape

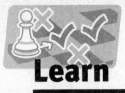

Learn

The States of Matter

The three states of matter we most commonly encounter are solids, liquids, and gases. Most substances can exist in all three states. A substance's current state depends on the temperature and pressure it is exposed to. Generally, a low temperature combined with a high pressure leads to a solid state (think about how water freezes at low temperatures under the weight of our atmosphere's pressure). As temperature rises or pressure falls, a substance will usually transition to a liquid form. As temperature rises or pressure falls further, that liquid can become a gas. But why do these changes happen?

The atoms or molecules inside most matter have weak attractions to one another (for simplicity's sake, we'll refer to atoms or molecules as *particles* from this point forward). These attractive forces lead to an ordered state, like in a solid. However, the inherent motion of particles leads to a disordered state, like in a gas. The current state of matter depends on whether the attractive forces are stronger than the motion trying to pull the particles apart. This is why substances change into more disordered states as temperatures rise; higher temperatures mean more molecular motion to break the attractive forces.

How is pressure involved? Pressure, such as the pressure exerted by Earth's atmosphere, pushes particles closer together and restricts their motion. Releasing the pressure can be like taking the lid off a can with a spring-loaded toy snake inside; attractive forces are broken and particles escape their confinement.

The most ordered state of matter is a *solid*. Solids generally have fixed shapes and volumes because their particles are strongly attracted to each other. The particles in a solid vibrate with motion, but generally stay put relative to one another. Some solids have more molecular order than others. The type of solid with the greatest amount of molecular order is called a *crystal*.

Liquids have less molecular order than solids. The particles in a liquid are attracted to each other strongly enough so that they stay together, but they have enough motion so that they slide around each other. This is why liquids can change shape so easily, even though they have fixed volumes.

Gases have the least molecular order. The particles in a gas move with so much energy that the attractive forces between them are completely overcome. The particles simply fly away from each other. This is why a gas will take on the shape and volume of its container, and if that container is opened, the gas will usually leave the container and spread randomly into the environment.

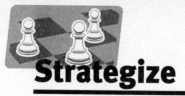

Strategize

This image shows how the particles behave in the three states of matter.

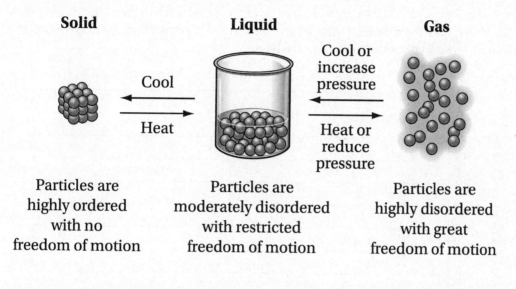

Solid

Particles are
highly ordered
with no
freedom of motion

Liquid

Cool

Heat

Particles are
moderately disordered
with restricted
freedom of motion

Cool or
increase
pressure

Heat or
reduce
pressure

Gas

Particles are
highly disordered
with great
freedom of motion

As shown in the figure above, the addition or subtraction of energy, such as heat energy, can cause a substance to go through a *phase transition*, or change of state. Examples of phase transitions include the melting of ice or the vaporization of water from a boiling pot. Both of these transitions involve the addition of heat energy because the energy causing the phase transition is related to a change in temperature. Water condensing onto a cool windshield on a humid day involves the removal of heat from the water vapor in the air. Evaporation is a special case; during evaporation, water changes from a liquid to a gas because of energy added when fast-moving gas molecules, such as those in Earth's atmosphere, collide with the surface of the water.

This figure shows all the types of phase transitions that matter can go through.

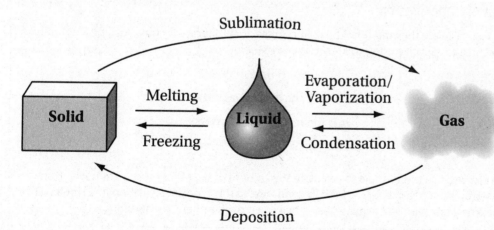

Sublimation

Solid

Melting

Freezing

Liquid

Evaporation/
Vaporization

Condensation

Gas

Deposition

Every substance requires a specific amount of heat to cause it to change from a liquid to a gas at a constant temperature. This amount is called its *latent heat*. For example, water has a latent heat of 540 calories per gram (cal/g). What does this mean? Well, you know that the boiling

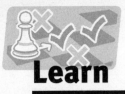
point of water is 100°C. However, a gram of water will not instantly vaporize when it reaches that temperature. It will vaporize when 540 additional calories of heat energy are added while its temperature is 100°C. It's important to note that the temperature of the water will not rise as it vaporizes, since the additional heat energy is being used to break bonds between the water molecules. The graph below shows how this works.

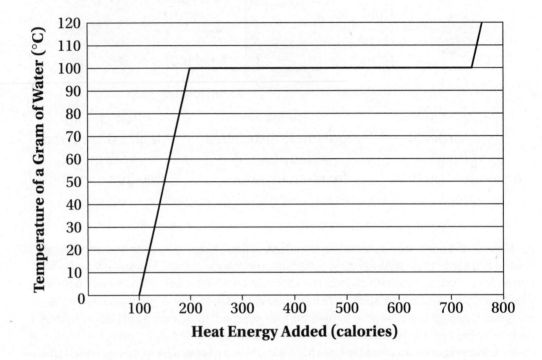

Up Close

Heat of Vaporization

You can calculate the amount of heat, in calories, that is necessary for a specific amount of a substance to vaporize using the formula shown here:

$$H = mL$$

where H is the heat of vaporization

m is the mass of the substance

L is the latent heat of the substance

You can also use this formula to calculate the amount of heat that must be removed from a given amount of a substance for it to condense. In this type of calculation, the result will have a negative sign (–) because heat is being removed rather than added.

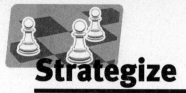

Strategize

Remember Water

We're all familiar with water in its various states. We slip on its solid form. We drink its liquid form. We feel it evaporate into its gaseous form when we sweat. The experiences you've had with water can help you remember how molecules behave in the different states. Solid water, or ice, is the easiest to hold in your hand because its molecules aren't moving much. Liquid water is more difficult to hold because the molecules slide around each other and can slip through your fingers; even still, you can hold some liquid water in a cupped palm and it will retain a bowl shape there. Gaseous water, or water vapor, is nearly impossible to hold in your hand since the highly mobile molecules will fly up and out of a cupped palm.

Read the Sign

When trying to figure out how a change in heat energy will affect a substance's state, the sign on the energy value will give you the hint you need. A positive sign means that the substance is gaining energy and will therefore progress from a solid to a liquid to a gas. A negative sign means the substance is losing energy and its state will change in the opposite direction.

A1. In which state do the particles of a substance have enough freedom of motion to slide around each other but not completely separate?

A) crystal

B) gas

C) liquid

D) solid

STEP 1: Reread and Realize

What is the question asking you to do?

Realize: You are being asked to identify the state of matter in which particles can slide around each other but not fly away from each other. Use the *Remember Water* strategy to help figure out the answer.

STEP 2: Remember Water

Remember that liquid water can slip through your fingers because its molecules can slide around each other. However, liquid water does not fly out of your palm because its molecules do not have enough energy to completely separate.

STEP 3: Rule Out

Eliminate the choices that do not involve the proper state of matter.

Choice A is incorrect because a crystal is the most ordered form of a solid. Particles have very little freedom of motion in this state.

Choice B is incorrect because the particles in a gas have enough energy to separate from one another in all directions.

Choice D is incorrect because the particles in a solid do not have enough energy to slide around one another.

This means the correct answer is C!

A2. Mercury is a liquid at room temperature. It has a boiling point of approximately 357°C and a latent heat of 70 cal/g. Approximately how much heat energy will be required to completely vaporize a 200g sample of mercury at 357°C?

A) 3 calories

B) 5 calories

C) 14,000 calories

D) 25,000 calories

STEP 1: Reread and Realize

What is the question asking you to do?

Realize: The question is asking you to figure out the heat of vaporization for a 200g sample of mercury.

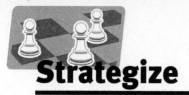

Strategize

STEP 2: Remember

You have been given an equation for this type of calculation. It is

$$H = mL$$

where H is the heat of vaporization

m is the mass of the substance

L is the latent heat of the substance

STEP 3: Calculate

Plug the values you have been given into the equation for heat of vaporization to figure out the answer. The correct calculation is shown here:

$$H = mL$$
$$H = (200g)(70cal/g)$$
$$H = 14,000 \text{ cal}$$

Based on this calculation, you can see that choice C is correct.

Choice A is the value you will get if you divide the mass of the mercury by its latent heat.

Choice B is the value you will get if you divide the temperature of the mercury by its latent heat.

Choice D is the value you will get if you multiply the temperature of the mercury by its latent heat.

 WATCH OUT!

Forgetting about pressure: Because we see it happen to water, it's easy to remember that changing temperatures can change the state of a substance. But don't forget about pressure. Changing the pressure on a substance can change its state even if the temperature is held constant. A very high pressure will cause a substance to be solid; continuously lowering the pressure will cause the substance to become a liquid and ultimately a gas.

Using the wrong numbers: Read questions involving calculations, such as the question in Example 2, very carefully. Be sure not to plug the wrong numbers into the equation. For instance, two of the incorrect answer choices in Example 2 are arrived at by plugging the mercury's temperature value into the equation instead of its latent heat value.

Guided Practice

1. **Which statement describes the solid state of matter?**

   A) It has a fixed shape and volume.

   B) It has a variable shape and volume.

   C) Its molecules have a high level of disorder.

   D) Its molecules have great freedom of motion.

STEP 1: Reread and Realize

Reread the Learn section of the text and write the details you find about solids on the lines below.

_____

_____

_____

_____

STEP 2: Remember Water

Relate the question to your personal experience regarding water. Which option clearly does not apply to water in its solid form?

_____

_____

_____

_____

STEP 3: Rule Out

Combine the information you wrote for Steps 1 and 2 and eliminate the answer choices that contradict that information.

_____

_____

_____

_____

2. Rubbing alcohol exists as a liquid at room temperature. A 10g sample of rubbing alcohol experiences a heat energy change of –2,050 calories while going through a single phase transition. Which phase transition most likely occurred?

A) liquid to gas

B) solid to gas

C) gas to solid

D) gas to liquid

STEP 1: Reread and Realize

Carefully reread the question to pick out the details. What is the sign on the value of the heat change? How many times did the phase change as the heat energy changed? Write these details on the lines below.

_____

_____

_____

_____

STEP 2: Read the Sign

What does the negative sign on the value of the heat energy change tell you? Did the alcohol gain or lose energy? What does this gain or loss mean for the order and motion of the molecules in the sample?

_____

_____

_____

_____

STEP 3: Rule Out

Which options can you eliminate based on your answers in Steps 1 and 2?

_____

_____

_____

_____

Guided Practice

3. Nitrogen has a boiling point of –200°C. Its latent heat is 48 cal/g. What will be the heat energy change in a 50g sample of nitrogen at –200°C as it transitions from a gas to a liquid?

A) 2,400 calories

B) –2,400 calories

C) 10,000 calories

D) –10,000 calories

STEP 1: Reread and Realize

Carefully reread the question to pick out the details. What is the latent heat of nitrogen? How much nitrogen is in the sample? What phase transition is the nitrogen going through?

_____

_____

_____

_____

STEP 2: Read the Sign

You can eliminate two of the answers based on their signs. You know that the nitrogen is changing from a gas to a liquid. Does this mean it will lose or gain energy? Which sign correctly indicates this gain or loss?

_____

_____

_____

_____

STEP 3: Use the Equation

Plug the appropriate values for mass and latent heat into the equation for heat of vaporization to calculate the answer. Don't forget to add the appropriate sign based on your answers in Step 2.

_____

_____

_____

_____

Independent Practice

1. Which statement describes matter in its gaseous state?

   A) Its temperature is high.

   B) It's under a lot of pressure.

   C) Its molecules are highly ordered.

   D) Its molecules are barely moving.

   HINT *Remember that the molecules in a gas have a lot of energy.*

2. Which statement about water molecules in a freezing sample of water is true?

   A) The molecules gain energy.

   B) The molecules become less ordered.

   C) The temperature caused by the molecules increases.

   D) The movement of the molecules decreases.

   HINT *Remember that while freezing, a sample of water becomes colder, and that temperature is essentially the measure of molecular motion.*

3. Hydrogen has a boiling point of –253°C. Its latent heat is 108 cal/g. What will be the heat energy change in a 10g sample of hydrogen at –253°C as it transitions from liquid to a gas?

   A) 1080 calories

   B) –1080 calories

   C) 27,320 calories

   D) –27,320 calories

   HINT *The correct answer should be positive, not negative, since the hydrogen is vaporizing and must therefore gain heat energy.*

ReKap

In this lesson, you learned the properties of three states of matter, how molecules behave in the states of matter, and how to calculate the transfer of heat that occurs during a phase transition. Remember the following:

- The three states of matter are solid, liquid, and gas.

- Changes in temperature and pressure can both cause phase transitions to occur.

- Molecules behave differently in the three states of matter.

- Matter must absorb or release heat energy to change between two states of matter; each substance has its own latent heat value.

- A negative result from a heat transfer calculation means that a substance has lost heat energy.

? **How will the information in this lesson help you explain to patients why maintaining a constant body temperature of 98.6°F is so important?**

_____

_____

_____

_____

Answers

Guided Practice

1. Step 1: Solids have a fixed volume, fixed shape, and molecules with a low level of disorder and almost no freedom of motion.

    Step 2: Choice B does not apply to water in its solid form.

    Step 3: Eliminate Choice B, C, and D. Choices C and D describe the levels of disorder and motion of gas molecules. Choice B was eliminated in Step 2.

    Answer: (A) It has a fixed shape and volume.

2. Step 1: The value has a negative sign and it has gone through one phase transition.

    Step 2: The negative sign means the sample lost heat energy. This would cause the molecule to lose motion and gain order.

    Step 3: Eliminate Choices A, B, and C. Choices A and B both of those transitions would require the sample to gain energy. Choice C involves two phase transitions: gas to liquid, then liquid to solid.

    Answer: (D) gas to liquid

3. Step 1: The latent heat is 48 cal/g. The sample has a mass of 50g. It is changing from a gas to a liquid.

    Step 2: Nitrogen will lose energy. A negative sign shows a loss.

    Step 3: $H = mL$

    $$H = -(50g)(48 \text{ cal/g})$$

    $$H = -2,400 \text{ cal}$$

    Answer: (B) -2,400 calories

Independent Practice

1. **Answer: (A) Its temperature is high.**

    Gases exist at relatively high temperatures and low pressures. Their molecules are highly disordered and have a high degree of movement.

2. **Answer: (D) The movement of the molecules decreases.**

    Molecules in a solid such as ice vibrate, but otherwise do not move. Matter loses energy and decreases in temperature as it freezes. Also, molecules in freezing matter become more orderly.

3. **Answer: (A) 1080 calories**

    Calculate the answer as follows:

    $H = mL$

    $H = (10g)(108 \text{cal/g})$

    $H = 1,080 \text{ cal}$

Answers

ReKap

The human body contains thousands of substances in various states. The proper functioning of the body requires that the complex interplay of solids, liquids, and gases not be disrupted by phase changes that could occur if the body's temperature fluctuated randomly. Even a small change in temperature can affect how some molecules in the body behave and interact with one another.

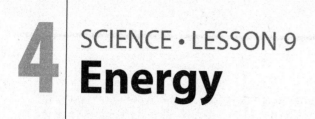

SCIENCE · LESSON 9
Energy

The concept of energy is interwoven throughout health care. A patient might have a temporary or permanent muscle weakness. Another patient might find that he is undernourished, even though he is overweight. Both of these conditions relate to energy in one way or another. To study these and other conditions, you will need a basic understanding of the various forms of energy, and the way energy can be transferred and converted between forms.

Common Uses in Health Care

- metabolic conditions, such as diabetes
- diet and weight loss or gain
- injuries caused by movement or impact

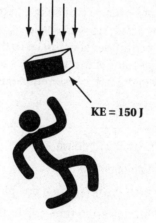

KE = 150 J

PE = 800 J

Key Terms/Formulas

- **calorie** – common unit for measuring energy, 1 cal = 4.2 J
- **energy** – the ability to do work
- **joule (J)** – standard unit for measuring energy
- **kinetic energy** – energy of motion
- **potential energy** – stored energy
- **velocity** – describes speed and direction

Formulas:

Kinetic Energy: $KE = \frac{1}{2} mv^2$

Potential Energy: $PE = mgh$

Total Energy = KE + PE

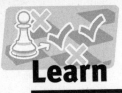

Learn

Energy and Energy Units

We use energy units in our daily conversations, but might not realize it. A common everyday energy unit is the dietary calorie. We check out the nutrition information on a granola bar and find out that it contains *140 calories*. What does this really mean?

Energy is basically the ability to do work. We do the work of exercise, for example, by converting the energy in food to power our muscles. We also store extra food energy to be converted later. Energy that is being used and energy that is being stored are measured using the same units. The most common units are joules (J) and calories.

Joules are based on units of force and distance; the greater the force or distance involved, the greater the energy. Because force is dependent on the mass and the acceleration, the energy involved in moving an object depends on its mass, how fast you get it moving, and how far you move it. Calories are based on units of heat. One calorie is that amount of heat required to raise the temperature of 1 gram of water by 1°C. The greater the temperature change, or the greater the mass of water being heated, the greater the number of calories needed.

We can convert energy units, such as calories to joules: 1 calorie equals about 4.18 J. This is important because we often want to figure out the total energy (heat, motion, and other types of energy) and therefore would want them to have the same units when we add them up. It is also important because all forms of energy can be converted to other forms—1 J of energy from food will be converted to a total of 1 J of motion, heat, and electrical energy.

According to the Law of Conservation of Energy, energy can neither be created nor destroyed. It can be transferred, and it can change form, however. For example, when we push a shopping cart, we transfer energy from our muscles to the cart. We also convert food energy to make our muscles move—some of that energy is also converted to heat energy. However, the total amount of energy in the cart, our surroundings, and us, remains the same.

Summarize:

- Energy is the ability to do work.
- Energy exists in many forms.
- Energy can be transferred from one place to another.
- Energy can be converted from one form to another.
- Energy is never lost within a system.

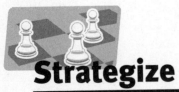

Strategize

Reread, Remember, Rule Out

To succeed on questions about energy in general:

Step 1: Always **reread** the question. Figure out what the question is asking you to do.

Step 2: **Remember** that energy can neither be created nor destroyed.

Step 3: Using the information you remembered, predict how the energy might be transferred or converted, and **rule out** the choices that do not match.

Apply

A1. A person is using a hand-cranked cell phone charger; the amount of electrical energy transferred to the cell phone battery is less than the amount of energy the person is burning by doing the cranking. What is the best explanation for this difference?

A) Some of the energy is being destroyed in the transfer.

B) Electrical energy is less powerful than cranking energy.

C) Some of the cranking energy is converted to a form other than electricity.

D) Cranking energy is measured in dietary calories, but electrical energy is measured in joules.

STEP 1: Reread and Realize

What is the question asking? Reread the question—it is asking what is happening to cause energy to appear to be lost.

STEP 2: Remember

Energy cannot be created or destroyed, only transferred and converted.

STEP 3: Rule Out

Based on what you remember, rule out any choice that does not fit—you can rule out choice A because it involves energy being destroyed. Since the total amount of energy must be the same, you can rule out choice B, because it implies that the total amount of energy is lower after cranking. You know that total energy is the same, no matter what units you use, so you can rule out choice D. The answer is choice C. The energy that isn't converted to electricity could be expressed as heat, or used to power the muscles used to turn the crank.

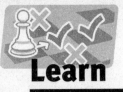

Learn

Kinetic Energy and Potential Energy

Kinetic energy (KE) is the energy related to motion. Mechanical energy (or movement energy) is the form of KE we are most familiar with—we instinctively know that a baseball traveling at 100 miles/hour will have more energy than one traveling at 50 miles/hour. Other forms of kinetic energy include electromagnetic energy (e.g., heat and light), electrical energy (movement of electrons), and nuclear energy.

Potential energy (PE) is related to the amount of energy that is stored in an object. Gravimetric PE is the form we are most familiar with—we instinctively know that an object falling from 10 feet above the ground will have more energy than one falling from 5 feet above the ground. Other forms of PE include chemical energy (e.g., energy stored in food or batteries) and elastic energy (e.g., energy stored in rubber bands or springs).

Problems involving KE and PE will use the following equations:

Kinetic Energy: $KE = \dfrac{1}{2} mv^2$

Potential Energy: $PE = mgh$

Total Energy = KE + PE

In these equations, m = mass (kg), v = velocity (meters/second or m/s), g = gravitational constant (10 m/s²), and h is height (m). The gravitational constant is also called the acceleration of gravity, because the velocity of a falling object will increase as it falls, due to the force of gravity.

In both equations, when the units kg, m, and s are used, the energy units will be Joules.

$$1J = \dfrac{1kg * m}{s^2}$$

Let's look at a ball rolling off the top of a wall. The height of the wall is 10 m. The mass of the ball is 0.20 kg. When the ball is 1 m above the ground, its velocity is about 13.4 *m/s*. What is the KE?

$$KE = \dfrac{1}{2} \cdot 0.2kg \cdot \left(13.4 \dfrac{m}{s} \right)^2 = 18.0J$$

What is the PE?

$$PE = 0.2kg \cdot 10 \dfrac{m}{s^2} \cdot 1m = 2J$$

What is the total energy?

The total energy is 18J + 2J = 20J.

Notice the relationship between *KE* and *PE* in the table, when we look at each value as it changes from the top of the wall to 1 meter above the ground.

Remember the importance of order of operations (PEMDAS) when using a calculator. In this last question, using the x^2 button on the calculator after multiplying the three numbers in the equation will produce an incorrect answer (1.8). The 13.4 m/s must be squared before you multiply anything else.

Since only the v is squared in the KE equation, the velocity/speed of the object has more impact on the KE than does the mass.

Height (m)	KE (J)	PE (J)	Total Energy (J)
10	0	20.0	20.0
9	2.0	18.0	20.0
8	4.0	16.0	20.0
7	6.0	14.0	20.0
6	8.0	12.0	20.0
5	10.0	10.0	20.0
4	12.0	8.0	20.0
3	14.0	6.0	20.0
2	16.0	4.0	20.0
1	18.0	2.0	20.0

The ball starts out with no KE, because it is not moving. As it falls, the PE decreases and the KE increases, as the ball height decreases and the ball velocity increases. Just as the ball hits the ground, it will have a KE of 20.0 J and a PE of 0 J.

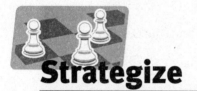

Strategize

Reread, Remember, Rule Out

To succeed on questions about KE, PE, and total energy:

Step 1: Always **reread** the question. Figure out what the question is asking you to do.

Step 2: **Remember** the equations for KE and PE, and that KE + PE = total energy.

Step 3: Using the information you remembered, predict the amount or type of energy asked for in the question, and **rule out** the choices that do not match.

A2. Which would have the most kinetic energy?

A) A 2-kg cart traveling at 50 m/s

B) A 1-kg cart traveling at 100 m/s

C) A 50-kg cart traveling at 2 m/s

D) A 100-kg cart traveling at 5 m/s

STEP 1: Reread and Realize

What is the question asking? Reread the question—it is asking about KE.

STEP 2: Remember

$$KE = \frac{1}{2} \, mv^2$$

STEP 3: Rule Out

Based on what you remember, rule out any choice that does not fit—since the question is asking about *most* KE, you can calculate them all and rule out the lowest three.

For choice A, $KE = \frac{1}{2} \cdot 2kg \cdot \left(50\,\frac{m}{s}\right)^2 = 2500J$.

For choice B, $KE = \frac{1}{2} \cdot 1kg \cdot \left(100\,\frac{m}{s}\right)^2 = 5000J$.

For choice C, $KE = \frac{1}{2} \cdot 50kg \cdot \left(2\,\frac{m}{s}\right)^2 = 100J$.

For choice D, $KE = \frac{1}{2} \cdot 100kg \cdot \left(5\,\frac{m}{s}\right)^2 = 1250J$.

You can rank the choices lowest to highest: C, D, A, B and rule out C, D, and A.

A3. Which would have the most potential energy?

A) A 2-kg rock at a height of 50 m

B) A 1-kg rock at a height of 100 m

C) A 50-kg rock at a height of 2 m

D) A 100-kg rock at a height of 5 m

STEP 1: Reread and Realize

What is the question asking? Reread the question—it is asking about PE.

STEP 2: Remember

$PE = mgh$

Remember, g is the gravitational constant (10 m/s^2)

STEP 3: Rule Out

Based on what you remember, rule out any choice that does not fit—since the question is asking about *most* PE, you can calculate them all and rule out the lowest three.

For choice A, $PE = 2kg \cdot 10 \, \frac{m}{s^2} \cdot 50m = 1000J$.

For choice B, $PE = 1kg \cdot 10 \, \frac{m}{s^2} \cdot 100m = 1000J$.

For choice C, $PE = 50kg \cdot 10 \, \frac{m}{s^2} \cdot 2m = 1000J$.

For choice D, $PE = 100kg \cdot 10 \, \frac{m}{s^2} \cdot 5m = 5000J$.

You can rule out choices A, B, and C—they are the same and are also smaller than choice D.

A4. You drop a 2-kg bag of sand from a height of 15 m. Assuming the total energy stays the same, what will the kinetic and potential energies be when the bag is 3 m above the ground?

A) KE = 200J and PE = 100J

B) KE = 240J and PE = 60J

C) KE = 290J and PE = 10J

D) KE = 300J and PE = 0J

STEP 1: Reread and Realize

What is the question asking? Reread the question—it is asking you to find KE and PE, which suggests you'll also need to find total energy.

STEP 2: Remember

$KE = \frac{1}{2} \, mv^2$, $PE = mgh$ and Total Energy $= KE + PE$

STEP 3: Rule Out

Based on what you remember, rule out any choice that does not fit—notice that the total energy is the same for all four choices, so you can't use that to rule any out. However, you know that the PE of an object 3 m above the ground can't be 0 J, so you can rule out choice D. The PE of a 2-kg object 3 m above the ground should be:

$PE = 2kg \cdot 10 \frac{m}{s^2} \cdot 3m = 60J$

You can rule out choices A and C because they have the incorrect PE. You can check your answer, however. The total energy just before you dropped the bag will be equal to the PE, since KE will be 0 J (the bag has a velocity of 0 m/s). At 15 m above the ground:

$PE = 2kg \cdot 10 \frac{m}{s^2} \cdot 15m = 300J$

At 3 m above the ground, total energy is still 300 J, so KE must be 300 J – 60 J = 240 J.

Guided Practice

Let's work through a few examples together. Look back at the lesson content as often as necessary to help you apply the concepts and strategies you learned.

1. You bounce a 0.5-kg basketball by letting it roll off your hand and fall to the ground. If the velocity of the basketball is 6.3 m/s just before it hits the ground, what is its kinetic energy at that point?

   A) 1.6 J

   B) 2.5 J

   C) 6.8 J

   D) 9.9 J

STEP 1: Reread and Realize

What is the question asking you to do? Reread the item and find the important details.

_____

_____

_____

_____

STEP 2: Remember

What is the equation to calculate KE?

_____

_____

_____

_____

STEP 3: Rule Out

Using your answer from Step 2, go through each answer choice. Which ones can you eliminate?

_____

_____

_____

_____

2. If you drop the 0.5-kg basketball from a height of 2 m, what will the potential energy of the ball be when it is 1 m above the ground?

    A) 1 J

    B) 2 J

    C) 5 J

    D) 10 J

STEP 1: Reread and Realize

What is the question asking you to do?

_____

_____

_____

_____

STEP 2: Read the Sign

What is the equation to calculate PE?

_____

_____

_____

_____

STEP 3: Rule Out

Which choices can you eliminate?

_____

_____

_____

_____

Guided Practice

3. When you drop the basketball from a height of 2 m, it hits the ground, but only bounces back up to a height of 1.9 m. This means that when you let the ball go, it had a PE = 10 J but when it returned, it had a PE = 9.5 J. What is the best explanation for the change in potential energy?

A) The ball gained mass.

B) About 0.5 J of the total energy in the ball was destroyed.

C) Some of the potential energy was converted into kinetic energy.

D) Some of the total energy was transferred to the ground when the ball hit it.

STEP 1: Reread and Realize

What is the question asking you to do? Reread the question and find the details that tell you.

_____

_____

_____

_____

STEP 2: Remember

How are PE and KE related, and what is always true about energy?

_____

_____

_____

_____

STEP 3: Rule out

Determine which answer choices can be eliminated. If more than one choice fits what you know about energy, look for the choice that makes more sense.

_____

_____

_____

_____

Independent Practice

1. A car on a roller coaster has a mass of 100 kg and a velocity of 7 m/s. What is the kinetic energy of the car?

   A) 350 J

   B) 700 J

   C) 2450 J

   D) 122500 J

   HINT *Remember that the order of operations in the KE equation is important.*

2. The 100-kg roller coaster car is at the top of a hill, with a height of 150 m. What is the potential energy of the car?

   A) 260 J

   B) 2600 J

   C) 15000 J

   D) 150000 J

   HINT *Remember that the gravitational constant is 10 m/s^2.*

3. The 100-kg roller coaster car rolls from the top of the 150-m hill and picks up speed. What is the kinetic energy of the car when it is 50 m above the ground, assuming no energy is transferred from the car to its surroundings?

   A) 25000 J

   B) 50000 J

   C) 100000 J

   D) 150000 J

   HINT *Remember that total energy will not change.*

ReKap

In this lesson you reviewed

- the concept of energy and forms of energy
- the law of conservation of energy
- common calculations of kinetic and potential energies

? **How will having knowledge about forms of energy help you to better understand a patient's diagnosis?**

_____

_____

_____

_____

Answers

Guided Practice

1. Step 1: Find the kinetic energy of the ball before it hits the ground.

   Step 2: KE = $\frac{1}{2}mv^2$

   Step 3: Eliminate Choice A, B, and C. Choice A is incorrect—it is the result obtained if the velocity is not squared. Choice B is incorrect—it is the result obtained if the entire product of 1/2mv is squared. Choice C is incorrect—it is the sum of the mass and the velocity.

   Answer: (D) 9.9J

2. Step 1: Find the potential energy of the ball when it is 1 m above the ground.

   Step 2: PE = mgh

   Step 3: Eliminate Choices A, B, and D. PE depends on the current height, and has nothing to do with a previous height. Choice A is incorrect—it is the value obtained by multiplying all the numbers given. Choice B is incorrect—it is the value for the initial height. Choice D is incorrect—it is the PE for the ball at the initial height.

   Answer: (C) 5J

3. Step 1: Explain why the potential energy of the ball changed.

   Step 2: PE and KE are both involved in the total energy of an object. Energy cannot be created nor destroyed.

   Step 3: Eliminate Choices A, B, and C. Choice A is incorrect because gaining mass would have increased PE. Choice B is incorrect because energy cannot be destroyed. Choice C is incorrect because if the ball still had any KE, it would have kept moving upward.

   Answer: (D) Some of the total energy was transferred to the ground when the ball hits it.

Independent Practice

1. **Answer: (C) 2450J**

   Choice A is incorrect because it is the answer obtained by not squaring the velocity. Choice B is incorrect because it is the answer obtained by not squaring the velocity and omitting the 1/2 in the equation. Choice D is incorrect because it is the answer obtained by squaring the product of all of the numbers.

2. **Answer: (D) 150000J**

   Choices A and B are incorrect because they are the result of adding the numbers in the equation (choice B also includes an extra 0). Choice C is incorrect because it is the result of omitting the gravitational constant.

3. **Answer: (C) 100000J**

   Choices A and B are incorrect because they are the result of using PE instead of KE (choice A includes multiplying by 1/2). Choice D is incorrect because it is the initial PE (or total energy).

ReKap

Example: a better understanding of the relationship between the height of a fall (or the mass of the person) and the amount of injury; an understanding of how calories in food are related to calories in exercise.

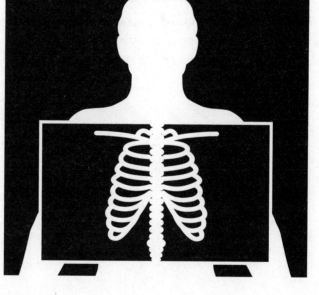

SCIENCE · LESSON 10
Energy and Population Changes

Health, energy, and population are all interrelated. Too much or too little exposure to the Sun's energy can threaten health; poor health care can affect population growth.

Common Uses in Health Care

- heat-related burns, sunburns, and x-ray exposure
- radiation for cancer treatment
- infant mortality and life expectancy trends

Key Terms/Formulas

- **conduction** – energy movement through matter
- **convection** – energy movement through the movement of matter
- **electromagnetic radiation** – energy that travels in waves
- **electromagnetic spectrum** – arrangement of electromagnetic radiation in order of wavelength or frequency
- **emigration** – movement of people out of a country or region
- **fertility rate** – number of births per woman living in a country or region
- **immigration** – movement of people into a country or region
- **radiation** – movement of energy through space in the form of waves

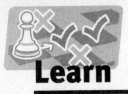

Energy from the Sun

Almost all of the energy on Earth comes from the Sun. How does it get from the Sun to Earth? How does the energy move around once it gets here? There are three basic ways to transfer energy:

- **Radiation**—waves of energy travel through space from one place to another; an example is how sunlight travels from the Sun to Earth through space.

- **Convection**—energy is carried by moving matter (usually air or water); an example is how hot air from the oven moves through the kitchen when you open the oven door.

- **Conduction**—energy moves through matter; an example is how heat moves through a pot, making the handle hot even though it is only the bottom of the pot that touches the heat source.

Note that radiation is the only type of energy transfer that does not require matter—energy from stars, like the Sun, can travel through the vacuum of space by radiation, but not by convection or conduction. We can therefore study the radiation emitted by the Sun and other stars and have found many stars similar to the Sun throughout the universe.

Energy transferred by radiation is also called Electromagnetic Radiation (EMR) and it travels in waves. The size of the wave determines its properties; when we arrange the types of radiation by length or by frequency (waves per second), we describe the Electromagnetic Spectrum:

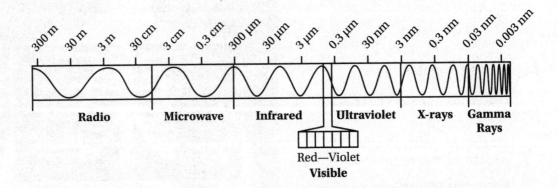

Gamma rays, x-rays, and ultraviolet rays can damage living cells because they are able to pass through the cell and break DNA strands. Ultraviolet radiation is often divided into UVA and UVB ranges. UVA rays are larger than UVB rays, and so are considered less dangerous.

Visible light is the most familiar type of EMR—most of us can distinguish different bands of visible light as color, starting with red, at about 700 nm through orange, yellow, green, blue, and then ending with violet at about 400 nm.

The wavelength of radiation is related to the energy being transmitted—the smaller the wavelength, the greater the number of waves per second, and the greater the amount of energy transmitted. This means that gamma, x-ray, and UV radiation, in addition to being the right size to damage the DNA in cells, also has more energy with which to damage.

If gamma, x-ray, and UV radiation is so dangerous, why are these three forms of radiation so important in health care?

- Gamma radiation is small enough to penetrate anywhere in the body. This means it can be used to shrink internal tumors without surgery. Because damage is dependent on the amount of exposure, the treatments are typically done by moving a focused radiation beam through a path that always passes through the tumor but only passes through each area of healthy tissue around the tissue part of the time.

- X-rays also pass through the tissues in our bodies, but they are partially or fully blocked by dense tissue so they can be used to study bones and skeletal structure. X-rays are also blocked by certain elements (such as barium) so they can be used to view functioning in softer tissues with the addition of those elements (by swallowing or injecting). Again, because damage is dependent on the amount of exposure, keeping the exposure low by using very short exposures and avoiding unnecessary x-rays is essential.

- UV rays do not pass deeper than skin cells, but are very useful for killing bacteria and fungi on surfaces that can't be treated easily with disinfectants or heat (such as paper and certain plastics). Controlled UV exposure can also help certain conditions (such as jaundice and vitamin D deficiency)—again the important factor is to keep the exposure to the minimum necessary.

The ultraviolet, visible, and infrared radiation that Earth receives from the Sun is essential for life. Plants use ultraviolet light to power photosynthesis and make food, infrared radiation warms Earth and drives our weather cycles, and we all depend on visible light to get around. The amount of radiation we get depends both on the amount put out by the Sun and on our distance from the Sun—the amount received decreases by the square of the distance. For example, a planet twice as far from the Sun as Earth is would get only one-fourth the amount of energy.

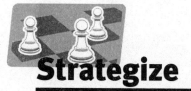

Strategize

Reread, Remember, Rule Out

To succeed on questions about energy transfer and energy from the Sun:

Step 1: Always **reread** the question. Determine what the question is asking you to do.

Step 2: **Remember** that energy from the Sun can be radiated, convected, or conducted.

Step 3: Using the information you remembered, predict the type of energy being radiated, convected, or conducted, and **rule out** the choices that do not match.

Apply

A1. Which statement best explains why we can get sunburned during the day but we do not get a similar burn from the stars at night?

A) The Sun is the only star that emits UV rays.

B) The other stars emit UV rays, but not infrared rays.

C) Earth is very far from the other stars, so receives very little UV energy from them.

D) We are too far from the other stars for their energy to travel to Earth by convection.

STEP 1: Reread and Realize

What is the question asking? Reread the question—it is asking you to compare the energy from the Sun with energy from other stars.

STEP 2: Remember

The wavelength of radiation determines its properties.

STEP 3: Rule Out

Based on what you remember, rule out any choice that does not fit—you can rule out choice B because infrared radiation does not cause sunburn, even though it makes us feel warm. You can rule out choice A because many stars are similar to the Sun, which emits UV radiation. You can rule out choice D because energy travels through space only by radiation, as there is no matter for conducting or convecting. Choice C is the correct answer.

A2. A medical imaging company is developing a way to reduce the amount of radiation exposure patients get during x-rays. Which proposal makes the most sense?

A) Convert the machinery to use gamma radiation.

B) Reduce the x-ray energy and supplement with UV rays.

C) Instead of a 10-second exposure, use 10 one-second exposures.

D) Develop a more sensitive way to record the x-rays after they pass through the patient.

STEP 1: Reread and Realize

What is the question asking? Reread the question—it is asking you to compare the proposals and choose the one that will reduce x-ray exposure while still producing useful x-ray images.

STEP 2: Remember

The wavelength of radiation determines its properties AND dose and duration determine amount of damage.

STEP 3: Rule Out

Based on what you remember, rule out any choice that does not fit—you can rule out choice A because gamma rays cause more damage than x-rays, so would not be a safer alternative. You can rule out choice B because UV rays don't penetrate deeper than skin. You can rule out choice C because the dose and cumulative duration are the same. You are left with D, which makes sense, because a more sensitive way to record the x-rays would mean you could use a shorter exposure.

Learn

Population Changes

If the Sun's energy were the only resource needed for life, living conditions might be similar throughout the world. Unequal access to other resources, such as land, water, and minerals, leads to different standards of living. Standard of living both affects and is affected by population growth in a region or country.

Population growth is an indication of the difference between the increase in number of people (birth rate plus immigration rate) and the decrease in number (death rate plus emigration rate).

Developed countries have more access to resources, so people living in developed countries tend to have better health care and nutrition. Infant mortality rate is low and average lifespan is high. The population growth in more developed countries, however, tends to be low, because of low birth rates.

Population growth in less developed, or developing countries (sometimes called third-world countries), tends to be high, because of high birth rates. The high birth rates overcome higher infant mortality and shorter lifespans. Health care can play a role in population growth: if lowering infant mortality and increasing lifespan lowers birth rate, then increased access to health care can slow the population growth in a country.

Emigration (moving out) can also slow population growth, just as **immigration** (moving in) can increase population growth. Most developed countries restrict immigration, so population growth stays low; consequently, emigration from developing countries probably can't occur fast enough to have a large effect on population growth.

Fertility rate is similar to birth rate—birth rate is usually measured in terms of births per person (often reported per thousand or million people) per year while fertility rate is measured in terms of births per woman. Typical fertility rates for more developed countries are low—1 to 2 births per woman, which translates to about 8-10 births per thousand per year in birth rate. While there are many factors that influence birth rate and fertility rate, health care is probably a main factor; access to birth control, as well as a woman's health and the health of her babies, would likely have a large effect.

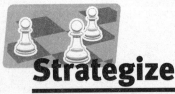

Strategize

Reread, Remember, Rule Out

To succeed on questions about population changes:

Step 1: Always **reread** the question. Determine what the question is asking you to do.

Step 2: **Remember** that population growth in more developed countries is low, and in less developed countries is high, due to many interrelated factors.

Step 3: Using the information you remembered, predict the level of development or population growth, and **rule out** the choices that do not match.

Apply

A3. Which set of birth rates is typical of a less developed country?

Birth Rate (births per thousand)							
Year	2003	2004	2005	2006	2007	2008	2009
Country X	10.99	10.88	10.78	10.71	10.67	10.65	10.65
Country Y	39.53	38.99	41.38	41.00	40.78	40.52	40.24

A) Country X

B) Country Y

C) Both Country X and Country Y

D) Neither Country X nor Country Y

STEP 1: Reread and Realize

What is the question asking? Reread the question—it is asking you to compare the birth rates: Country X has a birthrate of about 10-11 while Country Y has a birthrate of about 39-41 births per thousand people.

STEP 2: Remember

A typical birth rate in a more developed country is 8-10 per thousand.

STEP 3: Rule Out

Based on what you remember, rule out any choice that does not fit—you can rule out choice A because Country X fits in with the typical birth rate of a more developed country. You can also rule out choice C for the same reason. Country Y has a birth rate that is 4 times higher than that of Country X—this is a high birth rate and typical of a less developed country. Choice B is the correct answer.

Guided Practice

Let's work through a few examples together. Look back at the lesson content as often as necessary to help you apply the concepts and strategies you learned.

1. **The energy carried by radiation increases as the wavelength decreases. Which of these comparisons is correct?**

    A) X-rays are more energetic than gamma rays.

    B) UV rays are more energetic than visible rays.

    C) Infrared rays are more energetic than visible rays.

    D) Microwave rays are more energetic than gamma rays.

STEP 1: Reread and Realize

What is the question asking you to do? Reread the item and find the important details.

_____

_____

_____

_____

STEP 2: Remember

Which has the smaller wavelength of each pair?

_____

_____

_____

_____

STEP 3: Rule Out

Using your answer from Step 2, go through each answer choice. Which ones can you eliminate?

_____

_____

_____

_____

2. Which statement best describes population growth in less developed countries, compared to more developed countries?

A) Population growth is lower in less developed countries because infant mortality tends to be higher.

B) Population growth is higher in less developed countries because they tend to have higher immigration.

C) Population growth is higher in less developed countries because they tend to have less access to birth control.

D) Population growth is lower in less developed countries because they tend to have fewer resources to support the population.

STEP 1: Reread and Realize

What is the question asking you to do? Reread the item and find the important details.

_____

_____

_____

_____

STEP 2: Remember

Do less developed countries tend to have a higher or lower population growth than more developed countries?

_____

_____

_____

_____

STEP 3: Rule Out

Using your answer from Step 2, go through each answer choice. Which ones can you eliminate?

_____

_____

_____

_____

Independent Practice

1. An asteroid in our solar system receives four times as much energy from the Sun as Earth does. Which is the correct relationship between Earth and the asteroid?

    A) Earth is half as far away from the Sun as the asteroid.

    B) Earth is twice as far away from the Sun as the asteroid.

    C) Earth is four times as far away from the Sun as the asteroid.

    D) Earth is one-fourth as far away from the Sun as the asteroid.

    HINT *The relationship between distance and energy involves the square of one of the numbers.*

2. A nursing student spends a lot of time in a greenhouse, working with plants. She still wears sunscreen while she is in the greenhouse. Which statement best describes the reason using sunscreen is either necessary or not necessary?

    A) Wearing sunscreen in a greenhouse is necessary because it gets so hot in there.

    B) Wearing sunscreen in a greenhouse is not necessary because the plants absorb all the UV radiation.

    C) Wearing sunscreen in a greenhouse is not necessary because no UV radiation gets through the glass.

    D) Wearing sunscreen in a greenhouse is necessary because some UV radiation gets through the glass and the daily exposure can add up.

    HINT *Think about the source and type of radiation plants use.*

3. According to the data below, which country fits the profile of population growth for a less developed country?

Total population (in millions)					
Year	2008	2009	2010	2011	2012
Country A	302	305	308	311	314
Country B	25	24	23	22	21
Country C	21	23	25	27	29
Country D	327	326	325	324	322

    A) Country A

    B) Country B

    C) Country C

    D) Country D

    HINT *Growth rate is more important than total population.*

ReKap

In this lesson you reviewed

- Three main methods for transferring energy
- The composition and characteristics of sunlight and other energies
- Measurements of population growth and factors that affect it

> **? How will having knowledge of the relationship between health, energy, and population growth help you to better understand a patient's diagnosis?**
>
> _____
>
> _____
>
> _____
>
> _____

Answers

Guided Practice

1. Step 1: Compare types of electromagnetic energy.

   Step 2: A - gamma rays; B - UV rays; C - visible rays; D - gamma rays

   Step 3: Eliminate Choices A, C, and D. Choice A is incorrect—x-ray waves are longer than gamma ray waves. Choice C is incorrect—infrared waves are larger than visible waves. Choice D is incorrect—microwaves are larger than gamma ray waves.

   Answer: (B) UV rays are more energetic than visible rays.

2. Step 1: Compare population growth in developed and less developed countries.

   Step 2: Less developed countries tend to have higher growth rates than more developed countries.

   Step 3: Eliminate Choices A, B, and D. Choices A and D state that the growth rates are lower. Choice B, while immigration may happen in less developed countries, it is not likely to be greater than immigration to more developed countries.

   Answer: (C) Population growth is higher in less developed countries because they tend to have less access to birth control.

Independent Practice

1. **Answer: (B) Earth is twice as far away from the Sun as the asteroid.**

   Choices A and D are incorrect because the object receiving more energy would be closer to the Sun, not farther away. Choice C is incorrect because the energy decrease is proportional to the square of the distance.

2. **Answer: (D) Wearing sunscreen in a greenhouse is necessary because some UV radiation gets through the glass and the daily exposure can add up.**

   Choice A is incorrect because heat is due to infrared radiation and has nothing to do with UV. Choices B and C are incorrect, because some UV must pass through glass in order for plants to grow in a greenhouse, and UV radiation coming from the sun shines all around the room, not just on the plants, so plants absorbing UV in one location won't reduce the amount of UV in another part of the greenhouse.

3. **Answer: (C) Country C**

   Choice A is incorrect because, even though it is a large population (about the same as the U.S.), Country A has a growth rate of less than 1%. Choices B and D are incorrect because the populations are declining.

ReKap

Examples: understanding how too much sun exposure increases the risk of skin cancer, how radiation treatment for cancer can make a patient sick because of damage to normal cells, how burns can happen both from being in contact with a hot material or by being close to a heat source, how a patient's country of origin might affect basic health because of nutrition and health care differences.

UNIT
5
Grammar

Grammar Basics

Grammar rules may seem worlds away from learning to take a patient's vitals or how to start an IV line. But having a solid grasp of the basic rules of English grammar is an important skill you will use on a daily basis both as a nursing student and as a licensed nurse as you communicate with peers, doctors, and patients.

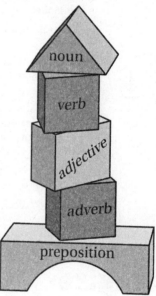

Common Uses in Health Care

- writing clear and accurate discharge instructions
- taking easy-to-read notes on a patient's care and progress
- putting together a list of clear steps for home care for a patient's caregiver

Key Terms/Formulas

- **adjective** – modifier that describes a noun
- **adverb** – modifier that describes an adjective, adverb, or verb
- **article** – word that limits a noun by making it specific or general
- **capitalization** – use of uppercase letters
- **direct object** – a noun or pronoun naming the receiver of an action
- **indirect object** – a noun or pronoun naming the person or thing for which the action was done
- **noun** – word that names a person, place, or thing
- **plural** – two or more
- **preposition** – word that shows relationships or locations
- **pronoun** – word that stands in for a noun or refers to a noun
- **singular** – one
- **subject** – a noun or noun phrase naming the doer or actor in a sentence
- **verb** – an action or state-of-being word

Words are the basic building blocks of language. Being able to properly identify and use parts of speech is critical to achieving a great score on the admissions test.

Part of Speech	Grammatical Functions	Examples
Noun	• Names a person, place, thing, or idea • Acts as subjects or objects in sentences • Can be common or proper	• Common nouns: textbook, classroom, nurse • Proper nouns: Dr. Lopez, Washington General Hospital
Verb	• Action words • Words showing a state of being	• He *beats* the egg. She *is* hot.
Adjective	• Modifies or describes a noun	• *yellow* bird, *ten* fingers
Adverb	• Modifies or describes a verb, adjective, or adverb	• ran *quickly*, *incredibly* difficult,
Pronoun	• A word that replaces and refers to a noun	• he, she, it, they
Article	• A word that limits a noun (tells whether it is general or specific)	• *a* feather, *an* apple (indefinite) • *the* bus, *the* doctor (definite)
Preposition	• Words that show relationship or location to another word	• *by* the house, *down* the stream, *over* the bridge, *through* the woods
Possessive noun or pronoun	• A word that shows ownership	• *Amanda's* uniform • *my* study guide

The parts of speech above can also function solo or in groups in key roles in a sentence, namely as subjects, verbs, and objects. Take a moment to look over these components. You will review how they work together in more depth later in the course.

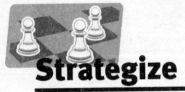

Strategize

Put the Sentence on Trial

How can you determine which parts of speech appear and how they function within a sentence? When you put the sentence on trial, you need to ask and answer some key questions:

Ask yourself...	...to Find
Who or what did it?	the subject
What did he/she/they/it do?	the verb
Who or what received the action of the verb?	the direct object
Who or what received the direct object?	the indirect object
Are there any words following prepositions?	objects of prepositions
What kind?	adjective
How many?	adjective
How/when/where?	adverb
Whose?	possessive noun or pronoun

Apply

Now let's put this strategy to use on a couple of questions like those that you would see on the admissions test.

A1. Which of the following correctly identifies the parts of speech in the underlined portions of the sentence below?

Running red <u>lights</u> demonstrates his complete and <u>total</u> disregard for the safety of others.

A) Noun; adverb

B) Noun; adjective

C) Verb; noun

D) Verb; adverb

STEP 1: Investigate

First, scan the options for the first underlined word. It can either be a noun or verb. Put the sentence on trial to find nouns and check for a match in the answer choices.

STEP 2: Ask and Answer

Who or what did it? (the subject)

Running red lights is our subject phrase.

Ask: Is lights is a person, place, or thing?

Answer: Yes, so we have a noun here!

STEP 3: Act

Eliminate choices C and D.

▶Now, repeat the steps to find the answer for the second half of the question.

STEP 1: Investigate

Scan remaining choices A and B to check the answer options for the second underlined word.

STEP 2: Ask and Answer

Which word does *total* modify?

Total is modifying "disregard."

Ask: Does *total* describe how/when/where?

Answer: No. *Total* tells answers the question *What kind of disregard?* so it must be an adjective!

Apply

STEP 3: Act

Select answer B!

Still unsure? When in doubt, plug the tested word into the sentence alone. Sentences make sense without modifiers, but they will not make sense if you take out a noun, pronoun, or verb!

 WATCH OUT!

Look at the first word in the sample question—*running*. This is a special type of word called a gerund (a verb + *ing*) that acts like a noun. Don't mistake gerunds for verbs on test day!

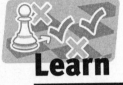

Learn

Remember that some types of words may also be **singular** or **plural**. Nouns, verbs, and pronouns all have singular and plural forms. Recall that singular words describe just one actor. Plurals identify or describe two or more.

While most nouns are made plural by adding *s* or *es*, irregular plural nouns frequently appear on the test. Review the examples below to help answer these items successfully.

Forming Regular and Irregular Plurals

Word Type	Action	Examples
Most words	• Add -*s*	• *doctor → doctors* • *ratio → ratios*
Words ending in –*ch, -j, –s, -sh, -x, or –z*; some words ending in -o	• Add –*es*	• *class → classes* • *rash → rashes* • *potato → potatoes*
Words ending in -*f* or -*fe*	• Add -*ves*	• *self → selves* • *knife → knives*
Words ending in -*y*	• Add -*ies*	• *baby → babies*
Words such as *man, woman, child, person*	• Know your irregular forms	• *man → men* • *woman → women* • *child → children* • *person → people*
Words with Latin or Greek endings	• Change -*us* to -*i* • Change -*on* to -*a* • Change -*is* to -*es* • Change -*um* to -*a* • Change -*a* to -*ae* • Change -*x* to -*ces*	• *nucleus → nuclei* • *crisis → crises* • *serum → sera* • *thorax → thoraces*

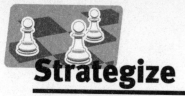

Strategize

Count!

Does the noun or subject phrase represent one or more than one actors/things? If it's just one, use the singular. If it's two or more, be sure to use the correct plural form.

- Identifying whether a subject is singular or plural is critical to succeeding on questions that test subject-verb agreement. You will review more on this topic later in the course.

- Determining whether the noun is singular or plural will help you decide whether to change the ending to the singular or plural form on irregulars.

Predict and Match!

After you have determined whether the word is singular or plural:

- Predict what form of noun or verb you will need.

- Match your prediction to the correct answer choice.

Apply

A2. Which of the following nouns is written in the correct plural form?

- **A)** womens
- **B)** tomatos
- **C)** knifes
- **D)** cacti

STEP 1: Count

Determine whether each noun shown is singular or plural. Any singular nouns could be eliminated immediately.

STEP 2: Work Backwards

Each of the words shown is a plural. But are the plural forms correct? To find out, first determine the singular form of each word—women, tomato, knife, and cactus.

STEP 3: Predict and Match

Use your knowledge of irregular plurals to predict the correct form for each word. Eliminate Choice A: the plural of woman is women, an irregular plural which does not add an *s* to the end. Choice B is incorrect: tomato adds an *es* in the plural form. Choice C neglects the *f* to *v* transformation. Only cacti follows these rules, so it must be the right answer!

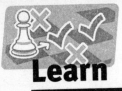
Everyone knows to capitalize the first word in a sentence, but the nursing admissions test will check your understanding on less common capitalization rules as well.

Capitalize a word if it's...	
...a proper noun, or the name of a specific person or place, such as the *White House*	...a title preceding someone's name, like *Senator* Lisa Murkowski
... a title standing in for a name. "Can you pass me the scalpel, *Doctor*?"	the first or last word in a title or an especially important word in a title, like *Atlas of Human Anatomy*
... the name of a specific class or course, like *Biology 101* or *Latin Poetry and Poets*	...the name of a scholarship, award, monument, or prize, like *National Merit Scholarship* or the *Caldecott Medal*
...the name of a ship, plane, rocket, like *Titanic* or *Apollo 13*	...a holiday, month, or day of the week, like *Wednesday*, *March*, or *Veteran's Day*
...a nationality, language, or ethnicity such as *Hinduism*, *Mandarin*, or *Swedish*	... a corporation, school, or government agency, like *General Electric*, *Beddow High School*, or the *Department of Health and Human Services*
... a direction being used as a place name, like *the South*, the *North Atlantic*	...a geographical location such as cities, states, countries, continents, bodies of water, beaches, or mountains, as in *Dallas*, the *Alps*, and the *Bay of Bengal*

WATCH OUT

Be careful not to make these common overcapitalization errors:

- seasons (*The winter was milder than usual.*)
- titles not standing in for names (*The secretary took notes.*)
- compass directions (*Proceed south on Main Street.*)
- general course topics (*I have to take a history class this year.*)
- geographical words that are not being used as proper nouns (*I live in a big city by the ocean.*)
- family relationships that are not part of a title or being used as a proper noun (*My cousin and I went to the store. Our fathers gave us some money.*)

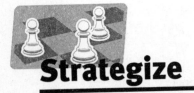

Strategize

Scan, Ask, Predict

To succeed on capitalization questions, follow these steps.

STEP 1: Scan

The answer choices to see which words in the sentence are being tested.

STEP 2: Ask

For each of these words, ask:

Is it a proper noun?

if not...

What is the role of the word?

STEP 3: Predict

Predict the correct form and eliminate choices that do not include that form.

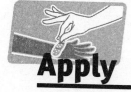

Apply

A3. Which of the following sentences uses capitalization rules correctly?

- **A)** Josie read an excerpt from *the sun also rises* to the judge at the drama competition.
- **B)** Josie read an excerpt from *the Sun Also Rises* to the judge at the drama competition.
- **C)** Josie read an excerpt from *The Sun Also Rises* to the judge at the drama competition.
- **D)** Josie read an excerpt from *The Sun Also Rises* to the Judge at the drama competition.

STEP 1: Scan

Which words are being tested?

Italics should always draw your attention!

You can also see that there are multiple options for the word *judge* in the answers.

Therefore, *the sun also rises* and *judge* are in play.

STEP 2: Ask

What are the roles of the tested words?

What does *the sun also rises represent*? Italics often show titles, in this case the title of a book.

Judge is being used as the title of a person, but it is not attached to a name or standing in for a name. No name means no caps!

STEP 3: Predict and Eliminate

Book titles require capitalization of the first and last words as well as any meaning words. Check the answers and eliminate those that do not correctly capitalize the title. Choices A and B are eliminated. Then, use the word *judge* to decide which answer is completely correct. *Judge* should not be capitalized since it is not standing in for or preceding a name. Eliminate Choice D. Choice C is correct.

Guided Practice

1. Which of the following correctly identifies a noun in the sentence below?

   Her retirement party was attended by twenty former colleagues.

   A) Her
   B) retirement
   C) party
   D) twenty

   STEP 1: Ask and Answer

   Find the verb first! Then ask: *Who or what was attended?* to locate the subject noun.

   _____

   STEP 2: Act

   Plug in each answer choice to the sentence.

   _____was attended.

   _____was attended.

   _____was attended.

   STEP 3: Eliminate

   Take away answer choices that do not make sense or change the meaning of the whole sentence. Which answers can we eliminate?

   _____

   _____

2. Which of the following is the correct completion of the sentence below?

   When two _____ collide, a nuclear reaction occurs.

   A) nucleus
   B) nucleuses
   C) nuclei
   D) nuclears

   STEP 1: Count!

   Does the sentence need a plural or singular noun form?

   The keyword *two* tells you which form you need.

STEP 2: Ask!

What type of word is nucleus?

_____

_____

STEP 3: Predict

Which of the irregular plural formation rules apply to the noun *nucleus*? Make your prediction. Then match it to the answer choices.

_____

_____

3. Which of the following correctly capitalizes the sentence below?

None of the students remembered to bring their copies of <u>kant's *critique of pure reason* to their german philosophers class.</u>

A) None of the students remembered to bring their copies of kant's *critique of pure reason* to their german philosophers class.

B) None of the students remembered to bring their copies of Kant's *critique of pure reason* to their German philosophers class.

C) None of the students remembered to bring their copies of Kant's *Critique of Pure Reason* to their German Philosophers class.

D) None of the students remembered to bring their copies of Kant's *Critique Of Pure Reason* to their German Philosophers class.

STEP 1: Ask

Is the sentence correct as written?

If not, eliminate A immediately.

STEP 2: Scan

Which words are being tested?

_____

STEP 3: Answer

Notice that B, C, and D have 3 different versions of the words "critique of pure reason."

What role do those words play?

_____

Independent Practice

You are ready to show what you know! Answer the questions below without looking back at the lesson content. Use the hints to help you.

1. Which of the following functions as an adverb in the sentence below?

   The howling wind gently rustled the dry autumn leaves.

   A) howling
   B) gently
   C) rustled
   D) dry

   HINT *Which word tells us how, when, or where?*

2. Select the correct version of the underlined portion of the sentence below.

   The <u>chairman of the committee mailed the report to chief Johnson</u> of the local police.

   A) chairman of the committee mailed the report to chief Johnson
   B) Chairman of the Committee mailed the report to chief Johnson
   C) Chairman of the committee mailed the report to Chief Johnson
   D) chairman of the committee mailed the report to Chief Johnson

   HINT *Which words are being tested?*

3. Which of the following is the correct completion of the sentence below?

   The researcher looked for trends by performing multiple statistical _____ of the data set.

   A) analysis
   B) analyses
   C) analysises
   D) analyzes

   HINT *Remember the pluralization rules for Latin and Greek words!*

ReKap

In this lesson, you reviewed basic grammar rules commonly tested on nursing admissions tests. You also learned a variety of strategies to deal with specific grammar topics on the tests. Make sure you practice and master the following basic grammar strategies prior to test day:

- Memorize grammar rules and definitions.

- Put the sentence on trial: Ask, Answer, Act! (parts of speech)

- Count! Predict and match. (singular/plural)

- Scan! Ask! Predict! (capitalization)

- On all questions, scan and eliminate to save time and increase your odds of getting the question right!

? **How will knowing the rules of grammar help you communicate more effectively as a nurse?**

_____

_____

_____

_____

Answers

Guided Practice

1. Step 1: Her retirement party was attended.

    Step 2: Her was attended.
    Retirement was attended.
    Party was attended.

    Step 3: Eliminate "her was attended" and "retirement was attended."

    Answer: (C) party

2   Step 1: The sentence needs a plural noun form.

    Step 2: Nucleus is a scientific word.

    TIP: Scientific and medical words often have Latin or Greek forms.

    Step 3: Change –us to –i

    Answer: (C) nuclei

3. Step 1: The sentence is not correct as written.

    Step 2: *Kant's critique of pure reason and german philosophers* are being tested.

    Step 3: Italics indicate the title of a work.

    TIP: There is no need to find the correct form of each word if there is one word or group of words that appears in different forms in each answer choice.

    Answer: (C) *Kant's Critique of Pure Reason*

Independent Practice

1. **Answer: (B) gently**

    Gently ends in an *–ly*, which is a clue that it is an adverb. *Howling* is a gerund, *rustled* is the verb, and *dry* is an adjective modifying *leaves*. Dry is a tempting answer for this question as it precedes another adjective. However, by pairing it with *autumn* and *leaves*, it becomes clear that it is modifying the noun *leaves* in this sentence.

2. **Answer: (D) chairman of the committee mailed to the report of Chief Johnson**

    The title *chairman of the committee* does not precede a name so it must remain lowercase. *Chief* is a title preceding a name so it must be capitalized.

3. **Answer: (B) analyses**

    Analyses correctly changes the *–is* ending to the plural *–es*. Choice A is singular. Choice C uses standard pluralization on an irregular noun. Choice D changes the word from a noun to a verb, rendering the sentence ungrammatical.

ReKap

Knowing the rules of grammar can help you explain in clear terms what you want a listener to understand. Good grammar and punctuation are important. Some people may not listen if the communication is vague or sloppy.

5 GRAMMAR · LESSON 2
Punctuation

Punctuation adds meaning and clarity to written English. We can use punctuation to emphasize a point, transcribe a conversation, or signal what kind of information is coming up in a sentence. On test day, the ability to properly recognize and use a variety of punctuation marks is a critical skill. A keen use of punctuation will allow you to communicate clearly and professionally.

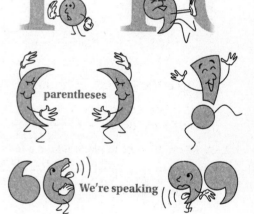

Common Uses in Health Care

- medical transcription
- keeping clear and accurate records of interactions with patients
- writing intake reports in a clinical setting

Key Terms/Formulas

- **apostrophe** –punctuation mark used to form possessives, contractions, or pluralize letters, numbers, or other words which have no plural form

- **colon** – punctuation mark signaling a list or information that adds to the idea before the colon

- **comma** – punctuation mark used for separating words or ideas

- **dialogue** – written versions of conversation or quotations

- **direct dialogue** – quotations; specific things someone said

- **hyphen** – punctuation mark used between spelled-out compound numbers or fractions

- **indirect dialogue** – description of what someone said; a paraphrase of a conversation

- **parentheses** – punctuation mark used to enclose additional information or explanations that would interrupt the flow of the sentence

- **punctuation** – symbols that give structure and organization to sentences

- **quotation marks** –punctuation that sets off direct dialogue and certain titles

- **semicolon** – punctuation mark used to link related independent clauses or a series of items containing commas

What is punctuation? Punctuation is a set of marks and symbols that give structure and organization to language. Punctuation serves as a code by which the author is able to convey meaning, intention, and emphasis.

Everyone knows that a period ends a sentence, an exclamation point shows a strong emotion, and a question mark signals a question. But some punctuation marks have more complex rules. Let's begin by reviewing these.

One of the most important punctuation marks is the comma. Commas tell the reader how to parse information, add emphasis, and create clear sentence structure.

Comma Usage	
Usage guideline or rule	**Example**
Commas can indicate a pause in a sentence, such as a comma placed after introductory information.	*Before the war,* architects rarely used concrete block construction.
Commas can indicate pauses to present non-essential phrases.	Asha, *who is a straight A student,* attends Roosevelt High.
Commas are used to show a direct address, or calling a person by name.	*Jake,* please put the roast in the oven.
Commas can separate items in a list.	Jodi put *bananas, pears, and oranges* in the fruit salad.
Commas divide series of words, phrases, or clauses.	Today we will *drive to swim practice, run to the grocery store, and make dinner.* (the comma before the conjunction is an optional comma, a.k.a., Oxford or serial comma)
Commas can separate adjectives that both describe a word equally. If you can separate the adjectives with *and,* then a comma is usually appropriate.	Pete visited the *old, crumbling* house one last time. Pete visited the *big green* house one last time. (no comma necessary)
Commas follow the salutation in an informal letter or note.	Dear Jaden, I can't wait to see you. Love, Mom
Do not use a comma to set off an essential phrase. Essential phrases often include the word *that.*	Monika ate the cake *that Annie made for her.* (no comma necessary)
Commas are used to separate the pieces in dates and place names.	June 12, 1979 Detroit, Michigan

 WATCH OUT!

Beware of comma splices! Do not use a comma to join two independent clauses together. Add a conjunction or use a semicolon.

Rules governing some other common punctuation marks are also frequently tested.

Common Punctuation Marks		
Punctuation mark	**Usage**	**Example**
Semicolon	Punctuation mark used to link related independent clauses or a series of items containing commas.	She scrubbed her hands; she prepared for the operation.
Colon	Punctuation mark signaling a list or information that adds to the idea before the colon. Colons may also be used after the salutation in formal letters or memos.	My mother told me to buy the following: a loaf of bread, a container of milk, and a stick of butter. To whom it may concern: Dear Sir or Madam:
Apostrophe	Punctuation mark used to form possessives, contractions, or pluralize letters, numbers, or other words which have no plural form.	Jim's golf clubs, Rosa's house Dot your i's and cross your t's!
Hyphen	Punctuation mark used between spelled-out compound numbers or fractions.	When I am sixty-five, I plan to retire. Three-quarters of the class went on the field trip.
Parentheses	Punctuation mark used to enclose additional information or explanations that would interrupt the flow of the sentence.	Karyn will (I assume) remember to bring the potato salad.

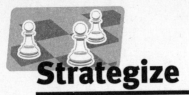

Strategize

Punctuation is a code that lets us know how to read a sentence correctly—where to breathe, where a new idea starts, how ideas relate to each other. For all types of punctuation questions, you should focus on breaking that code.

Identify the task:

Before beginning any punctuation question, quickly scan the question and answer choices to see what is being tested.

Are multiple punctuation marks in play? Is the question asking you to properly punctuate a sentence or choose a correctly punctuated version of a sentence? Does the question ask you to find one correctly punctuated sentence out of a group of different sentences? Make sure you perform this mini-analysis on every question to reduce confusion and to prevent unnecessary work. Once the task is clearly defined, the question can be approached strategically.

When tackling punctuation items on test day, it is important to Break the Code! Codebreaking is a multistep strategy which can be used flexibly with any punctuation question.

STEP 1. Break the code

Determine the author's meaning or intent.

STEP 2. What's my job?

Determine the role of the punctuation mark. Does it match the author's meaning as it is being used?

STEP 3. Use your ears

Read the sentence to yourself (silently), note places you take a breath or pause.

Often, you will follow these steps in order. But some questions may require you to use only some steps. Practicing this strategy will help you use the strategy flexibly on test day.

Apply

Now let's put this strategy to use on a question like ones you might see on test day.

A1. Which of the following punctuation marks correctly completes the sentence below?

Everyone is asked to bring the following items to school ____ pens, paper, a calculator, and some folders.

A) -

B) ;

C) :

D) !

STEP 1: Identify the task.

Read the question stem for clues. What is the task?

Insert the proper punctuation mark.

STEP 2: Break the code.

Read the sentence. What is the author trying to say?

The author is telling us what items we need to bring to school.

STEP 3: What's my job?

What comes after the missing punctuation mark?

A *list* of things to bring to school. Choice C, a colon, completes the sentence.

WATCH OUT!

A common error is using semicolons and colons interchangeably. These two punctuation marks may look similar, but they serve different roles!

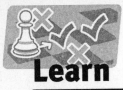

Often as a nurse, it is important to relay conversations with a patient. *Dialogue* is what we call the written version of conversation. Written dialogue has its own set of rules and conventions and also affects the way common punctuation marks are used in a sentence.

There are two types of dialogue:

Direct dialogue or *direct quotations* are the written representations of a person's exact words or conversation. Direct quotations rely on the use of quotation marks to show the dialogue. There are several rules governing the use of quotation marks.

Quotation Marks and Dialogue Rules	
Rule	**Example**
Quotation marks must come in pairs. If you open a quotation mark it must be closed at the end of the quote.	"Always remember to close the quote," the teacher said.
Capitalize the first letter of a direct quote if the quote represents a complete sentence.	Danny said, "You never told me it was your birthday!"
Do not capitalize the first letter of a direct quote if it is a fragment or incomplete sentence.	Jamie said the new car was "the cat's meow."
Do not capitalize the second part of a quote if it is interrupted mid-sentence.	"I don't know what it was," said Peter, "but it sure was big!"
Enclose a comma before closing the quote prior to attribution.	"I never tried chop suey before," said Kate.
A quote within a quote takes single quotation marks.	"And then she said, 'No way!' as she huffed off," Erin told me.
Short works such as chapters, songs, poems, short stories, and plays should have their titles enclosed in quotation marks.	We read "Ode to a Grecian Urn" in our English class.
The ending punctuation mark for the quote should be enclosed within the quotation marks. Use a comma to transition from quote to attribution.	Jerry said, "All's well that ends well."
	"She gave me the best present," said Karen

Indirect dialogue or *indirect quotations* are paraphrases or approximations of a person's words or conversation. For example: *Jose told Mateo that he would give him a ride home.* Indirect dialogue does not use quotation marks.

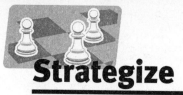

Strategize

For questions containing quotation marks, follow the same strategies used for other punctuation marks. However, add a step. When we Break the Code on a quotation marks item, we need to ask the following questions which relate to the author's intent:

- Who is talking?

- Is this a direct quote?

- Where does the direct quote start and end?

- Is there a quote within a quote?

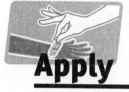

Apply

Let's practice our strategy on a quotation item.

A2. **How should we correctly punctuate the sentence below?**

Leslie said I know Alyssa really likes the song Mandy by Barry Manilow.

Step 1: Who is talking?

Leslie is the speaker.

Step 2: Is this a direct quote?

Read the sentence carefully. *Leslie said* is an attribution phrase. Whenever you see words like *said*, *stated*, or *exclaimed*, a direct quote is very likely.

Step 3: Where does the direct quote start and end?

Since this is a direct quote, you need to insert a comma and a double quotation mark after *Leslie said*. The quote continues on until the end of the sentence, so a double quotation mark needs to be added after the period.

Step 4: Is there a quote within a quote?

Reading carefully reveals a song title. Since song titles appear in quotation marks, and this song title appears nested within a direct quote, single quotation marks should enclose the song title. For example: Leslie said, "I know Alyssa really likes the song 'Mandy' by Barry Manilow."

Guided Practice

1. Which of the following punctuation marks correctly completes the sentence below?

   Bella went to the costume shop to buy Halloween supplies __ a tube of face paint, body glitter, vampire fangs, and some fake blood.

   A) ;

   B) -

   C) ...

   D) :

   STEP 1: Identify the Task.

   What is the question asking you to do?

   _____

   _____

   STEP 2: Break the code.

   What is the author trying to say?

   _____

   _____

   STEP 3: What's my job?

   Examine the blank and determine what function it needs to perform to maintain the author's meaning. Which punctuation mark is needed to do this job?

   _____

   _____

2. Which of the following sentences correctly applies the rules of punctuation?

A) Elizabeth purchased leeks, cheese, eggs, and bacon; she whipped up an omelet.

B) Elizabeth purchased leeks, cheese, eggs, and bacon, she whipped up an omelet.

C) Elizabeth purchased; leeks, cheese, eggs, and bacon: she whipped up an omelet.

D) Elizabeth purchased; leeks, cheese, eggs, and bacon, she whipped up an omelet.

STEP 1: Identify the task.

The question asks you to find the correctly punctuated sentence. Which punctuation marks are being tested in the answer choices?

_____

_____

STEP 2: Eliminate obvious wrong answers.

Concentrate on the first tested punctuation mark. Does the sentence need any type of mark after the word *purchased*?

_____

STEP 3: Break the code.

What is the author trying to say?

The author gives us two independent but related clauses. How should you separate the two clauses?

_____

Guided Practice

3. Which of the following sentences correctly punctuates direct dialogue?

   A) Eileen boasted, "I met the guy who sings 'Party Up' at the concert!"

   B) Eileen boasted; "I met the guy who sings 'Party Up' at the concert!"

   C) Eileen boasted, "I met the guy who sings "Party Up" at the concert!"

   D) Eileen boasted "I met the guy who sings "Party Up" at the concert!"

STEP 1: Identify the Task.

What type of question is this? What is the question asking us to do?

_____

_____

STEP 2: Break the code.

As soon as we spot direct dialogue in play, jump to the quotation mark questions. Where does the direct quote start and end?

_____

_____

STEP 3: Is there a quote within a quote?

_____

Independent Practice

1. Which of the following punctuation marks correctly completes the sentence below?

Spot fetched the paper for his owner_ he expected a bone.

A) ;

B) -

C) ,

D) :

> **HINT** *What's my job? What role should the missing punctuation mark play?*

2. Which of the following sentences correctly uses the rules of punctuation?

A) Last night Jamal requested multiple tools to complete the project: a hammer, a drill a sander.

B) Last night, Jamal requested multiple tools to complete the project: a hammer, a drill, a sander.

C) Last night, Jamal requested multiple tools to complete the project; a hammer, a drill a sander.

D) Last night Jamal requested multiple tools to complete the project; a hammer, a drill, a sander.

> **HINT** *Use your ears! Is there a natural pause that needs a comma?*

3. Which of the following sentences correctly punctuates direct dialogue?

A) Corinne said "You will not believe it, but she shouted "next customer!" at me!"

B) Corinne said, "you will not believe it, but she shouted "next customer!" at me!"

C) Corinne said, "You will not believe it, but she shouted, 'Next customer!' at me!"

D) Corinne said "You will not believe it, but she shouted 'Next customer!' at me"!

> **HINT** *Focus on one rule being tested and eliminate any answers that do not follow that rule. Then evaluate the remaining choices.*

ReKap

In this lesson, you learned about rules governing several types of punctuation marks. Commas, semicolons, colons, parentheses, hyphens, and apostrophes each have specific uses and are tools used by an author to convey meaning and emphasis.

You also learned about direct and indirect dialogue and the use of quotation marks.

You learned strategies to help you answer test items. The strategies can be used flexibly to answer any punctuation based test question. These strategies are:

- Identify the Task
- Break the Code
- What's My Job?
- Use Your Ears

? **Describe one common usage for each of the following punctuation marks: comma, semicolon, colon, parentheses, and quotation marks. Then, tell why using punctuation properly is important to helping readers understand your writing.**

_____

_____

_____

_____

_____

Answers

Guided Practice

1. Step 1: Fill in the correct punctuation mark.

   Step 2: Bella bought a bunch of Halloween supplies at the costume shop.

   Step 3: A colon is needed since it starts a list of items.

   Answer: (D) :

2. Step 1: A semicolon or nothing between purchased and leeks; a semicolon, comma, or colon between bacon and she.

   Step 2: No, the sentence does not need punctuation after purchased.

   Step 3: A semicolon is used to separate two independent but related clauses.

   Answer: (A) Elizabeth purchased leeks, cheese, eggs, and bacon; she whipped up an omelet.

3. Step 1: The question is asking one to use quotation marks to punctuate the dialogue correctly.

   Step 2: The direct quote starts after boasted; it ends after concert.

   Step 3: A song title in within the quotes.

   Answer: (A) Eileen boasted, "I met the guy who sings 'Party Up' at the concert!"

Independent Practice

1. **Answer: (A) ;**

   Correctly link two connected and related independent clauses with a semicolon.

2. **Answer: (B) Last night, Jamal requested multiple tools to complete the project: a hammer, a drill, a sander.**

   While both Choices B and C correctly insert a comma after the introductory phrase, the second punctuation mark between project and a hammer differs between the two answers. Eliminate Choice C since a semicolon is not the correct signal for a list of items.

3. **Answer: (C) Corinne said, "You will not believe it, but she shouted, 'Next customer!' at me!"**

   Choice C correctly adds a comma after the attribution. It also properly uses single quotation marks for the quote within a quote and encloses the exclamation point within the closing quotation mark.

ReKap

A comma is used to separate words or ideas. A semicolon is used to separate related independent clauses. A colon is used to signal a list. Parentheses are used to enclose additional information. Quotation marks are used to set up direct dialogue.

Proper punctuation conveys meaning and rhythm to writing. For example, using commas to offset items in a list slows the reader so that the items can be identified. A semicolon requires the reader to come to a near stop (i.e., slow). Colons introduce an item or series of items that illustrate what has come before the colon. Proper punctuation is to the written word what facial expressions are to verbal expression.

Intermediate Grammar

Basic subject-verb agreement is something used every day in casual speech and writing. But in formal writing—and even in public speaking—this can become tricky as sentences grow more complex. Pronouns keep spoken and written English from sounding choppy and repetitive. The ability to use pronouns and verbs correctly is critical for clear communication in health care settings as ambiguity can result in confusion during treatment and care.

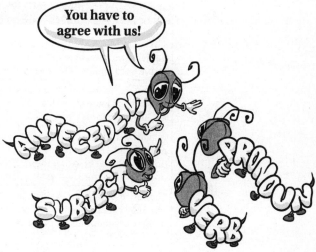

Common Uses in Health Care

- writing patient education materials
- keeping clear and accurate health care records
- composing accurate and precise patient histories

Key Terms/Formulas

- **antecedent** – the word to which a pronoun stands in for or refers back
- **collective nouns** – a number or collection of people or things spoken of as one whole unit
- **mass nouns** – uncountable nouns, nouns without discrete units
- **plural** – many
- **pronoun** – a word that stands in for a noun or refers to a noun
- **singular** – one
- **subject** – person, place, thing, or phrase that is acting or being
- **verb** – an action or being word

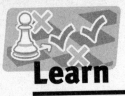

Learn

In English, both subjects and verbs have singular and plural forms. Subjects and verbs must agree with each other to produce a grammatical sentence. This means a singular subject must have a singular verb. A plural subject must have a plural verb. The conjugation of a simple verb such as *swim* illustrates how verbs change to match the subject.

Regular Verb Conjugations		
	Singular	**Plural**
First person	I swim	We swim
Second person	You swim	You swim
Third person	He/She/It swims	They swim

In casual or informal speech and writing, English sentences tend to follow a fairly simple subject + verb + object order, such as *Dante likes peaches*. For simple subject-verb-object sentences, matching the subject and verb is automatic for most English speakers. But in more complicated sentence structures—and in certain special cases—it can be difficult to *hear* correct agreement. In formal writing, sentences often are longer or more complicated.

Key Subject–Verb Agreement Rules	
Rules	**Examples**
Subjects with two or more nouns or pronouns joined by the word *and* must take a plural verb form.	Isaiah and Brianna are at the mall. She and her sister attend the same college.
Compound subjects with two or more singular nouns or pronouns joined by the word *or* or *nor* must take a singular verb form.	Colin or Marquis leads the stretches for the football team each practice. Neither he nor she likes oysters.
When a compound subject has two or more nouns of mixed number (at least one singular and one plural noun) joined by *or* or *nor*, the verb must match the number of the word nearest the verb.	The dog or the cats scratch the door each day. The cats or the dog scratches the door each day.
The verb must agree with the subject of the sentence. The subject of the sentence is not necessarily the noun or pronoun closest to the verb.	The *captain*, as well as all the sailors, is ready to set sail. The *lady* with all the cats wears a uniform to work.
In sentences beginning with *there*, the verb must match to the subject that follows.	There are four lights. There is only one soda left.
Most indefinite pronouns such as *each, anyone, anything, anybody, everyone, everything, everybody, either, neither, someone, somebody, no one, nobody, either, neither* must pair with a singular verb form.	Each of the children takes a prize home. Neither was elected to the city council. Nobody knows why the shop is closed. Someone has lost her earring.

Quantities, mass nouns, collective nouns, and grouping words can often cause confusion when it comes to subject-verb agreement. There are rules for these special cases.

Special Cases	
Fractional quantities take a singular or plural verb based on the noun they are connected to in the sentence.	One-third of the cherries were eaten by Joanna. One-third of the water flows out of the pool each hour.
Grouping words such as *most, more, many, all, none* take a singular or plural verb based on the noun they are connected to in the sentence, or on the meaning of the sentence.	All was not lost as there were still five minutes left in the game. All of the cows are grazing in the pasture. *Many* is *more* than *some*. Many of you are wondering who sold the most cookies.
Mass nouns, or nouns representing things that are not counted, take singular verbs.	Spaghetti is delicious. Wood is an excellent building material. Smoke fills the air.
Collective nouns group more than one person, animal, or item together but behave as singular subjects.	A flock of sheep was guarded by the dog. The team is going to the playoffs. The regiment of soldiers is marching to battle.

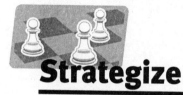

Strategize

Our ears can often let us down when a sentence does not follow simple subject-verb-object order, or in special cases such as the usage of mass or collective nouns. While using your ears was a key strategy in earlier lessons, you should not rely on this strategy for subject-verb agreement items on test day. Try to initially *turn off your ears* when you spot a subject-verb agreement question. Instead, rely on a methodical use of strategies.

1. Identify the subject.

Locate the subject of the sentence. Is it a one-word subject or a subject phrase? If it is a subject phrase, which word is the actor in the sentence?

2. Count.

Once the subject is identified, determine if the subject is singular or plural. Be on the lookout for special cases or nouns and pronouns behaving unusually.

3. Cut the clutter.

If you spot subjects separated from the verb by clauses or prepositional phrases, cut everything between the subject and the verb and reread the sentence. For this step only, turn your ears back on as you reread the amended sentence.

 WATCH OUT!

Beware of collective nouns! The "of _____" construction should make you suspect a collective noun. These nouns act as singular subjects—ignore the words after *of* when matching collective nouns to verbs.

Apply

Let's get some practice on each of the strategic steps. First, concentrate on locating and identifying the subject.

Identify the Subject

> **Circle the subject in each sentence.**
>
> **Bethany delivered a commencement speech at the high school.**
>
> **Torry and his friend Aaron clapped at the end of the speech.**

What did you pick? Remember, the subject is the sentence's main actor. In the first sentence, the main actor is *Bethany*. The second sentence has two actors to form a compound, plural subject—*Torry and his friend Aaron*.

Now let's move on to the second strategy. Count and determine whether the following subjects are singular or plural.

Counting Subjects: Singular or Plural?		
I	S	P
They	S	P
The team	S	P
The pack of wolves	S	P
Diego	S	P
Caroline and her friends	S	P
Everybody	S	P
Keisha or E.J.	S	P

Finally, cut the clutter by removing excess words in the following sentence. Let's rewrite the following sentence without the unnecessary words.

Alejandro, the owner of many vintage cars, drives a hybrid to work.

Decluttered: **Alejandro drives a hybrid to work.**

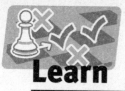

Learn

A pronoun is a word that stands in for or replaces a noun. In English, we use pronouns to avoid repeating a noun over and over. Some of the most commonly used pronouns are personal pronouns and possessive pronouns, but all pronouns must refer back to a noun called an antecedent.

Personal and Possessive Pronouns		
	Singular	**Plural**
First person	I, me, mine, my	we, us, our, ours
Second person	you, your, yours	you, your, yours
Third person	he, she, it, him, her, hers, his, its	they, them, their, theirs

What else should you know about pronouns? Pronouns must:

- Agree in number with the antecedent—either singular or plural

- Agree in person with the antecedent—first, second, or third person

- Agree in gender if the antecedent is a gendered noun—John = he, Isha = she

Ever wondered whether you should say *who* or *whom*? Pronouns may vary in form when they play different roles in sentences. Think back to what you learned about objects as you review the table below.

Pronoun Cases		
Pronouns as Subjects	**Pronouns as Objects**	**Possessive Pronouns**
I	me	mine, my
you	you	your, yours
he, she, it	him, her, it	his, her, hers, its
we	us	our, ours
they	them	their, theirs
who, whoever	whom, whomever	whose

 WATCH OUT!

Remember, *they*, *their*, and *them* should not replace singular pronouns just to avoid using gendered language. A genderless singular antecedent (such as *student*, *voter*, *person*) can be replaced either with *his* or *her* or *his or her* as a unit.

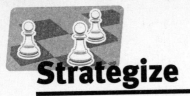

Strategize

Because pronoun items can appear in a variety of formats and are often used in combination with other topics such as subject-verb agreement, use these strategies flexibly. Assess each test question individually and then draw from the following strategies to answer the item correctly.

1. **Find the antecedent.**
   Locate and identify the antecedent. To which word is the pronoun referring? Often the antecedent will be the subject of the sentence.

2. **Count.**
   Once the antecedent is identified, determine if it is singular or plural. Quickly eliminate any answer choices that are not the correct number.

3. **Pick the person, the case, and the gender.**
   See if the pronoun is acting as a subject, an object, or possessive. Determine which person is needed based on the antecedent. Decide whether a gendered pronoun or neutral pronoun is needed.

 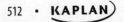

Apply

A1. For each of the following items, circle the antecedent and fill in the blank.

Damon quickly dialed _____ phone.

1. Find the antecedent.

What does the blank in the first sentence replace? Look back at the beginning of the sentence to find the antecedent *Damon*.

2. Count.

Is Damon one person or many? Just one, so you will need a singular pronoun.

3. Pick the person, the case, and the gender.

What is Damon doing in this sentence? He is performing an action, so he must be the subject. But the pronoun refers to the phone, so the pronoun requires the possessive case. Damon is just one person, and male, so the correct word is the singular possessive male pronoun *his*.

Now try these!

Melanie gave _____ brother a cookie.

The boy jumped up and down when _____ won first place.

The choir did not want to leave the stage as _____ continued to receive applause.

Marwan and Amira went to the store, but _____ could not find _____ favorite snacks.

Each boy received _____ diploma on graduation day.

The cows chewed _____ cud all day long.

Guided Practice

1. Which of the following sentences provides an example of correct subject-verb agreement?

   A) The flock of geese are flying south for the winter.

   B) The finance committee, a group of local business owners, meet once a month.

   C) The team rides to away games on a charter bus.

   D) The herd, made up of Holstein and Guernsey cows, are in the milking barn.

STEP 1: Identify the subject.

Find the subject in each of the answer choices.

_____

_____

STEP 2: Count.

Is each subject singular or plural?

_____

_____

STEP 3: Cut the clutter.

Cut any non-essential words so you have a one word subject next to the verb. Write each subject–verb pair and cross through any that are ungrammatical.

_____

_____

2. Which of the following is the correct pronoun to complete the sentence below?

My sister Harsha picked up Benji; then _____ gave him a ride to the pool party.

A) he

B) she

C) it

D) they

STEP 1: Find the antecedent.

This sentence uses a semicolon to split two related independent clauses. Often the antecedent for a blank after the semicolon will actually be in the clause prior to the semicolon. Who is giving someone a ride?

_____

Step 2: Count.

Is the antecedent singular or plural? Can we eliminate any answers now?

_____

STEP 3: Pick the person, the case, and the gender.

Should the pronoun be first, second, or third person? Why? Is the pronoun acting as a subject, object, or possessive? Is the antecedent gendered?

_____

_____

_____

Guided Practice

3. Which of the following is the correct pronoun and verb for the sentence below? The antecedent of the pronoun to be added is underlined.

We watched the <u>troupe</u> of dancers pirouetting across the stage; _____ performing a dance choreographed by Jerome Robbins.

A) they were

B) he was

C) its

D) it was

STEP 1: Count.

The introductory sentence identifies the antecedent. Is the antecedent singular or plural? How do you know?

_____

STEP 2: Match the pronoun to the antecedent.

Which pronoun should be used to refer to the word troupe?

_____

STEP 3: Eliminate incorrect answers and evaluate the remaining choices.

Which answers can be eliminated immediately based on the pronoun?

_____

Evaluate the remaining choices. Which one must be the correct answer? Why?

_____

Independent Practice

1. Which of the following is an example of a grammatically correct sentence?

A) Who was the first explorer to reach the South Pole?

B) Whom was the first explorer to reach the South Pole?

C) How was the first explorer to reach the South Pole?

D) Whose was the first explorer to reach the South Pole?

HINT Find the antecedent and determine which case the pronoun should be.

2. Which of the following correctly completes the sentence below?

Nichelle and Denise hosted _____ yearly birthday bash in Las Vegas.

A) her

B) they're

C) their

D) hers

3. Which of the following sentences provides an example of correct subject-verb agreement?

A) The herd of antelope trample the grass on the Kenyan plains.

B) The colony, after hours of debates, are finally voting on a name for the settlement.

C) The council, fearing the upcoming election, vote for a reduction in waste management fees.

D) The swarm of bees is chasing the greedy honey bear.

ReKap

In this lesson, you learned strategies to help you answer test items about subject-verb agreement and pronoun usage. Implementing these strategies will allow you to answer any test question focusing on subject-verb agreement or pronoun usage. These strategies are:

- Identify the subject

- Count

- Cut the clutter

- Identify the antecedent

- Pick the person and case

? **What are some of the most common errors found in subject-verb agreement questions? What are common errors found in test questions about pronouns? How will avoiding common grammatical errors help you communicate with patients and peers as you pursue your nursing career?**

_____

_____

_____

_____

_____

Answers

Counting Subjects Answers (page 510)

I	S
They	P
The team	S
The pack of wolves	S
Diego	S
Caroline and her friends	P
Everybody	S
Keisha or E.J.	S

A1 Answers

Melanie gave__her__brother a cookie.

The boy jumped up and down when__he__won first place.

The choir did not want to leave the stage as__it__continued to receive applause.

Marwan and Amira went to the store, but__they__could not find__their__favorite snacks.

Each boy received__his__diploma on graduation day.

The cows chewed__their__cud all day long.

Guided Practice

1. Step 1: The subject in each sentence is: The flock of geese; The finance committee; The team: The herd

    Step 2: flock = singular; committee = singular; team = singular; herd = singular

    Step 3: ~~The flock are flying~~; ~~The committee meet~~; The team rides; ~~The herd are~~

    Answer: (C) The team rides to away games on a charter bus.

2. Step 1: Harsha is giving someone a ride.

    Step 2: The antecedent is singular. Eliminate D because it is plural.

    Step 3: The pronoun should be third person. It is talking about another named person and does not refer to a you. The pronoun is the subject of the second clause. Harsha is a girl and needs a feminine pronoun.

    Answer: (B) she

3. Step 1: The antecedent is singular. It is a grouping or collective noun.

    Step 2: The pronoun *it* should be used to refer to the word troupe.

    Step 3: Choices A and B can be eliminated based on the pronoun. Choice C is a possessive pronoun and does not include a verb. Choice D is the correct answer.

    Answer: (D) it was

Answers

Independent Practice

1. **Answer: (A) Who was the first explorer to reach the South Pole?**

   Choice A correctly uses the subjective form of the pronoun *who*. The pronoun substitutes for the unknown explorer. If the sentence is turned into a factual statement, instead of a question, *who* would be replaced by *Amundsen was the first explorer to reach the South Pole.*

2. **Answer: (C) their**

   Choice C correctly identifies the plural antecedent *Michelle and Denise* by assigning a plural pronoun. Choice A incorrectly forms a feminine singular even though *and* joins the two feminine nouns in the subject.

3. **Answer: (D) The swarm of bees is chasing the greedy honey bear.**

   Choice D correctly matches a singular verb form with the collective noun *swarm*. The other choices incorrectly pair plural verb forms with collective nouns.

ReKap

Common errors found in subject-verb agreement questions include errors in number. For example, I *work*; he *works*. The kitchen or bedrooms *need* to be cleaned; the bedrooms or kitchen *needs* to be cleaned. One of the dogs *walks* slowly. The people who have dogs *walk* slow too.

One can avoid common grammatical errors by double-checking pronoun use (i.e., me, myself, and I); cut the clutter so you can clearly identify the subject and verb; and proofread, but do it later.

GRAMMAR · LESSON 4
Word and Sentence Structure

Word, sentence, and paragraph structure provide the clues readers need to make sense of written English. Forming clear and correct sentences will help you easily convey the information your future patients need in an accurate manner.

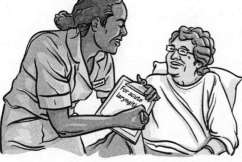

Common Uses in Health Care

- presentations or e-mail communications with co-workers

- providing clear and concise discharge or care instructions

- producing informational pamphlets and brochures for patients

Key Terms/Formulas

- **affixes** – a group of letters added to a root word to form a new word; includes prefixes and suffixes

- **complex sentence** – a sentence containing at least one dependent clause in addition to an independent clause

- **compound sentence** – a sentence containing two or more independent clauses

- **concluding sentence** – a sentence providing an analysis or conclusion based on the supporting information

- **paragraph** – a self-contained group of sentences about a similar theme, topic, or idea

- **prefix** – a group of letters added to the beginning of a root word

- **root word** – the simplest form of a word with no prefixes or suffixes

- **run-on sentence** – two or more independent clauses which have not been joined correctly

- **sentence fragment** – a phrase or clause punctuated as a sentence

- **simple sentence** – a sentence that only contains one independent clause

- **suffix** – a group of letters added to the end of a root word

- **supporting detail** – evidence, examples, and details that support or explain the topic of a paragraph

- **topic sentence** – a sentence introducing the main idea of a paragraph and linking that idea to the main theme of the piece of writing

- **word structure** – the pieces that make up a word, such as prefixes, roots, and suffixes

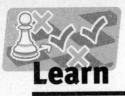

Learn

In English, words are built out of key pieces to produce the overall meaning of a word. The way these pieces join together to build words is called word structure. Words are primarily built out of root words and affixes, or word parts that are added to the root word. Take the time to be sure you understand each of these word parts now to prepare for this more advanced technique in later lessons. Clear understanding of how affixes function in English will allow you to correctly form words from root words.

Word Structure			
Word Part	**Location**	**Used To....**	**Examples**
Root word	Can be the beginning, middle, or end of a word. Can also be a stand-alone word.	Give the word's basic meaning	astro, audio, cardio, chron, derma, geo
Prefix	Attaches to the front of a root word	Change or extend a word's meaning	anti, epi, dis, un, post, peri
Suffix	Attaches to the end of a root word	Change or extend a word's meaning	itis, able, ible, ism, ology, ence, ance

Suffixes often alter the spelling of their root word. This will be covered in future lessons.

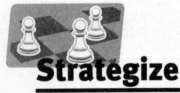

Strategize

Because word structure items can appear in word formation, spelling, and meaning questions, it is important to have a grab bag of strategies that can be used on any word structure item. We'll focus on applying these strategies to formation items today, but keep them in mind in future lessons as you encounter tricky spelling items or questions about meanings of unfamiliar words. As always, identify your task before selecting a strategy.

1. **Find the root.**
   In any word structure item, you should begin with the root word.

2. **Use caution while merging.**
   For formation and spelling questions, join the root with the affixes. Do not use hyphens or dashes. Roots should merge seamlessly with affixes.

Apply

Let's get some quick practice on forming words using roots and affixes.

Combine the root word with the prefix or affix to produce a correctly formed new word. Fill in the new word in the table.

Form a New Word			
Prefix	**Root**	**Suffix**	**New word**
	appendix	itis	
il	logic	al	
ab	duct	ion	

Use caution while merging.

appendix + itis = appendicitis

Il + logic + al = illogical

ab+duct+ion = abduction

Remember

Notice there are some spelling changes during final formation of the word appendicitis. The rules for suffix spelling changes will be reviewed in future lessons.

Learn

Sentence structure describes the composition of a sentence. Sentences are classified based on the grammar building blocks that make up their structure.

A simple sentence only contains one independent clause. An independent clause is a group of words that has a complete meaning. An independent clause must contain a subject and a predicate. To refresh, the subject is a person, place, thing, or phrase that is acting or being, what or whom the sentence is about. The predicate tells something about the subject or what the subject is doing.

In the most basic form, only a subject and predicate are needed to create a simple sentence.
Examples: He won. Kamala left. The dog barks. You'll be going.

Simple sentences may have other parts of speech such as objects, prepositions, adjectives, and adverbs.
Examples: Jaime ate the burger. I always complete each patient's chart by noon. Joaquin and Jenna drove to the party in the little blue car.

Compound sentences contain two or more independent clauses linked with a conjunction or semicolon. Conjunctions are linking words. There are two main types of conjunctions.

Coordinating Conjunctions						
For	And	Nor	But	Or	Yet	So

Correlative conjunctions must occur as pairs and join equal and parallel grammatical items. For example, a pair of singular nouns would be equal and parallel grammatical items, as would a pair of predicates.

Correlative Conjunctions	
Correlative conjunction pair	**Example**
either...or	Either Sue or Dulce will pick up the cake.
neither...nor	Neither Kaleb nor Jodi attended the party.
not only...but also	Not only did Fluffy knock over the vase, but he also spilled the kitty litter.
both...and	Both Annie and Kalil were at the fair.
whether...or	Whether it rains or shines the postal worker delivers the mail.

A complex sentence is a sentence containing at least one dependent clause in addition to an independent clause. Dependent clauses can be identified because they are marked with a subordinating conjunction.

Subordinating Conjunctions			
after	before	provided that	unless
although	even if	rather than	until
as	even though	since	when
as if	if	so that	whenever
as long as	if only	than	where
as soon as	in order that	that	whereas
as though	now that	though	wherever
because	once	till	while

Examples:

Before you leave, you should grab your coat.

After the class is over, we could all go out for coffee.

Carly will meet us as soon as she finishes all her homework.

Remember

A comma should follow a subordinate clause placed at the beginning of a sentence.

 WATCH OUT!

Some of the subordinating conjunctions can also be used as prepositions! A subordinating conjunction must precede a clause.

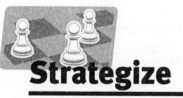

Strategize

Because structure items can appear in a variety of formats, use these strategies flexibly. Assess each test question individually and identify what your task is. Certain strategies are more applicable to items asking you to join sentences together or split them apart; others are better for identification of sentence structure items.

1. **Find the subject and predicate.**

   Locate the subject. Find the verb and anything attached to it.

2. **Locate or insert a conjunction.**

   If you are combining two simple sentences, look for answer choices that add a coordinating or correlative conjunction. If you are determining the type of structure, look for clues like commas. Then find coordinating or correlative conjunctions as signs of compound sentence structure.

3. **Locate or insert subordinating conjunction and clause.**

   Does the sentence use a subordinating conjunction to introduce a dependent clause? If so, it is complex. If you spot a subordinating conjunction, check to make sure it is introducing a dependent clause and is not acting as a preposition. If asked to create a complex sentence, find an item that inserts a subordinating conjunction and clause.

Apply

Let's put it all together! Read each sentence and follow the steps to see how different kinds of sentences are structured.

Carlotta left her purse in the car.

A1. Is the sentence above a simple sentence?

Find the subject and predicate.

The subject is Carlotta. What did Carlotta do? *She left her purse in the car.* This is the predicate. There are no conjunctions in this sentence, simply a subject + a verb + an object + a prepositional phrase. So, this is a simple sentence.

Carlotta left her purse in the car. Jada retrieved it.

A2. Create a compound sentence using the two simple sentences above.

Locate or insert a conjunction.

The task is to create a compound sentence so a conjunction must be inserted. Remember FANBOYS and select a conjunction that connects the two sentences above. Make sure you insert a comma prior to the conjunction. *Carlotta left her purse in the car, so Jada retrieved it.*

Carlotta left her purse in the car

A3. Which of the following additions to the sentence above creates a complex sentence?

   A) Carlotta left her bright red purse in the car, so Jada retrieved it.

   B) While she was hurrying into the airport, Carlotta left her purse in the car.

   C) Carlotta left her purse in the little red car after dark.

   D) Carlotta left her purse in the car, but she found it later.

Locate the subordinating conjunction.

The task is to identify a complex sentence. So for each sentence ask whether the sentence uses a subordinating conjunction to introduce a dependent clause. Choice A does not; it is the compound sentence we formed earlier. Choice B uses the subordinate conjunction *while* to introduce a dependent clause; therefore, it must be the correct answer.

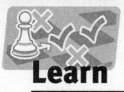

Learn

Paragraph structure describes the organization and composition of a paragraph. Each sentence in a paragraph plays a role and serves a function. Clearly structured paragraphs are easy to read and understand because information is presented logically. Paragraphs contain a group of sentences about the same topic or theme. Ideally, a well-written paragraph will contain at least five sentences, connect the point to the overall theme of the piece of writing, and be structured in such a way that each sentence has a clear purpose. Sentences in paragraphs can typically be divided into a few primary roles.

A topic sentence introduces the main idea of a paragraph and links that idea to the main theme of the piece of writing. Supporting details provide evidence, examples, and details that support or explain the topic of a paragraph. A concluding sentence provides analysis or a conclusion based on the supporting information.

topic sentence **Sharks often inspire fear or hatred; however, sharks' reputations as man-eating monsters are undeserved. [In reality, very few sharks are even capable of seriously harming humans, much less killing them. The bull, tiger, great white, and white tip sharks are the only species of sharks known to have fatally wounded people, but** *[supporting details]* **more than 400 species of sharks roam the oceans and waterways. Even among the species posing a danger to man, attacks on humans are incredibly rare. For example, only 11 confirmed shark bite fatalities occurred in the United States between 2000–2010. A swimmer is far more likely to drown than be bitten by a shark.] Ultimately,** *concluding sentence* **the facts and statistics do not support the reputation of sharks as man-eaters.**

Well-written paragraphs often provide keywords known as road signs to cleanly transition between ideas and sentences. These road signs tell readers what to expect from the sentence. Let's take a look at some examples from the paragraph above.

> *For example*, **only 11 confirmed shark bite fatalities occurred in the United States between 2000-2010.**

The writer uses the road sign *for example* to tell the reader that this is a supporting detail.

> *Ultimately*, **the facts and statistics do not support the reputation of sharks as man-eaters.**

In this sentence, the writer uses the road sign *ultimately* to signal a conclusion.

On test day, keeping an eye out for road signs will help you quickly spot the function of a sentence in a paragraph.

The principles of good paragraph structure also apply to longer essays. Without clear organization, essays are unfocused and present information in a way that is difficult for the reader to follow.

In an essay, each paragraph should function as a unit making a clear point.

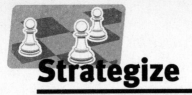

Strategize

Paragraph structure items will ask you to determine the functions of sentences within a paragraph. You may also be asked to select a sentence to add to a paragraph to fulfill a certain role. These strategies will allow you to move quickly through paragraph structure items without wasting unnecessary time.

1. **Identify the task before reading the paragraph.**
   What is the question asking? Tailor the way you read the paragraph to meet the demands of the question.

2. **Find the topic of the paragraph.**
   Figure out what the paragraph is about. All of the sentences must relate back to this in some way, so determine this as part of your first read. The topic sentence is frequently the first sentence in a paragraph.

3. **Skim for road signs and structure.**
   On function identification items, look for road signs that give you clues about the function of the sentence. Skimming based on typical structure can also be helpful. Topic sentences and concluding sentences are rarely buried in the middle of a paragraph. Use this knowledge to guide you in locating them in a passage.

Apply

A4. Read the following paragraph. Then answer the questions.

As baby boomers age, the shortage of qualified health professionals will become increasingly critical. Baby boomers are beginning to enter their senior years, a time of life in which health issues increase and health care needs rise. In addition to increased health care needs, baby boomers are projected to outlive all prior generations in terms of average life expectancy. By 2030, a projected 70 million baby boomers will be senior citizens. This increased longevity means there will be sustained demands for long-term health. Shortages of health care professionals, particularly those dealing with routine health care needs and geriatrics, are already problematic in many parts of the United States. The economic and social impacts of an unprecedented boom in the senior population are not yet fully known. Given the projected doubling of the senior population by the year 2030, it is clear that as baby boomers grow older, changes in public policy are needed to guarantee accessibility to adequate health care.

What is the topic of this paragraph?

> The passage is about health care shortages as baby boomers age.

Which sentence is the topic sentence of the paragraph?

> The first sentence clearly establishes the problem and clues the reader that the paragraph will explain or analyze this problem in some way.

What supporting details does the author give?

- Health care needs increase with age; boomers are aging

- Increased lifespans for boomers

- More demand for health care

- Existing shortages

Which sentence is the concluding sentence?

> The last sentence is the conclusion. The author gives us clues via placement at the end and through the keywords *it is clear*.

Remember

Supporting details tend to cluster in the middle of paragraphs. If tasked with finding a topic or concluding sentence, read the opening and closing sentences carefully but just skim the paragraph's middle.

Guided Practice

1. Which of the following words is written correctly?

   A) peri-carditis

   B) anti-virals

   C) anti-biotics

   D) epidemiology

   STEP 1: Find the root.

   Find the root in each of the items.

   _____

   _____

   STEP 2: Hunt for prefixes and suffixes.

   Find the prefixes and suffixes in each answer choice.

   _____

   _____

   STEP 3: Use caution while merging.

   Which of the items perform a correct merger of the roots and the affixes? Why?

   _____

   _____

2. Which of the following is an example of a compound sentence?

A) Tariq sold the car because he was moving out of state.

B) While you were swimming, Allie set up the beach volleyball net and some umbrellas.

C) Colleen and J.J. drove to the store after running out of chips.

D) Manuel enjoys going for a short jog on trails, but Anya prefers running laps on the track.

STEP 1: Identify the task.

What is the question asking you to find?

_____

STEP 2: Locate a comma.

Remember a compound sentence normally will have a comma before the conjunction. Quickly eliminate any answers missing commas. Which answers can you eliminate?

_____

STEP 3: Locate a coordinating conjunction.

Remember a compound sentence must have a conjunction. Do any remaining sentences use a FANBOYS conjunction?

_____

Guided Practice

3. Which of the following sentences would be the most appropriate topic sentence for the paragraph below?

> Jerome Robbins began his career as a soloist with the American Ballet Theater. He used his training as a dancer to inspire some of his most famous choreographed works, such as *On the Town* and *The King and I.* Robbins did not limit himself to dancing, however, and went on to earn acclaim as a director. *West Side Story* is perhaps the work Robbins is best remembered for, but he produced, directed, and choreographed numerous popular shows during his lengthy career. Robbins passed away in 1998, but his work lives on in the dancers and stars of musical theater he inspired.

A) Jerome Robbins also choreographed and produced the show *Gypsy.*

B) Described by many as an American legend, Jerome Robbins left a lasting legacy in the world of American theater and dance.

C) Bob Fosse was an influential choreographer who occasionally worked with Jerome Robbins.

D) As a ballet master of the New York City Ballet, Jerome Robbins was able to train emerging stars.

STEP 1: Identify the task before reading the paragraph.

What do we need to find? How does this task affect the way you should read the paragraph?

_____

STEP 2: What is the topic of the paragraph?

Read the paragraph. In general, what is the paragraph about?

_____

STEP 3: Skim for road signs and structure.

Which answer directly concerns the overall topic of the paragraph and introduces that topic to the reader?

_____

Independent Practice

1. Which of the following words is written correctly?

   A) post-operative

   B) re-distributed

   C) psychopathology

   D) dis-solution

   HINT *Isolate the roots. Which answer correctly merges an affix with the root?*

2. Which of the following is a simple sentence?

   A) The aggravated woman pushed and shoved her way through the throngs of holiday shoppers.

   B) Once you finish the book, I will return it to the library for you.

   C) Every time I try to nap, the telephone rings.

   D) Kelsey has always enjoyed physics, but she has decided to major in economics instead.

   HINT *Eliminate any sentences with dependent clauses.*

3. A clinical study recently examined the effectiveness of a new beta blocker. The clinical trial tracked patients using the new drug for a period of eighteen months and found no serious side effects. All side effects noted were similar in frequency to side effects reported by the control group taking a placebo. Preliminarily, the trial should be expanded to include more patients and compare efficacy to existing beta blockers available by prescription. Additionally, the trial should explore the use of this beta blocker in comparison to other commonly prescribed hypertension drugs.

   Which of the following sentences provides an example of a concluding sentence?

   A) Over five hundred patients participated in the clinical study.

   B) The new beta blocker outperformed the placebo on all measures.

   C) Finally, if the expanded trial succeeds, the FDA should approve the new drug based on the results of the study.

   D) Existing beta blockers do not show similar results in patients over age 35.

   HINT *Look for words that act as conclusion road signs.*

ReKap

In this lesson, you learned strategies to help you answer items about word structure, sentence structure, and paragraph organization. Implementing these strategies will allow you to correctly answer test questions focusing on structure or organization. These strategies are:

- Find the root.
- Hunt for prefixes and suffixes.
- Merge the pieces.
- Find the subject and predicate.
- Locate or insert a conjunction.
- Locate or insert subordinating conjunction and clause.
- Find the topic of the paragraph.
- Skim for road signs and structure.

? Why is it important to write clearly structured sentences and paragraphs? How will attention to structure and organization help you communicate with patients and peers as you pursue your nursing career?

_____

_____

_____

_____

_____

Answers

Guided Practice

1. Step 1: The root of each item: card, vir, bio, dem

   Step 2: The prefixes and suffixes for each answer choice are: peri/itis, anti/als, anti/ics, epi/olgy

   Step 3: Epidemiology. It is the only choice that does not insert a hyphen at one of the merges.

   Answer: (D) epidemiology

2. Step 1: The question is asking one to find the example of a compound sentence.

   Step 2: Eliminate sentences that do not have commas: Choices A and C

   Step 3: D uses the conjunction *but*.

   Answer: (D) Manuel enjoys going for a short jog on trails, but Anya prefers running laps on the track.

3. Step 1: We need to find the topic sentence that fits with the paragraph. This task necessitates one read the paragraph for the main idea or topic.

   Step 2: The paragraph is about Jerome Robbins, who was a great theater director and choreographer.

   Step 3: Answer B concerns the overall topic. The other answers are unrelated to the main topic or supporting details.

   Answer: (B) Described by many as an American legend, Jerome Robbins left a lasting legacy in the world of American theater and dance.

Independent Practice

1. **Answer: (C) psychopathology**

   Choice C correctly omits the use of a hyphen to join the affix to the root.

2. **Answer: (A) The aggravated woman pushed and shoved her way through the throngs of holiday shoppers.**

   Choice A is a simple sentence, as it does not include multiple independent clauses or any dependent clauses. Choice B and C are complex sentences, and choice D is a compound sentence.

3. **Answer: (C) Finally, if the expanded trial succeeds, the FDA should approve the new drug based on the results of the study.**

   Choice C offers the road sign *finally* as a clue that it is a concluding statement. Choice C also presents analysis. The other choices offer supporting details about the clinical study and the drug.

ReKap

Clearly structured sentences are paragraphs are necessary to convey clear meaning to the reader. Clearly structured paragraphs are easy to read and understand because information is presented logically. Without clear structure, the information that is presented can be difficulty to follow and understand.

5 GRAMMAR • LESSON 5
Spelling and Usage

Many words in English are borrowed or modified from a variety of language families, so spelling can be challenging. On the test, expect to see multiple items testing your ability to correctly spell both common and less common words that may have health care applications.

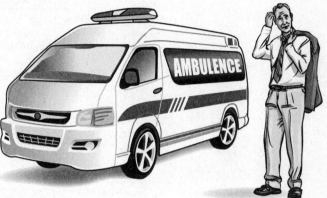

Common Uses in Health Care

- professional written communication with supervisors or colleagues

- writing clear and precise notes on patient care and progress

- producing informational pamphlets and brochures for patients

Key Terms/Formulas

- **homophone** – a word that sounds the same as another word but has a different meaning

- **root word** – the simplest form of a word with no prefixes or suffixes

- **stress** – emphasis placed on a syllable while saying a word

- **suffix** – a group of letters added to the end of a word to change or extend the meaning of the root word

- **syllable** – a unit of spoken language; each syllable must include a vowel sound but may also include consonant sounds

- **word structure** – the pieces that make up a word, such as prefixes, roots, and suffixes

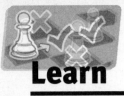

Many spelling errors occur when suffixes are added to words incorrectly. It is important to understand the rules and guidelines that dictate whether the endings of a root word should change when merged with a suffix.

Common Spelling Rules and Exceptions			
Word that...	**Rule**	**Examples**	**Exceptions**
ends in *e* + suffix starting with a consonant	Keep the *e* if it is silent and the suffix you are adding begins with a consonant.	state + ment = statement peace + ful = peaceful encourage + ment = encouragement	judge + ment = judgment awe + ful = awful
ends in *e* + suffix starting with a vowel	Drop the silent *e* ending if you add a suffix beginning with a vowel.	change + ing = changing move + ing = moving	Keep the *e* if the word ends in *ce* or *ge* and the suffix is *able* or *ous*. change + able = changeable outrage + ous = outrageous like + able = likeable
ends in *ay, ey, oy, uy*	Keep the *y* when adding a suffix.	relay + ed = relayed survey + ing = surveying destroy + er = destroyer buy + er = buyer	
ends in *y* preceded by a consonant	Change the *y* to *i* and add the suffix.	injury + ous = injurious carry + er = carrier pity + ful = pitiful hurry + ed = hurried	Keep the *y* when adding the suffix *ing*. steady + ing = steadying study + ing = studying
ends in a consonant-vowel-consonant and is only one syllable	Double the final consonant to add a suffix beginning with a vowel.	rub + ing = rubbing bag + ing = bagging tag + ed = tagged knit + ed = knitted	Omit the double consonant if the word ends in *w*. sew + ing = sewing mow + ed = mowed plow + ed = plowed snow + ing = snowing plow + ed = plowed snow + ing = snowing
ends in a consonant-vowel-consonant but has more than one syllable AND the last syllable is stressed	Double the final consonant to add a suffix beginning with a vowel.	control + er = controller refer + al = referral occur + ing = occurring defer + ed = deferred patrol + ing = patrolling	Omit the double consonant if the word ends in w. allow + ing = allowing
ends in *c*	Add a k when adding a suffix beginning with *e*, *i*, or *y*	garlic + y = garlicky frolic + ed = frolicked panic + ing = panicking	

 WATCH OUT!

Beware of *ie/ei* words! The best guideline is *i* before e except after c or when sounding like *a* as in **neighbor** or **weigh**. For example, **believe** and **friend** keep the *i* before e, but **sleigh** and **receive** take e before *i* due to this guideline. However, there are several exceptions to this rule such as: **weird, science, seize, protein, policies.**

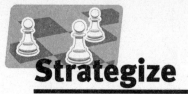

Strategize

Because word structure items can appear in word formation, spelling, and meaning questions, it is important to have a grab bag of strategies that can be used on any word structure item. We'll focus on applying these strategies to formation items today, but keep them in mind in future lessons as you encounter tricky spelling items or questions about meanings of unfamiliar words. As always, identify your task before selecting a strategy.

1. **Find the root.**
   In almost all spelling items, the first task should be finding the root word of the final word. Remember, during merge, endings often change, so it is important to find the original root word.

2. **Pay attention to REBS (root ends and beginnings of suffixes)**
   For formation and spelling questions, join the root with the affixes. Do not use hyphens or dashes. Roots should merge seamlessly with affixes.

3. **Can the root stand alone?**
   When deciding between suffix options, it is often important to see whether the root is a stand-alone word. Look at your isolated root and ask whether it is a complete word.

Apply

Now let's get some practice quickly identifying misspelled words.

First, underline the root of each word. Pay special attention to REBS (root ends and beginnings of suffixes) and which rules should apply. Then circle the word if it is misspelled.

Spelling Speed Drill			
rebelion	beding	gloryous	concurred
perceive	colicy	injurred	conceive
wiring	enforcing	neice	
shiped	delaying	veil	

Now let's correct the misspelled words.

Correct spelling	What rule triggered the change?
rebel + ion = rebellion	ends in consonant-vowel-consonant, last syllable stress
ship + ed + shipped	ends in consonant-vowel-consonant, root is only one syllable
bed + ing = bedding	ends in consonant-vowel-consonant, root is only one syllable
colic + y = colicky	ends in a hard *c*, suffix starts with *y*
glory + ous = glorious	root ends in *y*, suffix is *ous*
injure + ed = injured	root ends in e, suffix begins with a vowel
niece	i before e except after c

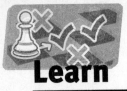

Some suffixes have multiple variations. For these suffixes, there are guidelines for which version of the suffix should be added to the root word.

Choosing the Right Suffix Form			
Suffix	**Rule**	**Examples**	**Exceptions**
able	If the root word can stand alone as a complete word, then add the suffix *able*. Make sure you drop the e if the root word ends in e.	convey + able = conveyable imagine + able = imaginable afford + able = affordable depend + able = dependable	digestible responsible flexible accessible combustible contemptible sensible
ible	If the root word cannot stand alone as a complete word, then add the suffix *ible*.	divis + ible = divisible invis + ible = invisible terr + ible = terrible horr + ible = horrible	inevitable irritable
ance, ancy, ant	If the root word ends in a hard *c* or *g* sound, ends in *ure*, or ends in *y*, add *ance/ancy/ant*.	elegant significant alliance dalliance variance reliance insurance endurance	defendant
ence, ency, ent	If the root word ends in a soft *c* or *g* sound, ends in *ist*, or ends in *id*, then add *ence/ency/ent*.	innocent absent intelligence persistence confidence independence	avoidance assistance resistance
tion	Most root words that end in a *t* add *ion*.	addiction position exception direction	
sion	If the root word ends in *s*, *l*, or *r*, then add *sion*.	compulsion revulsion diversion excursion permission discussion depression	
cian	If the final word names a person or profession, add *cian*.	musician physician politician electrician	

A good approach is to use this root word guideline and memorize common exceptions

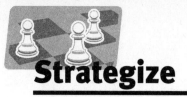

Strategize

Use the same strategic steps to work through suffix variation items.

1. Find the root.
Remember, the root will help guide you to the correct addition of affixes.

2. Pay attention to REBS (root ends and beginnings of suffixes)
Ask: *What letter or pattern of letters does the root word end with? Does the suffix begin with a vowel or a consonant?*

3. Can the root stand alone?
Spelling patterns may vary if the root can stand as a complete word or if it must have an affix.

Apply

Let's get some quick practice on choosing the correct suffixes.

Spelling with Suffixes		
Root	**Which suffix?**	**Complete word**
assure	ance/ence	assurance
comply	ant/ent	compliant
distract	tion/sion/cian	distraction
dimen	tion/sion/cian	dimension
inver	tion/sion/cian	inversion
techni	tion/sion/cian	technician
horr	able/ible	horrible
enjoy	able/ible	enjoyable

Step 1: Find the root.

In this exercise you are given the root. Jump straight to Step two and pay attention to REBS.

Step 2: Pay attention to REBS (root ends and beginnings of suffixes).

Examine the ending of each root and refer back to the chart if needed to find the relevant rule. For example, the first item has the root *assure*. The *ure* ending triggers a rule about *ance/ence* suffix choice. The rule tells us we need an *ance* suffix, and the silent *e* drops off when we merge the root with that suffix.

Step 3: Can the root stand alone?

You may not always need this step. For the word *assure*, you do not need to use the third step of the strategy because paying attention to REBS was enough to confirm the complete word spelling based on the rules.

Check the rest of your answers now. Review rules for any words you missed.

comply + ant = compliant	inver + sion = inversion	enjoy + able = enjoyable
distract + tion = distraction	techni + cian = technician	
dimen + sion = dimension	horr + ible = horrible	

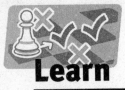

Learn

Homophones are words that sound the same but have different spellings and meanings. Homophone errors are often very common for people who rely on spellcheck. Spellcheck rarely catches homophone errors because they are not technically misspelled. Instead, they are errors in word usage. Let's review some of the most commonly confused homophones.

Homophones		
Homophone	**Meaning**	**Part of speech**
accept except	to answer affirmatively, receive; to regard as true other than, but	verb preposition
affect affect effect	to have an effect or influence on mood or disposition a result; something brought about by a cause or agent	verb noun noun
ascent assent assent	a climb or upward slope to agree to something, concur an agreement	noun verb noun
altar alter	raised structure for worship to change	noun verb
bare bare bear bear	lacking covering, exposed to expose an animal to tolerate, carry, support	adjective verb noun verb
capital capital capitol	a governing city; assets or gains excellent; a type of letter; grave or serious a lawmaking building	noun adjective noun
complement compliment	something that fills up, completes, makes perfect praise, an appreciative remark	noun noun
coarse course	rough duration, class	adjective noun
descent dissent dissent	a downward slope to object to, disagree with a disagreement or objection	noun verb noun
die die	to cease to live a numbered object rolled in games	verb noun
dye dye	to change the color a colored pigment	verb noun
discreet discrete	modest, prudent behavior a separate thing	adjective adjective
its it's	possessive form of *it* contraction of *it is*	possessive contraction
principal principal principle	leader or head most important a belief or moral code	noun adjective noun
stationary stationery	not moving, fixed paper	adjective noun
their there they're	possessive form of they that place contraction of they are	possessive adverb/pronoun contraction
to too two	towards, moving towards also, more than enough the number, two units	preposition adverb adjective, noun

vain	conceited; fruitless	adjective
vane	blade or sail	noun
vein	a blood vessel	noun
whose	possessive form of *who*	possessive
who's	contraction of *who is*	contraction
your	possessive form of *you*	possessive
you're	contraction of *you are*	contraction

Homophones are not the only words that are commonly used incorrectly or misspelled. The list below includes many words that are common in health care settings and are often misspelled. Review this list and memorize the correct spelling for any terms that seem difficult to spell.

Commonly Misspelled Words				
accessible	conception	excellent	legitimate	preferred
accidentally	decide	exercise	leisure	prejudice
accommodate	dehydration	exhalation	liable	psychiatrist
address	diarrhea	exhaustion	maintenance	psychologist
anxiety	diphtheria	fatigue	mattress	radiological
annual	disastrous	febrile	medicinal	referral
arterial	discipline	February	menstrual	rhythm
attendance	disease	federal	noticeable	salary
benefited	efficient	financial	nucleus	schedule
business	eligible	forehead	obstetrics	science
cardiology	environment	government	occasion	temperament
cafeteria	equip	gynecology	operate	temperature
calendar	equipment	hygiene	pamphlet	transferred
cemetery	equipped	imminent	perseverance	urology
committee	equivalent	instant	practically	unusual
conscientious	especially	intelligible	prescription	Wednesday

⚠️ **WATCH OUT!**

Some of these tricky words involve the rules for suffixes! Words that are commonly misspelled due to suffix rules are quite likely to appear in test items.

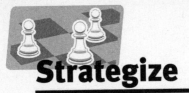
With homophones, it is impossible to rely on your ears to hear the correct spelling. In fact, our ears are typically the reason for homophone misspellings! Instead, when we identify a task in a test item as a homophone selection item, immediately proceed to a strategic approach to find the correct answer.

1. **Identify the part of speech.**

   Analyze the function of the word in the sentence. Ask whether it is being used as a noun, a verb, or a modifier. Identifying the part of speech will sometimes be enough to find the correct answer.

2. **Check the context.**

   Some homophones share the same part of speech. In these instances, read for the context or meaning of the word in the sentence and select the homophone that corresponds with the author's intent.

3. **Analyze apostrophes.**

   Apostrophes can serve as a tiebreaker on many of the trickiest homophone groups. It is helpful to break a word with an apostrophe into its two-word form, "_____ is." For example, "who's" becomes "who is," and "She's" becomes "she is."

Apply

Let's put the strategy into practice with a homophone selection drill. Use the strategic steps on each sentence to help you select the correct word.

Read the sentences below. Select the correct homophone to complete the sentence. Write the word in the blank.

The drug produced few serious side _____ and was recommended for over the counter sales by the FDA. (affects/effects)

Step 1: Identify the part of speech.

First, determine what part of speech the missing word must be. The right answer will be a noun. Looking at our answer choices, we can see that *affects* and *effects* can both serve as nouns, so move on and check the context.

Step 2: Check the context.

Affects and *effects* have different meanings. This author is clearly talking about something that resulted from the drug, not someone's moods, so *effects* must be the answer.

I don't know _____ coat this is, so I will drop it off at lost and found. (who's/whose)

Find the part of speech first. The right answer must be possessive. Context doesn't matter since only one of our answer choices is possessive, *whose*.

Now try a few more. Remember to use the strategies to find the right homophone.

Homophone Selection Drill

Althea ordered every topping _____sardines for the pizza. (accept/except)

The patient will _____the responsibility for full payment of the bill. (bare/bear)

The doctor wrote a letter of recommendation full of praise and _____ for the hardworking nurse. (complements/compliments)

_____ good friend would be flying into the airport for a long visit. (There/Their/They're)

Guided Practice

1. Which of the following options correctly completes the sentence below?

   Kelly's car was old, but it was very _____ and always got her to work in the morning.

   A) relyable

   B) relyible

   C) reliable

   D) relible

   STEP 1: Identify the task.

   Read the sentence, the question stem, and the answer choices. What is the task?

   _____

   _____

   STEP 2: Find the root. Does the root stand alone?

   Look carefully at the answer choices. What is the root of the word being formed in each answer choice? Can that root stand alone? Which suffix does it take?

   _____

   _____

   STEP 3: Pay attention to REBS (root ends and beginnings of suffixes).

   With what letter does the root word end? Recall previous rules about spelling changes for affixes. Does the root need alteration before merging with the suffix? Which answer is correct?

   _____

   _____

2. Which of the following options correctly completes the sentence below?

In her _____ practice, Dr. Portillo sometimes prescribed patients medication to treat depression.

A) psychyatric

B) psychiatric

C) psyciatric

D) psychiatrick

STEP 1: Identify the task.

Read the sentence, the question stem, and the answer choices. What is the task?

_____

STEP 2: Find the root.

Eliminate the suffixes to find the root word. Which is the correct version of the root, *psych* or *psyc*? Can you eliminate any incorrect answers?

_____

_____

STEP 3: Pay attention to REBS (root ends and beginnings of suffixes).

What suffix is being added? Which answer must be correct?

> **Remember**
>
> The suffix *–iatric* is a very common health care suffix meaning *relating to medical treatment.*

_____

_____

Guided Practice

3. Which of the following options correctly completes the sentence below?

As a strict vegetarian, it went against Ricardo's _____ to wear leather shoes with his school uniform.

A) principals

B) principles

C) principal's

D) principle's

STEP 1: Identify the task.

Read the question. Skim the answers. What type of question is this? What is the task?

_____

_____

STEP 2: Identify the part of speech.

Read the sentence and find the function of the missing word. What part of speech should the correct answer be? Can any answers be eliminated?

_____

STEP 3: Check the context.

The sentence tells us that Ricardo is a vegetarian and therefore does not want to wear leather shoes. Is the meaning of the missing word closer to *beliefs* or *leaders*? Which answer must be correct?

_____

_____

Independent Practice

1. The phlebotomist was unable to find any usable _____ for an IV in the severely dehydrated patient's arm.

   A) vanes

   B) vains

   C) veins

   D) vain's

   HINT *Check the context. Which homophone matches the meaning the author intends?*

2. Which of the following options correctly completes the sentence below?

   Jerome kept working diligently to learn how to play guitar, and eventually his _____ paid off.

   A) persistants

   B) persistents

   C) persistance

   D) persistence

   HINT *Find the root. Is there a guideline for suffixes being added to roots ending in ist?*

3. Which of the following words corrects the spelling of the underlined word in the sentence below?

   The stormy sky looked promising, but the amount of rain that fell on the dry crops was <u>negligble</u>.

   A) negligible

   B) negligable

   C) negligeable

   D) negligeible

   HINT *Find the root. Can it stand alone?*

ReKap

In this lesson, you learned strategies to help you correctly answer test items about spelling and word usage. Implementing these strategies will allow you to answer any test question about spelling correction or properly spelled word selection. These strategies are:

- Find the root.
- Pay attention to REBS (root ends and beginnings of suffixes).
- Can the root stand alone?
- Identify the part of speech.
- Check the context.
- Analyze apostrophes.

? Why is it important to have a good grasp on spelling rules and guidelines? How can strong spelling skills help you as you pursue your studies and nursing career?

_____

_____

_____

_____

_____

Answers

Homophone Selection Drill

except

bear

compliment

Their

Guided Practice

1. Step 1: The task is to find the correctly spelled word.

   Step 2: The root of the word formed in each answer choice is rely. Yes, the word root can stand-alone. The suffix *–able* is attached to stand-alone words.

   Step 3: The root ends in *y*. The *y* must change to an *i* before merging with the suffix. Therefore, Choice C is spelled correctly.

   Answer: (C) reliable

2. Step 1: The task is to select the correctly spelled word.

   Step 2: The root word is *psyche/psych*. Eliminate Choice C because it does not have the *h*.

   Step 3: The suffix *–iatric* is being added. Choice B is correct, as it correctly merges the root with the correct form of the suffix.

   Answer: (B) psychiatric

3. Step 1: The question is a homophone question. The task is to select the correctly spelled word.

   Step 2: The function of the missing word is a noun (a plural noun). Eliminate Choices C and D because they are possessive, not plural nouns.

   Step 3: The meaning of the missing word is closer to beliefs. Choice B is the correct answer.

   Answer: (B) principles

Independent Practice

1. **Answer: (C) veins**

   Choice C correctly uses the plural noun *veins*. The context tells us that a phlebotomist is looking for a blood vessel for the IV.

2. **Answer: (D) persistence**

   Choice D correctly uses the guidelines for adding an *ance/ence* suffix by adding *–ence* to a root that ends in *–ist*.

Answers

3. **Answer: (A) negligible**

Choice A correctly adds the suffix *–ible* to the root, which cannot stand alone as a complete word.

ReKap

It is important to have a good grasp on spelling rules and guidelines so that you can write grammatically correct notes. The written word should be free of error and convey a clear and concise message.

5

GRAMMAR · LESSON 6
Advanced English Techniques

As you embark on your career in health care, you may encounter difficult health care terminology. But both word structure and context clues offer ways to quickly interpret unfamiliar words. In this lesson, you will also examine point of view and advanced style elements you may encounter on test day.

Common Uses in Health Care

- quickly comprehending challenging health care terminology

- writing professional correspondence

- composing well-written and clear patient care instructions and informational materials

Key Terms/Formulas

- **active voice** – a sentence in which the subject performs or does the verb action

- **antonym** – a word opposite in meaning to another word

- **context clues** – additional words in a text which help the reader understand the meaning of an unfamiliar word

- **passive voice** – a sentence in which the subject is acted upon by the verb

- **point of view** – the way the author allows you to see and hear what is going on

- **synonym** – a word having nearly the same meaning as another word

- **word structure** - the pieces that make up a word, such as prefixes, roots, and suffixes

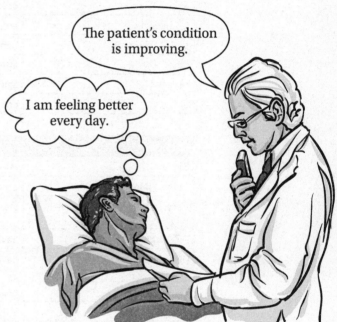

Point of View

Learn

On test day, you will be asked to find definitions or approximate meanings of unfamiliar words. Think back to what you learned about word structure, or the roots and affixes of a word. Analyzing word structure can be a valuable tool in deciphering the meaning of unknown words on test day.

In the charts below, you can see how common prefixes and suffixes can change or extend the meaning of the root word.

Frequently Used Prefixes		
Prefix	**Meaning**	**Example**
anti–	against	anticlimactic
dis–	not	disappear
epi–	on, upon	epidermis
in–, im–, il–	not, lack of	insignificant, imperfect, illegal
peri–, pre–, pro–	before	perinatal, preterm, prologue
post–	after	postmortem
re–	again	remake
un–	not	unkind, unhelpful

Frequently Used Suffixes		
Suffix	**Meaning**	**Example**
–able, –ible	capable of being	culpable, edible
–acy, –ance/–ence, –ant/–ent, –ity, –ty	state or quality of	privacy, maintenance, lividity, entirety
–ic, –ical, –al, –ac	having to do with	limbic, chemical, radial, cardiac
–ish, –ive, –y	having the quality or characteristic of	peevish, active, lazy
–ism	believing in	feminism
–itis	inflammation	tonsillitis
–ology	the study of	biology, theology
–or, –er	one who	sailor, trainer

You are likely to see these prefixes on test day. Note that prefixes can both make a root word more specific (*peri-*) or negate or form an antonym of the root word (*dis-*).

Being able to identify the meaning of some common root words can instantly give you a ballpark definition of the whole word.

Common Root Words		
Root	**Meaning**	**Example**
audio	sound	audiology, auditory
cardio	heart	cardiology, pericarditis
chron	time	chronic, chronology
demos	people	democracy, epidemic
derma	skin	dermatologist, epidermis
geo	earth	geography, geology
graph	writing	autograph, biography
man(u)	hand	manual, manuscript
mono	one	monotonous, mononucleosis
nat/nasc	birth	natural, perinatology, nascent
ortho	straight, correct	orthopedic, orthodox
ped/pod	foot	pedestrian, podiatrist
psycho	mind	psychology, psychiatric
sci	to know	science, conscience
script	written	manuscript, prescription
therm	heat	thermal, geothermal

In addition to word structure, context clues can be used to determine the meaning of an unfamiliar word. Context clues are the words around the unknown word which help shed light on its meaning. Some words can serve as road signs alerting you to the meaning of a word. These keywords can tell you whether to go straight ahead from other words in the text or detour from the other words to find the meaning of the unknown word.

Context Clues and Road Signs			
Context Clue	**Road Sign**	**Function**	**Keywords**
definition/description explanation	straight ahead	defines or describes the unfamiliar word	is, are, was, were, like, because, since
example/comparison	straight ahead	gives examples of the unfamiliar word	such as, like, for example, as, as is
synonym	straight ahead	gives a synonym of the unfamiliar word	or, also known as
contrast	detour	contrasts the unfamiliar word to other known words	unlike, in contrast, different, whereas, however, while
antonym	detour	gives an antonym of the unfamiliar word	not, unlike, opposed to, but, never

 WATCH OUT! Incorrect answers on test day often stem from missed road signs and keywords. Pay attention to both descriptive words and examples in the sentence and the keywords that tell you how to apply those descriptive words and examples to the unknown word's meaning.

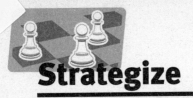

Strategize

1. **Find the root.**

   In any word structure item, you should begin with the root word. If provided with scratch paper on test day, transcribing the word and boxing off the root word is helpful in breaking apart words or forming new ones. Practice this technique on scratch paper as you prepare for the test so you will be able to quickly and easily spot root words on test day.

2. **Hunt for prefixes and suffixes.**

   Examine the word for prefixes and suffixes if the task is a word meaning task. For formation or spelling tasks, isolate the correct prefix or suffix in the word or select the necessary prefix or suffix to produce the desired meaning.

3. **Check the context clues.**

   Read the sentence carefully looking for descriptive or specific words (often modifiers), and examples. Pay careful attention to any road signs and keywords that tell you whether to go straight ahead or detour from those descriptive words when forming a definition for the unknown word.

Apply

Let's get some quick practice on finding the meaning of an unknown word in a couple of different test day formats.

A1. Which of the following is the best definition of the word *prescience*?

1. **Find the root.**

   To find the root we are going to need to eliminate the affixes. This word has a prefix and a suffix, and eliminating them leaves the root word *sci*. Sci means *to know* so we have a good starting point.

2. **Hunt for prefixes and suffixes.**

   Pre on the front end of the word means *before* and the *ence* on the end of the word means *state of*.

   Combine all the pieces:

Pre	+	sci	+	ence
before		to know		state of = state of knowing before

   Let's check the meaning "state of knowing before" with the answer choices.

   A) classes taken before science class

   B) knowing something before it happens

   C) a written order for medicine

   D) the study of the earth

   Choice B matches the definition made from the structure of the word.

   Let's practice using context clues now.

   The girl slowly got up to answer the phone because the summer heat made her feel torpid and lethargic.

A2. Which of the following is the meaning of the underlined word above?

   A) nervous

   B) bored

   C) lazy

   D) overworked

You can see there is not much to work with structurally in the short underlined word; therefore, read the sentence for context clues. Right away, the keyword *because* should serve as a road sign signaling an explanation. The sentence tells us the girl moved *slowly* because the heat made her feel *torpid*. The word *torpid* must somehow relate to the word *slowly*. There is also the road sign *and* signaling that *torpid* and *lethargic* are synonyms. Let's look for a match for the definition slow and lethargic. Choice C is the best match.

Learn

While many items on test day ask you to identify correct usage of the English language, some focus on style choices. For example, you may be asked to distinguish between active and passive voice.

In active voice, the subject performs or does the action in the verb:

Example: The dog licked the mailman.

In passive voice, the object moves to the front of the sentence and is acted upon by the verb or receives the action in the verb. The verb in passive voice is typically marked by a form of the verb *be* and adds this to the past participle. For example, the passive voice version of the prior sentence would be:

Example: The mailman was licked by the dog.

Let's look at some more examples.

Active: Robert ate the t-bone steak.
Passive: The t-bone steak was eaten by Robert.

Active: The red truck ran over the soda can in the middle of the road.
Passive: The soda can in the middle of the road was run over by the red truck.

 WATCH OUT! Just because a sentence has a form of the word *to be* does not automatically make it passive. It must also include a past participle.

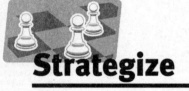

Strategize

1. **Find the verb.**
   The first step on an active or passive voice item should be locating the verb.

2. **Watch the W words.**
   One key indicator of passive voice can be the use of a "W" word (*was* or *were*) with a past participle. Quickly scan to locate "W" words in a sentence and check for a past participle if you are asked to identify or eliminate passive voice in an item.

3. **Ask about the actor.**
   To identify or change a sentence into active voice, ask the question "Who or what_____?" by inserting an active verb. For example "Who ate?" or "What jumped?"

Apply

Let's put the strategy into practice with a test day item about passive voice.

A3. **Which of the following changes the sentence below so that it is written in the active rather than in the passive voice?**

The care package was received by Jaylah three days after she wrote an email to her mother to ask her to send it.

A) Three days after she wrote an email to her mother to ask her to send it, the care package was received by Jaylah.

B) The care package was received by Jaylah three days after writing an email to ask her mother to send it.

C) Jaylah received the care package three days after she wrote an email to her mother to ask her to send it.

D) An email was written to Jaylah's mother three days before the care package was received by Jaylah.

1. Find the verb.

Examine the original sentence. Look closely at the front of the sentence as verbs often occur early in a sentence. The verb is *was received*. Who received something? Jaylah. This shows us we have a passive construction as the care package is the thing being received, not the receiver. This will need to change in the correct answer.

2. Watch the W words.

Skim the answer choices looking for W words (*was/were*) attached to verbs. Quickly eliminate choices A, B, and D as a W word occurs next to a verb.

3. Ask about the actor.

Finally, check the remaining answer choice to make sure it is in active voice by asking who received the care package and confirming that person is in subject position. Jaylah received it, and she is in the subject position in answer choice C.

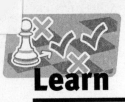

Another way to use style techniques to write well is to vary sentence structure and length. Recall what you have already learned about sentence structure. You know that sentences may have one or more independent clause as well as dependent clauses. Mixing up the arrangement and connections among these sentence pieces can make your overall writing more lively and engaging.

Style and format are also ways to emphasize certain parts of a sentence. The way a sentence is structured can convey the chronology of actions, the importance of events, or focus on a particular descriptive element.

Let's examine a couple of sentences that convey information accurately but are not particularly well written.

Choppy and overly simple:
I went to the store to get items for a meal. I bought yams at the store. I took the yams home. I made a meal.

Long, wordy, and hard to follow:
I went to the store and bought yams at the store and took the yams home to make a meal.

Easy to read with emphasis on the most important elements:
Using the yams I bought at the store, I made a meal at home.

On test day, you may be asked to combine or rewrite sentences using better fluency and style. On such items, you should eliminate redundant words. Also, pay attention to parallelism. Parallelism means being careful to use the same pattern of words to show that two or more ideas have the same level of importance. Parallel structures are typically linked by conjunctions. Read the following sentences:

Lance enjoys going for a run, biking, and taking a swim.

Lance enjoys running, biking, and swimming.
Or
Lance enjoys going for a run, riding his bike, and taking a swim.

The second and third versions maintain parallel structure and are much easier to read.

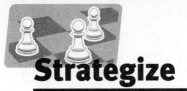

Strategize

1. **Match the meaning.**
   Read the sentence to determine whether the meaning is clear.

2. **Use your ears.**
   Often poorly written sentences will sound incorrect or very clunky when you read them to yourself.

3. **Combine with care.**
   Make sure you pay attention to maintaining parallel structure when combining sentences. Also, use structure to emphasize key elements of the sentence. Finally, avoid passive voice whenever possible.

Apply

Let's put the strategy into practice with a test day item about style and fluency.

A4. **To improve sentence fluency, which of the following states the information below in a single sentence?**

Javahnee dropped the laptop. The laptop was expensive. Then the whole group turned around. Everyone in the cafeteria stared at him.

A) The expensive laptop was dropped by Javahnee and the whole group made of people sitting in the cafeteria turned around and stared.

B) The laptop, which was expensive, was dropped by Javahnee, and the whole group, who sat in the cafeteria, turned around.

C) After Javahnee dropped the expensive laptop, everyone in the cafeteria turned around and stared at him.

D) When Javahnee dropped the laptop, then the whole group in the cafeteria turned around and stared at him because it was expensive.

1. **Match the meaning.**

   Read the original sentences carefully. The correct answer needs to convey the same meaning as the originals. Choice D changes the meaning by adding "because it was expensive." The original sentences did not tell us that was the reason people turned around.

2. **Use your ears.**

   Eliminate any sentences that sound awkward or clunky. Choice A uses "the whole group made of people sitting in the cafeteria" which is very awkward sounding. Get rid of this answer choice.

3. **Combine with care.**

   Look at choices B and C. Choice B uses passive voice and you want to avoid passive whenever possible. Choice C conveys the information clearly and fluently and is the correct answer.

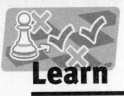

Point of view is the way the author allows you to see and hear what's happening. On test day, you will be asked to identify the point of view in texts. Writing can be in first, second, or third person point of view. Different pronouns and formal or informal tones help determine a piece's point of view.

The use of first person pronouns such as *I, me, my, mine,* or *we* indicates first person point of view. Although first person is sometimes considered a more casual form of writing, it is often used in professional writing as well. For example:

> I have been working as a health care professional for twenty years. I still find my job as rewarding as the day I started and plan to retire as an ICU nurse.

The use of *you* indicates second person point of view. Second person is less commonly used and less frequently seen in test day items or professional writing. Second person may be used in informational pamphlets or patient instructions.

> You should keep a log of the baby's feedings and bowel movements and bring it with you to the appointment with the pediatrician.

Third person tends to sound more formal than first person. In third person, a narrator refers to other people and will sometimes reference others' thoughts and actions. The author acts as an outsider relaying the action to the reader. Markers of third person point of view are third person pronouns such as *he/she/it/they,* the pronouns *everyone/one,* and indirect nouns such as *people.*

> Dr. Smith heads the emergency department of a busy hospital. People say he is one of the most effective managers to have held the position in many years.

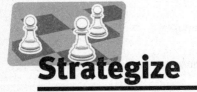

Strategize

Items on test day will ask you to identify the point of view of a text. Alternatively, they may ask you to pick which sentence in a group is written from a particular voice or point of view.

1. **Look for pronouns.**
   Quickly scan for the pronouns I (first person) and you (second person).

2. **Whose perspective?**
   First person is characterized by a personal perspective. Third person is characterized by an outsider perspective. Ask yourself which perspective the author is writing from.

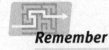

Remember

Watch out for quotations! Ignore pronouns within dialogue as these are not markers of point of view.

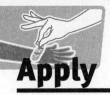

Apply

Let's put the strategy to use with a test day example.

A5. **Which of the following is an example of third person point of view?**

    A) You should never run a car engine while your garage door is closed.

    B) The waiter showed us the menu and we selected our main courses.

    C) I glanced at Quentin and whispered, "Do you think he saw us?"

    D) The two friends skipped down the street hand in hand.

1. Look for pronouns.

Right away you can spot *you* and *I* at the beginning of choices A and C. Eliminate these choices and move on.

2. Whose perspective?

Read choices B and choice D carefully. In choice B, the author is a character and is relaying the information from her point of view. The pronouns *us* and *we* are also clues that this is first person. Choice D is in third person, as the author is an outsider observing the scene indicated by the author's description of the two friends skipping down the street.

Guided Practice

1. Which of the following is the meaning of the underlined word below?

   Marcus attempted to <u>disentangle</u> the fawn from the snare designed to catch rabbits.

   A) free

   B) hunt

   C) observe

   D) trap

   STEP 1: Find the root.

   Examine the underlined word. What is the root?

   _____

   STEP 2: Hunt for prefixes and suffixes.

   Look carefully at the underlined word. Are there any prefixes or suffixes attached to it? What do they tell you about the meaning of the word?

   _____

   _____

   STEP 3: Check for context clues.

   Are there any context clues that help you find the meaning of the word? Combine this information with the meaning you produced in Steps 1 and 2. Which answer is correct?

   _____

   _____

   _____

2. To improve sentence fluency, which of the following best states the information below in a single sentence?

The dog chased the cat. The cat was a tabby cat. The chase occurred in the living room. The living room was empty.

A) The tabby cat was chased by the dog in the empty living room.

B) After the cat was chased by the dog, the living room was empty.

C) The dog chased the tabby cat around the empty living room.

D) The cat, which was a tabby cat, was chased in the living room, which was empty, by the dog.

STEP 1: Match the meaning.

Read each sentence in the answer choices and eliminate any choices which change the meaning of the original sentences. Which choice can you eliminate? Why?

_____

_____

STEP 2: Use your ears.

Reread the remaining choices. Do any sound awkward or ungrammatical? Which ones?

_____

_____

STEP 3: Combine with care.

Look at the remaining choices. Is either in passive voice? Which answer is correct?

_____

_____

Guided Practice

3. Which of the following is an example of third person point of view?

   A) On my trip to Kyoto, I ate sushi almost every day of the week.

   B) Before hammering the legs into the desk, you should attach the felt pads to the feet.

   C) After the snow melted, the pioneer family ventured out to hunt for food.

   D) Frequently we found poison ivy growing in the woods behind our house.

STEP 1: Identify the task.

What is the question asking you to find?

_____

STEP 2: Look for pronouns.

Skim the answer choices looking for the pronouns *I* or *you*. Which choices include these pronouns? Can we eliminate them?

_____

_____

STEP 3: Whose perspective?

Read the remaining answers carefully. Whose perspective is each choice written from? Is the author a character in either sentence? Which choice is the correct answer?

_____

_____

Independent Practice

1. Which of the following is the meaning of the underlined word below?

   The senator <u>disclaimed</u> any knowledge of improper use of funds by his campaign.

   A) admitted

   B) blamed

   C) proclaimed

   D) denied

   HINT *Use the word's structure for clues to meaning.*

2. Which of the following changes the sentence below so that it is written in the active rather than in the passive voice?

   It was long believed by paleontologists that dinosaurs became extinct after a meteor hit the earth.

   A) The earth was hit by a meteor which made dinosaurs extinct.

   B) Paleontologists believed that dinosaurs became extinct after a meteor hit the earth.

   C) After a meteor hit the earth, it was believed by paleontologists that dinosaurs became extinct.

   D) The theory of a meteor causing the extinction of dinosaurs was long believed by paleontologists.

   HINT *Watch out for W words.*

3. Which of the following options best uses grammar for style and clarity to combine the sentences below?

   Rocio received a survey after school was over. Rocio then filled out a survey about her interests. Rocio said she enjoys running on the beach. She also likes going to the movies. She likes to play basketball with her friends.

   A) After school, Rocio filled out a survey about her interests and said she enjoys running on the beach, going to the movies, and playing basketball with her friends.

   B) After school, the survey was filled out by Rocio. She said she enjoys running on the beach, going to the movies, and playing basketball with her friends.

   C) The survey, which was filled out by Rocio, said she enjoyed running on the beach, going to the movies, and she likes to play basketball with her friends.

   D) Rocio filled out an interest survey. In it she said she enjoys running on the beach, going to the movies, and to play basketball with her friends.

   HINT *Use your ears. Pay attention to parallelism.*

4. Which of the following sentences is an example of second person point of view?

   A) The shade of the lamp must be attached to the base with the screws provided.

   B) You should tighten the screws using a Phillips screwdriver.

   C) The cord should be threaded through the small hole in the base.

   D) Insert a forty watt bulb and tighten it by turning clockwise.

   HINT *Which pronoun signals second person?*

ReKap

In this lesson, you learned strategies to help you correctly answer test items about word meaning, active and passive voice, and point of view. Use the following strategies to efficiently move through test items on these topics.

- Find the root.

- Hunt for prefixes and suffixes.

- Check the context clues.

- Find the verb.

- Watch the W words.

- Ask about the actor.

- Look for pronouns.

- Whose perspective?

- Match the meaning.

- Use your ears.

- Combine with care.

? **Why is it important to understand elements of writing style? How will understanding difficult terminology help you in your nursing studies and career?**

_____

_____

_____

_____

_____

Answers

Guided Practice

1.   Step 1: The root of the underlined word is tangle.

     Step 2: The prefix *dis-* and the prefix *en-* are attached to the root word *tangle*. En + tangle means in tangle or tangled up. Dis + tangle means we want the opposite, not tangled up.

     Step 3: The words *snare* and *catch* show us that the fawn is trapped. Choice A must be correct because Marcus is undoing the fawn from the snare, or freeing it.

Answer: (A) free

2.   Step 1: Choice B can be eliminated. The word *after* added to choice B imposes a timeline to the events that is not clear in the original sentences.

     Step 2: Choice D awkwardly inserts clauses that break the flow of the sentence. It can be eliminated.

     Step 3: Choice A is passive. Active voice is stylistically preferable to passive voice. Choice C, with active voice, better conveys the action in the original sentence.

Answer: (C) The dog chased the tabby cat around the empty living room.

3.   Step 1: The question asks us to find a sentence written in third person.

     Step 2: Choice A has the pronoun *I*. Choice B has the pronoun *you*. Eliminate both choices because they are first and second person.

     Step 3: Choice C is written by an outsider. The author is part of Choice D, as evidenced by the word *we*. Choice C is correct.

Answer: (C) After the snow melted, the pioneer family ventured out to hunt for food.

Independent Practice

1. **Answer: (D) denied**

    Choice D correctly matches the meaning of the word as used in the sentence. Word structure indicates the meaning will be close to the opposite of claim.

2. **Answer: (B) Paleontologists believed that dinosaurs became extinct after a meteor hit the earth.**

    Choice B correctly moves paleontologists into the subject position in the sentence and eliminates the passive construction "was believed."

3. **Answer: (A) After school, Rocio filled out a survey about her interests and said she enjoys running on the beach, going to the movies, and playing basketball with her friends.**

    Choice A maintains parallel structure and active voice.

Answers

4. **Answer: (B) You should tighten the screws using a Phillips screwdriver.**

    Choice B is marked with the second person pronoun *you*. The other answer choices are written in third person point of view.

ReKap

Understanding difficult terminology will allow you to determine the definition or approximate meanings of unfamiliar words.

UNIT
6

Plan for Success

School Success

Once you've studied, taken the entrance exam, and applied to the program of your choice, it will feel like you're at the end of a long process. The reality, though, is that you're at the beginning of your journey towards an exciting career!

You were proactive about preparing for the TEAS V. Now it's time to build on that momentum and actively plot for longer-term success.

To succeed in a rigorous and unique academic environment, you must develop habits that will support the things you learn inside and outside of the classroom. Being a student isn't easy – you will be required to synthesize a large amount of information in a relatively short period of time. Learning how to manage your time and study effectively will make sure that school is an exciting and enjoyable experience.

Critical Thinking

In their daily activities, professionals are required to think critically. To think critically, one must listen actively, identify what's important, and gather necessary information by asking questions. These skills are also the keys to understanding all of the information you'll be responsible for learning in nursing school.

As a nursing student, you'll be gathering information from several sources, including textbooks, professors, and peers. The keys to thinking critically about information presented to you are:

1) Active Listening

2) Identifying What's Important

3) Asking the Right Questions

Gathering Information

Attending a class involves more than attendance and casual listening and note taking. Before class, read over the material that you professor will be covering that day. Being already familiar with the basics will help you understand what's important.

If your professor has made notes or outlines available to you, make sure you print them and bring them along to class. Having a jumping off point for your own note taking will give you more time for listening.

Active Listening

Listening is a very important skill for anyone to have. Being a good listener improves the quality of relationships and work. During your career, you will be required to listen to and process information quickly and accurately. School is an excellent time to practice this skill, as actively listening to your professors will ensure that you understand and remember the information they present to you in a classroom setting.

Many people are passive listeners, meaning that, when spoken to, they absorb about half of the information presented. For some, it is less than half. With so much to stimulate our senses, listening is something that is usually done subconsciously. To become an active listener, you must be mindful of distractions and make a conscious decision to pay close attention to the message being delivered to you.

Here are a few steps to active listening in the classroom:

1) Make a conscious decision to listen.

2) Although you will be tempted to take notes, looking at your professor will help you better grasp what he or she is saying. Instead of scribbling quick notes, ask your professor for permission to record his or her lecture. This will free you to listen slowly and carefully.

3) Don't jump ahead by trying to anticipate what your professor will say next – focusing on one thought at a time will allow you to listen to and organize information at the same time.

4) Avoid distractions. If you need to ask someone in your class to please quiet down – go ahead and do that. Your memory will thank you when it comes time to study!

Identifying What's Important

Active listening is an excellent tool, but it doesn't help you to discern which information, of all that's being provided to you, is the most important. If you're being tested on an entire unit of information, how do you filter the contents down to what's most important?

To pick out the most important pieces of information:

1) Start with the who, what, when, where, and why of the material.

2) Summarize what you've learned in the unit and write it out for yourself in a brief paragraph. This will distill the information down to its most succinct form.

3) Make a list of key words from the unit. Make sure that you are familiar with their definitions. This is a good place to start closing any gaps in your knowledge. It may also tip you off to a section of the unit you may need to review more than others.

4) Identify an organizational pattern for the unit. For example, if you're studying symptoms of diseases, sequence of events may be an organizational pattern to listen for. Words like "first" and "later" are cues that signal a timeline. Breaking the information out into a timeline may make it easier for you to memorize the details. Another structure you may find is cause and effect. Be mindful of words like "before" and "after," which commonly indicate cause and effect. You may wish to make a chart as a way of identifying important information presented in this format.

Asking the Right Questions

Let's face it – the content covered in school is difficult. Communicating with your professor when you do not understand something will be key to your success. Remember, there is never a down side to asking, and sometimes asking is the only way you can get to the bottom of what's most important. If, at the end of a lecture, you're confused about what you should take away from it, ask your professor to briefly summarize the main idea for the class. As a student, one of the most important things you'll do is ask questions – get comfortable with it now and don't be shy!

Applying What You've Learned

Now that you've listened, identified the important information, jotted down notes, and asked follow-up questions, it's time to draw conclusions about what you've learned. Being able to draw conclusions and communicate them effectively will be very important in graded presentations and papers. Your professors will depend on you to not only draw the right conclusions from information, but then to also communicate it to them in a way they understand.

Drawing Conclusions and Communicating Them Clearly

To draw an accurate conclusion, you must process all of the information you've gathered. Crosscheck your notes with the recording of your professor's lecture, or any notes your professor has made available to your class. Read your notes in conjunction with your textbook – does the information align, or is there something you need to clarify with your professor?

Even when answering a straightforward multiple-choice question, you must analyze the information you're given and draw the correct conclusion. This application is the starting point to the other, more complicated, assignments you'll be required to complete. Experiments, research papers, and presentations will all require analysis and a conclusion.

When taking an exam, writing a paper, or giving a presentation, you will need to present your conclusions, or, in other words, a summary of your findings. The following steps will help you communicate your findings in a functional way:

1) Consider your audience – are you speaking to or writing for someone who has the same level or more experience than you do?

2) Use appropriate vocabulary or define terms for your audience.

3) Provide a summary of your findings as well as a list of your supporting details before addressing the finer points of your conclusions.

4) Reiterate your findings several times to keep your audience or reader on track.

Managing Your Coursework

Long-Term Studying

At the beginning of most courses, a syllabus is distributed which outlines the subject matter you'll be learning and any important dates. Pairing the syllabus with your calendar, you should be able to map out rough study timelines.

Only you know which classes will require more of your attention. Use your best judgment to decide how many times a week you should plan to review your notes and coursework for each class. Develop a weekly schedule and stick to it. When it comes time for exams, you'll be prepared and ready to focus on your short-term study strategies, like doing practice tests.

Implementing a long-term study plan will not only help prepare you, but it will help you manage the stress of nursing school, as well. When content is broken down into lessons, and studying is broken down into hourly blocks, there is no need to panic.

Taking Notes

In school, some of your courses will be strictly lecture-based, meaning there won't necessarily be a workbook or textbook for you to follow along with. For that reason, it is important to master active listening for the classroom setting.

As you learned in a previous lesson, active listening involves making a conscious decision to focus and minimize distractions while identifying the most important information being presented. Classroom lectures are often long and encompass a range of details on a specific topic. Even if you are a fast note-taker, it's not possible to write down everything being said for study or paper-writing purposes.

As you listen, jot down the main idea of the lecture, which should be presented early on. The lecturer will give you clues by way of introduction, such as "Today, we'll be speaking about…" Later in the lecture, listen for words like "symptoms" or "causes" – these words signal the coming of a list that you'll want to write down.

Listen for how the speaker appears to be organizing the lecture – this will help you identify an outline for your notes and give you an idea of how much detail you should be trying to capture.

Define a set of abbreviations for yourself at the beginning of your course – a type of personal shorthand – and stick to them throughout your note taking. For example, instead of writing "symptoms" in its entirety every time it's mentioned, simply write "Sym" instead.

After class, re-read your notes, filling in any details that you recall next to their overall concept. Doing this right away will ensure that you have complete notes to review when you study.

Finding Your Study Style

Think about how you've studied in the past. Did you make flash cards, re-write your notes, speak them out loud? You might have a good idea of what works best for you and what type of learner you are, but the odds are that you haven't yet taken courses quite like college level courses.

Don't be afraid to try new study tactics. Striking a balance between your long-term study plan and short-term studying will ensure optimal performance on test days and in practical scenarios. Consider re-writing your notes and also making flash cards. Going through the exercise of re-writing will force you to concentrate on the subject matter at hand, while writing lists onto flash cards will make it easy for you to commit them to memory. Flash cards are also a good tool because you can keep them in your pocket and review them in your free time.

Another option is reading your notes to yourself out loud. If you learn by listening, a good option would be to make a recording of yourself speaking your notes. You can do this with a computer or a smart phone. Listen to your notes regularly – if this style of learning works well for you, you might be more likely to recall information heard in your own voice.

Keeping Cool Under Pressure

One simple way to regain your calm in a challenging academic situation is to be mindful of how your anxiety manifests in your body. Does your stomach knot or do your fists clench? Do the muscles in your back feel tired? Take a second to take stock of your own vitals. Is your heart racing?

Sometimes, a simple stretch or deep breathing can calm you significantly. Spending a moment to acknowledge your body will also help to refocus your mind. Check in with yourself several times a day, and you will be more prepared for times of great exertion.

Another quick way to reduce stress is to find a quiet place and stand there for a moment. The lack of stimulation to your senses will give your brain a break. With less to analyze, your mind can shut down and restart, in a matter of speaking.

If you are a visual person, carry an image in your mind or on your person, that calms you. It can be a photo of your family, a postcard from a vacation you took, or just a memory of a beautiful view. Consider how it makes you feel, and use that to keep calm in stressful situations.

If you find yourself unable to relax before an exam, you are not alone! Exercise is the easiest way to blow off steam while doing something great for your health. As a future health care professional, it will be your responsibility to set a good example for your patients. Getting into the habit of exercising when you feel stressed will help you recharge your mind and focus better on your studies.

Talking about what stresses you out is also a source of comfort. If you're not comfortable talking about school with your peers or professors, join an anonymous online forum. Support, even from strangers, can be surprisingly helpful! Knowing that other people understand you and the situations that you face every day will ease your mind and help you to feel a part of an important, global team.

Sharing and Receiving New Knowledge

Always remember that your fellow students are an excellent resource to you. Never be afraid to ask a question!

The Internet can be an amazing resource, but you must keep in mind that what you read online is not always official, current, relevant, or accurate. Your school can recommend trusted online resources. It's important to keep abreast of discoveries and recent developments, and the Internet is the fastest way of doing so. It is important for you to read your field's prominent publications, if only to be able to combat misinformation you may encounter online.

6 PLAN FOR SUCCESS · LESSON 2
Studying

Studying is a reality for students – there are many tips for going about studying in the best possible way, but there are no tricks. Studying takes time, dedication, and planning.

Studying is different than preparing for an exam. Studying should be done daily, where preparation for an exam should take place in the week preceding the test. You should have a weekly study schedule that sets aside time to review each of the courses you take. When it comes time for an exam, you should only need to review the information you've already studied in detail.

You've probably heard of "cramming" for an exam. This type of frantic review of material before an exam will only leave you with a superficial understanding of content that you'll need throughout your career. Do not shortchange your career for short-term success on an exam.

In-depth studying includes the following activities:

1) Memorizing facts

2) Focusing on understanding the content

3) Looking deeper to understand "why"

The outcome of using this approach will be better grades and a greater understanding of how the pieces of the nursing curricula fit together as a whole.

While studying is often a dreaded activity, do not procrastinate. Remind yourself why you wanted to study nursing and how hard you've worked to that point. Do what you need to do to succeed – your future will be an excellent reward.

A Few Things to Remember

Once you have been accepted into school and you have an idea of how to approach thinking about your coursework, consider the following helpful reminders:

1) It's important to have goals. Decide what it is that you want to get out of nursing school, and actively participate in your quest to fulfill that goal. Once you've settled on an objective, the path to meeting that objective will become easier to see.

2) Consider how you spend your time. Are you feeling stressed and rushed? The odds are, there are ways you can restructure your time so that you can complete your work while feeling more relaxed. If things or people in your life are intruding on valuable study time, make changes and communicate to the people in your life that part of being a support system is helping you to not be distracted.

3) Be organized! Taking just a few minutes a day to review your notes and organize them in a way that will make them easy to re-read will cut down on wasted study time before an exam.

4) Find a study group. Even if you are not struggling with your work, having a study group is extremely valuable. Studying can be an isolating activity – having a group to participate in will help round out your life and cut down on stress.

5) Don't fall behind. Be honest with yourself about what you understand and what you don't. The earlier you acknowledge a problem, the more time you have to sort it out before an exam.

KapSnap

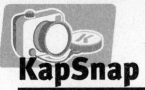
KapSnap

Reading Fundamentals

Skills

- understanding the differences between various kinds of texts
- determining what kinds of text you are reading
- determining how a text is structured

Key Terms/Formulas

- **cause-effect** – text structure that discusses an events and its results
- **compare-and-contrast** – text structure that compares two or more things, people, events, or ideas
- **expository text** – text that explains a topic
- **fiction** – made-up text
- **informational text** – factual text
- **narrative** – text that tells a story
- **persuasive text** – text that tries to convince
- **problem-solution** – text structure that presents a problem and then resolves it
- **sequence** – text structure that organizes text in chronological order
- **technical text** – text that contains precise and technical information
- **text features** – headings, subheadings, italicized or boldfaced words
- **text structure** – way in which text is organized

Strategies

- Scan and Skim
- Predict Before You Peek
- Analyze and Decide

Quick Steps

1. What kind of text is this?
2. What information do the text features give me?
3. What are the key words?
4. How is this text structured?

Common Errors

- Not looking for key words
- Forgetting to ask yourself what kind of text a passage is
- Mixing up text structures with similar key words

READING • LESSON 2

Paragraph and Passage Fundamentals

Skills

- understanding an author's purpose
- understanding how to identify the topic and main idea of a text
- understanding the purpose of supporting details
- understanding how to identify the theme of a text

Key Terms/Formulas

- **author's intent** – what the author hopes to accomplish with the text
- **author's purpose** – why the author writes a text
- **main idea** – what a text is specifically about
- **supporting details** – information that tells more about the main idea
- **theme** – a subject that the text touches upon more than once
- **topic** – what a text is generally about

Strategies

- Scan and Skim
- Check Your Response
- Read and Decide
- Make a Chart

Quick Steps

1. Why did the author write this text?
2. What is the text generally about?
3. What is the text specifically about?
4. What information tells more about the main idea?
5. What subject is frequently touched upon?

Common Errors

- Confusing a main idea with a detail
- Confusing a persuasive text with an informational one
- Incorrectly identifying a topic as a theme

READING • LESSON 3

Informational Fundamentals

Skills

- understanding what functional texts are and their purpose
- understanding how to determine the reliability of a text
- understanding the difference between statements based on fact and those based on opinion
- recognizing primary sources

Key Terms/Formulas

- **fact** – information that can be proven
- **functional text** – text that contains everyday information
- **index** – text in the back of a book that lists topics in a book alphabetically
- **instructions** – step-by-step directions on how to do something
- **label** – text that tells you what is in food or medication, or tell you how to use a product
- **opinion** – a personal statement or feeling that cannot be proven
- **primary source** – text that is original
- **reliability** – extent to which content is from a credible source
- **table of contents** – text in the front of a book that outlines what is in the book

Strategies

- Scan and Skim
- The Learning Curve
- Read and Decide
- Organize

Quick Steps

1. Why did the author write this text?
2. What purpose does it serve?
3. Are the sources reliable?
4. Is this statement based on fact or opinion?
5. Is this a primary source?

Common Errors

- Not understanding the components of nutritional labels
- Not recognizing an opinion in a statement

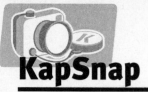

KapSnap

Reading Technical Documents and Tools

Skills

- determining how to use graphs, charts, and tables to compare information
- understanding how to read information in graphs, charts, tables, and other types of visual passages
- understanding how to read information from a map

Key Terms/Formulas

- **bar graph** – graph that presents numerical information by the length of lines or rectangles
- **compass rose** – graphic that shows directions on a map
- **distance scale** – a means to measure distance on a map
- **legend** – explanation of the symbols on a map
- **line graph** – graph that presents numerical information by using a line
- **map** – diagrammatic representation of an area showing cities, roads, and other sites
- **pie chart** – circle divided into sectors that each represent a portion of the whole
- **scale** – instrument that weighs items or people
- **scientific instruments** – tools used in science and medicine
- **table** – graphic that organizes and displays information
- **visual information** – image such as a chart, graphic, or map used to present

Strategies

- Study the Visual
- Find a Purpose
- Figure Out How It Works
- Pay Attention to Details
- Read the Question Carefully

Quick Steps

1. Identify what the visual tells you.

2. Decide what is being compared.

3. Determine what information the question is asking for.

Common Errors

- Confusing numbers on a scale
- Not focusing on the details of a visual image

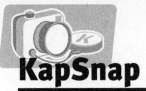

READING • LESSON 5

Advanced Paragraph and Passage Techniques

Skills

- understanding how to find evidence to support an inference, conclusion, or prediction
- understanding how to recognize bias in a text
- understanding how to recognize historical and cultural context
- understanding how to use context clues to figure out the meanings of words

Key Terms/Formulas

- **bias** – prejudice in favor of or against one thing, person, or group
- **context** – information in a text that offers clues to help you understand the meaning of a word
- **historical and cultural context** – clues that help you understand the period when a text was written
- **inference** – a judgment made that is based on evidence that comes from the text
- **logical conclusion** – a theory based on the inferences in a text
- **prediction** – a logical inference about what might be true or occur in the future based on evidence in the text

Strategies

- Scan and Skim
- Look for Evidence
- Test the Conclusion's Logic
- What Will Most Likely Happen or Be True?
- Check for Opinions
- Check for Hints
- Trust Your Instincts

Quick Steps

1. What evidence supports the conclusion?
2. Do context clues support a word's meaning?
3. Does a text have historical or cultural context?

Common Errors

- Confusing conclusions with evidence
- Not paying attention to context clues
- Judging a text without understanding its context

READING · LESSON 6

More Informational Techniques

Skills

- understanding more complex texts
- interpreting tables and yellow pages
- understanding directives

Key Terms/Formulas

- **appropriate source** – a source that can be trusted
- **critical reading skills** – skills that allow you to analyze and judge the credibility of a text and the author's intention
- **locating information** – the process of determining the most appropriate sources and finding specific information
- **recognizing bias** – analyzing whether an author has a prejudice in favor or against a thing, person, or group

Strategies

- Analyze
- Interpret
- Cite Evidence
- Make an Inference or Make a Prediction
- Analyze the Text for Context Clues
- Substitute the Word or Phrase For Another
- Check for Appropriateness
- Determine the Purpose of a Text
- Decide What Is Being Compared

Quick Steps

1. What kind of text is this?

2. What does it compare?

3. What inference is being made?

4. What word or words can be substituted for the unknown word or words?

Common Errors

- Jumping to conclusions about information in tables
- Confusing directives in communications

MATH • LESSON 1

Numbers

Skills

- working with negative numbers
- comparing fractions
- working with absolute values
- finding square roots

Key Terms/Formulas

- **absolute value** – the distance in units of a number from zero on a number line
- **negative number** – a number less than zero
- **number line** – a line with numbers marked as units
- **square root** – the square root of a number is a number that, when multiplied by itself, gives you the first number

Strategies

- Visualize
- Use the X-method
- Count
- Estimate and Adjust

Quick Steps

1. Visualizing on the number line to compare negative numbers
2. Counting on the number line to find absolute values
3. Using estimation and trial and error to calculate square roots

Common Errors

- Comparing negative numbers by comparing the numerals
- Carrying out calculations with absolute values in the wrong order
- Confusing squares and square roots

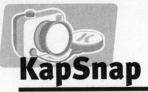

MATH • LESSON 2

Evaluating Numerical Expressions

Skills

- carrying out the correct order of operations
- adding and subtracting with regrouping
- using multiplication, division, and powers

Key Terms/Formulas

- **difference** – the result of subtracting one number from another
- **evaluating** – the process of finding the value of an expression by carrying out different operations
- **expression** – a combination of numbers with symbols for operations [such as 2 + 2, 5 × (8 – 3)]
- **operations** – any calculation you use to combine two numbers
- **order of operations** – the rules for the order in which to apply the operations while evaluating an expression
- **powers** – an expression where a number is multiplied by itself a given number of times
- **product** – the result of multiplying two numbers
- **quotient** – the result of dividing one number from another
- **regrouping** – the process of rearranging numbers in an addition or subtraction problem
- **sum** – the result of adding two numbers

Strategies

- Substitution
- PEMDAS
- Regrouping
- Estimation
- Powers and Exponents

Quick Steps

1. How do I determine the order of operations?
2. When should I regroup?
3. When should I just move from left to right?

Common Errors

- Adding/subtracting before multiplying/dividing
- Overlooking parentheses

KapSnap

Operations with Fractions and Decimals

Skills

- operations with fractions
- operations with decimals
- converting fractions and decimals

Key Terms/Formulas

- **common denominators** – a denominator shared by given fractions
- **denominator** – the lower part of a fraction
- **least common multiple (LCM)** – the smallest number that is a multiple of two given numbers
- **mixed number** – a fraction greater than one that is written as a combination of a whole number and a fraction
- **numerator** – the upper part of a fraction
- **place value** – the values expressed by a given decimal place; for instance, the first decimal place represents tenths, and the second represents hundredths
- **quotient** – the number that results from dividing one number by another
- **reciprocal** – the fraction that results from swapping the numerator and denominator
- **simplest form** – a fraction is in simplest form when the numerator and denominator can't both be divided by any number other than 1
- **whole numbers** – a set of numbers that contains the numbers you count with and zero (0, 1, 2, 3, 4, ...)

Strategies

- Using Common Denominators
- Converting Mixed Numbers
- Writing in Simplest Form
- Line Up Decimal Points
- Keep Track Of Decimal Places
- Use Long Division
- Identify Decimal Places

Quick Steps

1. How should I convert?
2. What values do I combine?
3. How do make my result simpler?

Common Errors

- You can't add or subtract fractions until you have common denominators
- You can't always add or subtract decimals by lining up the last digits
- You need to adjust your decimal points with you multiply or divide decimals

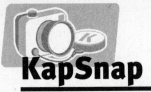
KapSnap

Ratios and Proportions

Skills

- understanding ratios, proportions, rates, and unit rates
- writing a ratio in simplest terms
- cross-multiplying to solve a proportion
- solving word problems involving proportions by cross-multiplying or using a unit rate

Key Terms/Formulas

- **cross-multiply** – multiply the numerator of one ratio in a proportion by the denominator of the other ratio
- **proportion** – a mathematical statement equating two ratios
- **rate** – a comparison of two quantities with different units
- **ratio** – a comparison of two quantities
- **unit rate** – the number of units of the first quantity in a rate that correspond to one unit of the second quantity

Strategies

- Identify Parts and Wholes
- Find the Unit Rate
- Set Up a Proportion with a Variable
- Cross-Multiply
- Use a Unit Rate

Quick Steps

1. What are the parts? What is the whole?

2. What quantities should the ratio compare?

3. How should the proportion be set up? Which quantities go in the numerator and which go in the denominator?

4. Can I use a unit rate to solve this problem? What is the unit rate?

Common Errors

- Comparing the wrong quantities
- Setting up the proportion incorrectly
- Cross-multiplication errors

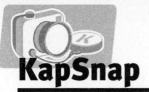
KapSnap

Applications of Percents

Skills

- finding a part given a percent and the whole
- finding a percent given a part and the whole
- finding the whole given a percent and a part
- finding the percent increase or decrease

Key Terms/Formulas

- **percent change equation** –

  $$\% \text{ change} = \frac{\text{amount of change}}{\text{original amount}} \times 100 \text{, where amount of change} = |\text{original} - \text{final}|$$

- **percent decrease** – percent change from the initial quantity to the final quantity, where the final quantity is greater than the initial quantity
- **percent equation** – percent · whole = part
- **percent increase** – percent change from the initial quantity to the final quantity, where the final quantity is greater than the initial quantity

Strategies

- Write Percents as Decimals to Make Calculations
- Use the Percent Equation
- Translate from Words to Equations
- Organize
- Use the Percent Change Equation

Quick Steps

1. Identify the whole, the part, and the percent.
2. Identify the original amount, the final amount, and the amount of change.
3. Write an equation.

Common Errors

- Incorrectly identifying the whole and the part
- Failing to write the percent as a decimal
- Choosing the incorrect amount as the original amount

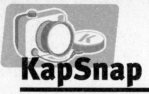

KapSnap

MATH • LESSON 6

Measurement Conversions

Skills

- converting customary units
- converting metric units
- converting from one system to the other

Key Terms/Formulas

- **conversion rate** – an equation that compares a measurement into two different units
- **conversion ratio** – an expression that presents a conversion rate in the form of a fraction; you can multiply a measurement by a conversion factor to convert it into a measurement with a different unit
- **customary system** – the measurement system used mainly in the United States, which uses units such as feet, miles, pounds, and gallons
- **dimensional analysis** – a process used to guide the steps of converting from one unit to another
- **metric system** – a measurement system used in most parts of the world (and by scientists in the United States), based on the decimal system; it uses units such as centimeters, kilograms, and liters

Strategies

- Use Dimensional Analysis to Convert
- Use Multiple Conversion Ratios

Quick Steps

1. How do I apply the UMCS strategy?
2. How do I identify units and conversion rates?
3. How do know how to arrange a conversion ratio?
4. How do I combine rates to make less common conversions?

Common Errors

- Converting with the wrong ratio

MATH • LESSON 7

Operations with Polynomials

Skills

- adding and subtract polynomials
- multiplying a polynomial by a monomial
- multiplying two binomials
- dividing polynomials

Key Terms/Formulas

- **binomial** – a polynomial with two terms
- **coefficient** – a number that is multiplied by a variable
- **constant** – a quantity that is not a variable
- **exponent** – the number that shows how many times a base is multiplied by itself in a power, shown as a superscript
- **like terms** – terms that have the same variable raised to the same power
- **monomial** – a polynomial with one term
- **polynomial** – a mathematical expression made up of terms that are variables, constants, or the product of variables and constants
- **term** – a variable, constant, or product of variables and constants
- **variable** – a quantity that changes, usually represented by a letter like x or y

Strategies

- Group Like Terms
- Distribute the Factor
- Use FOIL
- Break Apart the Numerator

Quick Steps

1. Rewrite subtraction as addition.
2. Identify the operation(s) you will need to use.
3. Distribute factors as needed.
4. Multiply or divide.
5. Combine like terms.

Common Errors

- Be careful of the signs when adding, subtracting, multiplying, or dividing integers.
- Distribute the negative sign to each term in the second polynomial when subtracting.
- Only combine like terms. Like terms have the same variable raised to the same power.
- Be sure to multiply each term in the first polynomial by each term in the second polynomial. Use FOIL to help you keep track.

KapSnap

Expressions, Equations, and Inequalities

Skills

- solving equations and inequalities
- writing and solving word problems
- solving absolute value equations and inequalities

Key Terms/Formulas

- **addition principle** – a principle that allows you add the same amount to both sides of an equation or inequality
- **algebraic equation** – an equation that includes at least one algebraic expression
- **algebraic expression** – an expression that includes at least one variable
- **equation** – a mathematical statement that says that two expressions have equal values
- **inequality** – a mathematical statement that says that one expression is less than, less than or equal to, greater than, or greater than or equal to another expression
- **multiplication principle** – a principle that allows you multiply by the same amount on both sides of an equation or inequality
- **solution** – the solution(s) of an algebraic equation or inequality is the set of values that make the statement *true*

Strategies

- Work Backwards
- Clear Fractions and Decimals
- Identify Unknowns
- Translate the Comparison
- Translate Operations
- Converting Absolute Value Equations and Inequalities

Quick Steps

1. Isolating the variable
2. Interpreting operations and signs
3. Converting absolute value expressions

Common Errors

- confusing addition and subtraction when solving
- confusing multiplication and division when solving
- confusing addition and subtraction when translating equations and inequalities
- forgetting to reverse inequality signs when multiplying by negative numbers

MATH • LESSON 9

Representations of Data

Skills

- understanding of the different ways in which data can be represented and the types of data typically represented in each way
- reading line graphs, circle graphs, bar graphs, and histograms
- interpreting representations of data

Key Terms/Formulas

- **bar graph** – a representation of data in which each category is shown as a bar, the height of which indicates the number of data values in the category
- **circle graph (pie graph)** – a representation of data in which each category is shown as a sector of a circle, the size of which indicates the part of the whole that the category represents
- **dependent variable** – the variable whose values are the outputs that result from inputting the independent variable
- **independent variable** – the variable whose values are the inputs
- **frequency** – the number of times a data value occurs in a set
- **histogram** – a representation of data in which the data values are arranged in intervals and each interval is shown as a bar, the height of which indicates the number of data values in the interval
- **interval** – a range of data values
- **line graph** – a representation of data in which each data value is plotted as an ordered pair and the points are joined with lines
- **ordered pair** – a set of coordinates in the order (x, y) that describe the location of a point
- **sector** – a section of a circle graph

Strategies

- Analyze the Graph
- Use the Percent Equation
- Predict Before You Peek
- Eliminate

Quick Steps

1. Read the question to determine the information you will need.
2. Analyze the graph to identify the information.
3. Use the information to solve the problem.

Common Errors

- reading the scale of a graph incorrectly
- reading the wrong set of data on a double-line or double-bar graph

MATH • LESSON 10

Other Topics

Skills

- estimating the answers to problems
- using estimation to check the reasonableness of an answer
- writing standard numbers using Roman numerals and write Roman numerals as standard numbers
- solving problems that involve working with money

Key Terms/Formulas

- **Arabic numerals** – the numerals we use in the modern world; also referred to as *standard* numerals
- **digit** – a single number, 0-9; digits make up numbers with multiple decimal places
- **estimation** – finding an approximate answer to a computation
- **place value** – the value of a digit in a number, given by the position of the digit relative to the decimal point
- **Roman numerals** – ancient numeric system that uses Latin letters

Strategies

- Rounding
- Compatible Numbers
- Process of Elimination
- Align Decimal Points
- Choose the Sign
- Roman Numerals
- Use Expanded Form
- Stop at Three
- Break Apart and Translate

Quick Steps

1. Round or choose compatible numbers to use to estimate the answer
2. Determine which operations to use to solve problems involving money
3. Use place value to translate between standard numbers and Roman numerals

Common Errors

- Choosing inappropriate numbers with which to estimate
- Confusing debits/credits and deposits/withdrawals
- Always using addition for Roman numerals instead of using subtraction for the digits 4 and 9

SCIENCE • LESSON 1

Scientific Reasoning

Skills

- identifying the steps of the scientific method
- recognizing and constructing a well-designed experiment
- analyzing and interpreting models built from experimental data

Key Terms/Formulas

- **conclusion** – a statement that analyzes the data
- **control** – the group that does not receive the experimental protocol
- **data** – measurements and observations
- **experiment** – a carefully designed procedure
- **hypothesis** – a testable statement
- **inference** – a conclusion based on the assumption of something being true
- **model** – usually a graph, chart, or diagram
- **observation** – a problem that needs to be solved

Strategies

- Reread and Realize
- Remember
- Rule Out

Quick Steps

1. Reread the question and figure out what it is asking you to do.
2. Remember the parts of a scientific investigation.
3. Rule out incorrect answers.

Common Errors

- Assuming that science is a body of knowledge instead of a method of investigation.
- Designing experiments without adequate controls, sample sizes, and randomization.
- Misinterpreting or overgeneralizing the predictions made by experimental models.

SCIENCE • LESSON 2

Cells

Skills

- understanding of the differences between the structures found in prokaryotes and eukaryotes, and the functions of each structure
- determining if substances are moving by active or passive transport, and to relate direction of movement to concentration of solutions
- understanding of the processes of cellular respiration and photosynthesis and how they are related

Key Terms/Formulas

- **active transport** – movement of substances against the concentration gradient
- **autotroph** – organism that makes its own food
- **cellular respiration** – process used by cells to release energy from glucose
- **heterotroph** – organism that cannot synthesize its own food
- **organelles** – *small organs* or functional parts of a cell
- **passive transport** – movement of substances with the concentration gradient
- **photosynthesis** – process used by cells to form glucose, using energy from the sun

Strategies

- Reread and realize
- Remember
- Visualize
- Rule out

Quick Steps

1. Passive = downhill, active = uphill
2. hypo = under, hyper = over
3. Photosynthesis and cellular respiration are the reverse of each other

Common Errors

- Confusing concentration of water with concentration of solute
- Confusing cellular respiration and photosynthesis

SCIENCE • LESSON 3

Heredity

Skills

- understanding the structure and function of DNA
- understanding cell division by mitosis and meiosis
- predicting the probability of inheriting characteristics or genetic diseases

Key Terms/Formulas

- **allele** – one of two or more variations of a single gene
- **amino acid** – the building block of a protein
- **chromosomes** – large strands of DNA in the nucleus that each contain several genes
- **deoxyribonucleic acid (DNA)** – the primary genetic material inside human cells
- **gene** – a short segment of DNA that codes for a single protein, or trait
- **genotype** – the gene combination present in a cell for a given trait
- **heterozygous** – having two different alleles for a trait
- **homozygous** – having two of the same alleles for a trait
- **meiosis** – reproductive cell production process
- **mitosis** – cell replication process
- **phenotype** – the visible characteristic determined by genotype
- **Punnett square** – a graphical tool used to calculate the probabilities of inheritance

Strategies

- Reread and Realize
- Remember
- Rule Out
- Use Squares!

Quick Steps

1. Determine what the question is asking you to do.
2. Remember the facts related to the question and eliminate incorrect answers.
3. Use Punnett squares to determine probabilities.

Common Errors

- Confusing DNA with RNA, purines with pyrimidines, genotypes with phenotypes
- Not separating alleles properly to start a Punnett square problem
- Forgetting the steps of mitosis and meiosis.

SCIENCE • LESSON 4

Human Body Systems

Skills

- determining the location of a part or substance within the hierarchy of structure
- knowing the various body systems, their parts, and their functions
- understanding how the various body systems interact

Key Terms/Formulas

- **circulatory** – system of organs and tissue that distribute substances throughout the body
- **digestive** – system of connected organs and tissue that breaks down food and expels solid waste
- **endocrine** – system of tissue that releases chemicals that control functions
- **excretory** – system of organs and tissue that collects and expels chemical waste
- **integumentary** – system of skin, hair, and nails to contain and protect the other systems
- **lymphatic** – system of tissues that distributes white blood cells and excess fluid throughout the system
- **muscular** – system of muscles and connective tissue for moving the body
- **nervous** – system of tissue that senses and controls the body
- **reproductive** – system of organs and tissue for producing offspring
- **respiratory** – system of organs and tissue that supplies oxygen and removes carbon dioxide from the body
- **skeletal** – system of bones and connective tissue for supporting the body

Strategies

- Reread and Realize
- Remember
- Rule Out

Quick Steps

1. Identify the system or systems that are the subject of the question.
2. Match the parts or functions of that system to the main focus of the question.
3. Base your answer on the main function of that system or set of systems.

Common Errors

- Confusing types of *waste*—digestive waste is processed in the large intestine; waste from the rest of the body functions passes through the blood and is processed by the liver and kidneys.
- Forgetting multiple names for systems, e.g., cardiovascular and circulatory, or pulmonary and respiratory.

SCIENCE • LESSON 5

Biological Classification

Skills

- knowing the hierarchy of taxonomic levels
- understanding binomial nomenclature
- knowing the three domains and six kingdoms of living things

Key Terms/Formulas

- **binomial nomenclature** – the use of an organism's genus and species as its scientific name
- **taxonomic hierarchy** – domain, kingdom, phylum, class, order, family, genus, species
- **taxonomy** – the system biologists use to classify organisms

Strategies

- Use a Mnemonic
- Identify
- Reread and Realize
- Remember
- Rule Out

Quick Steps

1. Reread the question to determine what it is asking you to do.
2. Remember the names of the domains, the names of the kingdoms, and the hierarchy of taxonomic levels.
3. Rule out incorrect answers.

Common Errors

- Using an old system of classification—for example, the five-kingdom system used several decades ago
- Not writing scientific names correctly
- Assuming that all higher taxonomic levels are larger groups of organisms than lower taxonomic levels

KapSnap

Atomic Structure

Skills

- predicting properties of elements
- predicting bonds, structure, and properties in molecules
- reading the periodic table

Key Terms/Formulas

- **atom** – the smallest unit of an element that still retains the properties of that element
- **atomic number** – number of protons in an atom; all atoms of any one element have the same atomic number
- **average atomic mass** – average of the mass numbers of all the atoms in an element; often close to the mass number of the most abundant isotope
- **bond** – an attraction between elements caused either by sharing or by transferring electrons
- **electron** – negatively charged atomic particle located in shells around the nucleus
- **ion** – an atom that has gained or lost electrons, giving it a negative or positive charge
- **isotope** – a specific atom of an element with a certain number of neutrons; changing the number of neutrons will form a different isotope
- **mass number** – total number of protons and neutrons in an atom
- **molecule** – a group of atoms bonded together in a specific ratio
- **neutron** – neutral atomic particle found in the nucleus
- **proton** – positively charged atomic particle found in the nucleus
- **valence electrons** – outermost electrons in an atom

Strategies

- Reread and Realize
- Remember
- Rule Out

Quick Steps

1. Use the periodic table to identify the elements involved and their properties.
2. Use your knowledge about the elements to determine what compounds are involved.
3. Use your knowledge about bonding to predict the structure and properties of the compound..

Common Errors

- Confusing ions and isotopes
- Confusing atomic number, mass number, and average atomic mass

SCIENCE • LESSON 7

Chemical Reactions

Skills

- balancing chemical equations
- recognizing oxidation and reduction
- understanding acids, bases, and salts

Key Terms/Formulas

- **acid** – a solution that contains more free hydrogen ions than water (pH < 7)

- **base** – a solution that contains fewer free hydrogen ions than water (pH > 7)

- **chemical reaction** – the creation of new substances through the rearrangement of atoms and molecules

- **metabolism** – the sum of all chemical reactions inside a living thing

- **oxidation** – the donation of electrons to another atom or molecule

- **pH** – the measure of how acidic or basic a solution is; ranges from 0 to 14

- **products** – matter that is produced during a chemical reaction

- **reactants** – matter that is consumed during a chemical reaction

- **reduction** – the acceptance of electrons by an atom or molecule

- **salt** – a substance produced by the reaction of an acid with a base

Strategies

- Reread and Realize
- Quick Steps for Counting Atoms
- Seek Clues
- Rule Out

Quick Steps

1. Reread the question to figure out what it is asking you to do.

2. Balance equations by counting the atoms on each side and adding coefficients to molecules to make the amounts of each atom equal.

3. Look for atoms trading electrons to identify oxidation and reduction. Look for the reactants H^+ or OH^-, or water as a product, to identify an acid-base reaction.

4. Rule out incorrect answers.

Common Errors

- Balancing only one type of atom in a chemical equation and leaving the others unbalanced.
- Confusing oxidation and reduction with one another.
- Not recognizing the individual components of a neutralization reaction.

SCIENCE • LESSON 8
States of Matter

Skills

- distinguishing between the states of matter
- understanding why phase transitions occur
- calculating heat energy transfer during phase transitions

Key Terms/Formulas

- **crystal** – a type of solid with highly ordered atoms or molecules
- **gas** – a state of matter with a variable shape and volume
- **heat** – a type of energy that is transferred during changes in temperature
- **latent heat** – the amount of heat energy a substance must release or absorb to transition between the liquid and gas states
- **liquid** – the state of matter that has a fixed volume but a variable shape
- **phase transition** – the changing of a substance from one state of matter to another
- **solid** – the state of matter that has a fixed volume and shape

Strategies

- Reread and Realize
- Remember Water
- Read the Sign
- Rule Out
- Calculate

Quick Steps

1. Reread the question to figure out what it is asking you to do.
2. Think about how the behavior of water molecules makes ice, liquid water, and water vapor behave.
3. Plug latent heat and mass values into the heat of vaporization equation.
4. Rule out incorrect answers.

Common Errors

- ignoring the role of pressure in phase transitions
- using temperature values instead of latent heat values while calculating heats of vaporization
- missing a negative sign on a heat of vaporization value

KapSnap

Energy

Skills

- describing forms of energy
- calculating potential and kinetic energy
- using the law of conservation of energy to calculate energy transfer

Key Terms/Formulas

- **calorie** – common unit for measuring energy, 1 cal = 4.2 J
- **energy** – the ability to do work
- **joule (J)** – standard unit for measuring energy
- **kinetic energy** – energy of motion
- **potential energy** – stored energy
- **velocity** – describes speed and direction

Formulas:

Kinetic Energy: $KE = mv^2$

Potential Energy: $PE = mgh$

Total Energy = KE + PE

Strategies

- Reread and Realize
- Remember
- Rule Out

Quick Steps

1. Choose the correct formula if a calculation is needed.
2. If both KE and PE are involved, look for where PE = total energy (zero velocity).
3. Check to make sure all energy is accounted for.

Common Errors

- math errors (especially with velocity in the KE equation)
- confusing energy transfer or conversion with energy being created or destroyed

SCIENCE • LESSON 10

Energy and Population Changes

Skills

- identifying the three main methods for transferring energy
- understanding the composition and characteristics of sunlight and other energies
- analyzing measurements of populations growth and factors that affect it

Key Terms/Formulas

- **conduction** – energy movement through matter
- **convection** – energy movement through the movement of matter
- **electromagnetic radiation** – energy that travels in waves
- **electromagnetic spectrum** – arrangement of electromagnetic radiation in order of wavelength or frequency
- **emigration** – movement of people out of a country or region
- **fertility rate** – number of births per woman living in a country or region
- **immigration** – movement of people into a country or region
- **radiation** – movement of energy through space in the form of waves

Strategies

- Reread and Realize
- Remember
- Rule Out

Quick Steps

1. Determine if the question deals mostly with energy or mostly with population.
2. If the question deals with energy, determine if it relates to energy transfer or parts of the spectrum.
3. If the question deals with population, look for key terms such as fertility, growth, or emigration.

Common Errors

- Confusing convection and conduction
- Confusing wavelength and frequency
- Confusing population size with population growth rate

GRAMMAR • LESSON 1

Grammar Basics

Skills

- determining parts of speech in a sentence
- correctly forming irregular plural nouns
- demonstrating knowledge of capitalization rules

Key Terms/Formulas

- **adjective** – modifier that describes a noun
- **adverb** – modifier that describes an adjective, adverb, or verb
- **article** – word that limits a noun by making it specific or general
- **capitalization** – use of uppercase letters
- **direct object** – a noun or pronoun naming the receiver of an action
- **indirect object** – a noun or pronoun naming the person or thing for which the action was done
- **noun** – word that names a person, place, or thing
- **plural** – two or more
- **preposition** – word that shows relationships or locations
- **pronoun** – word that stands in for a noun or refers to a noun
- **singular** – one
- **subject** – a noun or noun phrase naming the doer or actor in a sentence
- **verb** – an action or state-of-being word

Strategies

- Scan and Eliminate!
- Put the sentence on trial! Ask, Answer, Act!
- Count! Predict and Match
- Scan! Ask! Predict!

Quick Steps

1. Read the sentence and identify the task. What is the question asking you to find/do?
2. Scan and eliminate any obvious wrong answers.
3. Use your rules and strategies to find the correct answer.

Common Errors

- Misidentifying parts of speech
- Adding s/es to pluralize all nouns
- Overcapitalization

GRAMMAR • LESSON 2

Punctuation

Skills

- correctly using the rules of punctuation
- quickly identifying and correcting incorrect use of punctuation
- relaying spoken conversation accurately in writing

Key Terms/Formulas

- **apostrophe** – punctuation mark used to form possessives, contractions, or pluralize letters, numbers, or other words which have no plural form
- **colon** – punctuation mark signaling a list or information that adds to the idea before the colon
- **comma** – punctuation mark used for separating words or ideas
- **dialogue** – written versions of conversation or quotations
- **direct dialogue** – quotations; specific things someone said
- **hyphen** – punctuation mark used between spelled-out compound numbers or fractions
- **indirect dialogue** –description of what someone said; a paraphrase of a conversation
- **parentheses** – punctuation mark used to enclose additional information or explanations that would interrupt the flow of the sentence
- **punctuation** – symbols that give structure and organization to sentences
- **quotation marks** – punctuation that sets off direct dialogue and certain titles
- **semicolon** – punctuation mark used to link related independent clauses or a series of items containing commas

Strategies

- ID the Task
- Break the Code
- What's My Job?
- Use Your Ears

Quick Steps

1. Identify the task: what is the question asking me to do?

2. Take it a step at a time. For questions with multiple tested punctuation marks, make a decision on one of the marks and eliminate wrong answers before evaluating the others completely.

3. Find the author's intent. Then follow grammar rules that match that purpose.

Common Errors

- Overusing commas or using them incorrectly, especially comma splices
- Using double quotation marks for quotes within a quote
- Placing end punctuation outside of quotation marks

Intermediate Grammar

Skills

- pairing subjects and verbs based on agreement rules
- understanding agreement rules for special cases such as mass or collective nouns
- identifying and properly match pronouns with their antecedents

Key Terms/Formulas

- **antecedent** – the word to which a pronoun stands in for or refers back
- **collective nouns** – a number or collection of people or things spoken of as one whole unit
- **mass nouns** – uncountable nouns, nouns without discrete units
- **plural** – many
- **pronoun** – a word that stands in for a noun or refers to a noun
- **singular** – one
- **subject** – person, place, thing, or phrase that is acting or being
- **verb** – an action or being word

Strategies

- Identify the subject
- Count
- Cut the clutter
- Identify the antecedent
- Pick the person and case

Quick Steps

1. Identify the task: what grammar topic is being tested?
2. Pick a strategy and take it a step at a time. Eliminate wrong answers after you apply a strategic step.
3. Predict what markers (singular/plural, case, gender) the correct answer will need to demonstrate.

Common Errors

- Using plural verb forms with collective nouns
- Verb errors when subject is split from the verb by a clause
- Using plural pronouns with singular antecedents

GRAMMAR · LESSON 4

Word and Sentence Structure

Skills

- identifying word parts, including prefixes, suffixes, and root words
- understanding and analyzing different types of sentence structures
- identifying and properly organizing information in a paragraph

Key Terms/Formulas

- **affixes** – a group of letters added to a root word to form a new word; includes prefixes and suffixes
- **complex sentence** – a sentence containing at least one dependent clause in addition to an independent clause
- **compound sentence** – a sentence containing two or more independent clauses
- **concluding sentence** – a sentence providing an analysis or conclusion based on the supporting information
- **paragraph** – a self-contained group of sentences about a similar theme, topic, or idea
- **prefix** – a group of letters added to the the beginning of a root word
- **root word** – the simplest form of a word with no prefixes or suffixes

- **run-on sentence** – two or more independent clauses which have not been joined correctly
- **sentence fragment** – incomplete sentences, a phrase, or clause punctuated as a sentence even though it does not form a complete grammatical sentence
- **simple sentence** – a sentence that only contains one independent clause
- **suffix** – a group of letters added to the end of a root word
- **supporting detail** – evidence, examples, and details that support or explain the topic of a ragraph
- **topic sentence** – a sentence introducing the main idea of a paragraph and linking that idea to the main theme of the piece of writing
- **word structure** – the pieces that make up a word, such as prefixes, roots, and suffixes

Strategies

- Find the Root
- Use Caution While Merging
- Find the Subject and Predicate
- Locate or Insert a Conjunction

- Locate or Insert Subordinating Conjunction and Clause
- Find the Topic of the Paragraph
- Skim for Road Signs and Structure

Quick Steps

1. Identify the task: what grammar, spelling, or structure topic is being tested?
2. Pick a strategy and take it a step at a time. Eliminate wrong answers after you apply a strategic step.
3. Predict what markers (lack of hyphens, commas, conjunctions, road signs) the correct answer will need to demonstrate.

Common Errors

- Using hyphens to attach affixes to word roots
- Confusing complex and compound sentences
- Mixing up subordinating conjunctions and prepositions

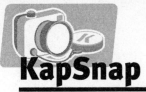
KapSnap

Spelling and Usage

Skills

- identifying word parts, such as suffixes and root words
- demonstrating knowledge of spelling and word structure guidelines, rules, and exceptions
- identifying misspelled words and correct them
- understanding proper usage of common homophones

Key Terms/Formulas

- **homophone** – a word that sounds the same as another word but has a different meaning
- **root word** – the simplest form of a word with no prefixes or suffixes
- **stress** – emphasis placed on a syllable while saying a word
- **suffix** – a group of letters added to the end of a word to change or extend the meaning of the root word
- **syllable** – a unit of spoken language, each syllable must include a vowel sound but may also include consonant sounds
- **word structure** – the pieces that make up a word, such as prefixes, roots, and suffixes

Strategies

- Find the Root
- Pay Attention to REBS
- Can the Root Stand Alone?
- Identify the Part of Speech
- Check the Context
- Analyze Apostrophes

Quick Steps

1. Identify the task.
2. Look for obvious differences in the answer choices such as apostrophes or changes in the root word.
3. Tackle the item strategically. Eliminate wrong answers as you make strategic judgments.

Common Errors

- selecting the wrong suffix
- confusing homophones
- leaving a silent e during merge

GRAMMAR · LESSON 6
Advanced English Techniques

Skills

- quickly comprehending challenging health care terminology
- writing professional correspondence
- composing well-written and clear patient care instructions and informational materials

Key Terms/Formulas

- **active voice** – a sentence in which the subject performs or does the verb action
- **antonym** – a word opposite in meaning to another word
- **context clues** – additional words in a text which help the reader understand the meaning of an unfamiliar word
- **passive voice** – a sentence in which the subject is acted upon by the verb
- **point of view** – the way the author allows you to see and hear what is going on
- **synonym** – a word having nearly the same meaning as another word
- **word structure** – the pieces that make up a word, such as prefixes, roots, and suffixes

Strategies

- Find the Root
- Hunt for Prefixes and Suffixes
- Check the Context Clues
- Find the Verb
- Watch the W Words
- Ask About the Actor
- Look for Pronouns
- Whose Perspective?
- Match the Meaning
- Use Your Ears
- Combine With Care

Quick Steps

1. Identify the task.

2. Look for key markers such as pronouns or W words in the answer choices.

3. Proceed with care. Read closely and combine carefully to create fluent and stylish sentences.

Common Errors

- Ignoring road signs and context clues
- Not paying attention to prefixes that change the word's meaning
- Mixing up past tense and passive voice